LGAM.M

Handbook of
Gynecologic Oncology

MSKCC–MDACC Handbook of Gynecologic Oncology, 2nd edition
Barakat RR, Bevers MW, Gershenson DM, Hoskins WJ (eds).
London, Martin Dunitz Publishers, Ltd.

Please help us improve the next edition of this handbook. If you find omissions in material that should be added, complete this page and mail or fax it to:

Gynecology/Breast Academic Office
Memorial Sloan-Kettering Cancer Center
1275 York Avenue, Room MRI-1027
New York, NY 10021
Phone: (212) 639-8125
Fax: (212) 717-3214

Chapter: _____

Topic: _____

Recommendations: _____

_____

_____

_____

_____

_____

Or e-mail us at gynbreast@mskcc.org.

Handbook of Gynecologic Oncology

Second Edition

Edited by

Richard R Barakat, MD
Gynecology Service, Department of Surgery
MSKCC, New York, USA

Michael W Bevers, MD
Department of Gynecologic Oncology
UT MDACC, Houston, USA

David M Gershenson, MD
Department of Gynecologic Oncology
UT MDACC, Houston, USA

William J Hoskins, MD
Formerly Gynecology Service, Department of Surgery
& Disease Management Teams, MSKCC;
Curtis and Elizabeth Anderson Cancer Center
Memorial Health University Medical Center
Savannah, USA

MARTIN DUNITZ

© 2000, 2002 Martin Dunitz, a member of the Taylor & Francis Group

Although every effort has been made to ensure that all owners of copyright material have been acknowledged in this publication, we would be glad to acknowledge in subsequent reprints or editions any omisions brought to our attention.

First published in the United Kingdom in 2000
by Martin Dunitz, Taylor & Francis Group plc, 11 New Fetter Lane, London, EC4P 4EE.

Tel: +44-(0)20 583 9855
Fax: +44-(0)20 842 2298
E-mail: info.dunitz@tandf.co.uk
Website: http://www.dunitz.co.uk

Second edition 2002

Reprinted 2003

Although every effort has been made to ensure that drug doses and other information are presented accurately in this publication, the ultimate responsibility rests with the prescribing physician. Neither the publishers nor the authors can be held responsible for errors or for any consequences arising from the use of information contained herein. For detailed prescribing information or instructions on the use of any product or procedure discussed herein, please consult the prescribing information or instructional material issued by the manufacturer.

A CIP catalogue record for this book is available from the British Library

ISBN 1-84184-166-8

Distributed in the USA by
Fulfilment Center
Taylor & Francis
10650 Tobben Drive
Independence, KY 41051, USA
Toll Free Tel.:   +1 800 634 7064
E-mail: taylorandfrancis@thomsonlearning.com

Distributed in Canada by
Taylor & Francis
74 Rolark Drive
Scarborough, Ontario M1R 4G2, Canada
Toll Free Tel.:   +1 877 226 2237
E-mail: tal_fran@istar.ca

Distributed in the rest of the world by
Thomson Publishing Services
Cheriton House
North Way
Andover, Hampshire SP10 5BE, UK
Tel.:   +44 (0)1264 332424
E-mail: salesorder.tandf@thomsonpublishingservices.co.uk

Composition by Wearset Ltd, Boldon, Tyne and Wear
Printed and bound in Great Britain by Biddles Ltd, Guildford and King's Lynn

Contents

Appendices

Preface to the First Edition

MD Anderson Cancer Center (MDACC) and Memorial Sloan-Kettering Cancer Center (MSKCC) both have long had training programs in gynecologic oncology. At MDACC, Felix Rutledge established a program to train obstetricians and gynecologists that predated the official recognition of the subspecialty of gynecologic oncology, and their official fellowship program began the first year such fellowships were approved by the American Board of Obstetrics and Gynecology. At MSKCC, Alexander Brunschwig established the Pelvic Cycle, which combined training in gynecology, urology, and colorectal surgery. This program was open to general surgeons, gynecologists, and urologists. With the approval of official fellowship programs in gynecologic oncology, John L Lewis, Jr, Dr Brunschwig's successor at MSKCC, converted the Pelvic Cycle into a fellowship in gynecologic oncology. Dr Lewis was the first Director of the Division of Gynecologic Oncology of the American Board of Obstetrics and Gynecology and Felix Rutledge was a member of this first Division. Both institutions have had continuous fellowship programs since the initiation of gynecologic oncology as a subspecialty.

Given the backgrounds of MDACC and MSKCC and their continuing interest in fellowship training, it is fitting that the faculty of these two institutions combine their efforts to produce a handbook in gynecologic oncology. This handbook is directed towards fellows in gynecologic oncology, medical oncology, and radiation oncology. It is also a valuable resource for residents in obstetrics and gynecology, internal medicine, general surgery, and radiation oncology, as well as for anyone else – from medical students to practicing physicians – who cares for women with gynecologic cancer.

The disease chapters are concise and easy to read, and we have included chapters on breast cancer and colorectal cancer. The remaining contributions are designed to be a ready resource to any physician who cares for women with gynecologic cancer, and consist of chapters on biostatistics, pharmacology, principles of chemotherapy and radiation therapy, critical care, perioperative care, procedures, nutrition and TPN, and supportive care. In addition, there are many illustrations and extensive appendices for quick reference. To ensure that the information contained in this handbook is always current, we plan to update it every two years.

The editors and faculties of MDACC and MSKCC are pleased with this handbook, and hope it proves to be of use to a wide range of physicians and students of gynecologic oncology.

Richard R Barakat, MD

Michael W Bevers, MD

David M Gershenson, MD

William J Hoskins, MD

Acknowledgments

The editors are grateful to Martin Dunitz and Alison Campbell at Martin Dunitz Publishers in London for their help and guidance throughout the development of this book. Thank you to the editorial and graphics staff at Memorial Sloan-Kettering Cancer Center, Denise Haller-Buckley, George Monemvasitis, K Alexandra MacDonald, and Terry Helms, for their dedication and organizational skills.

Contributors

Faculty of Memorial Sloan-Kettering Cancer Center
1275 York Avenue, New York, NY 10021

Carol A Aghajanian, MD
Solid Tumor Service
Department of Medicine

Kaled M Alektiar, MD
Department of Radiation Oncology

Richard R Barakat, MD
Chief, Gynecology Service
Department of Surgery

Carol L Brown, MD
Gynecology Service
Department of Surgery

Dennis S Chi, MD
Gynecology Service
Department of Surgery

Penny Damaskos, CSW
Department of Social Work

Jakob Dupont, MD
Developmental Chemotherapy Service
Department of Medicine

Mary L Gemignani, MD
Breast and Gynecology Services
Department of Surgery

José G Guillem, MD, MPH, FACS
Colorectal Service
Department of Surgery

Andrea B Hamilton, PhD
Psychiatrist, Private Practice
128 East 91st Street, Suite A
New York, NY 10128

Martee L Hensley, MD, MSc
Solid Tumor Service
Department of Medicine

William J Hoskins, MD
Formerly Gynecology Service
Department of Surgery & Disease
Management Teams, MSKCC;
Director, Curtis and Elizabeth
Anderson Cancer Center
Memorial Health
University Medical Center
Savannah, GA 31404

Harvey G Moore, MD
Colorectal Service
Department of Surgery

Richard Payne, MD
Chief, Pain and Palliative Care Service
Department of Neurology

Elizabeth A Poynor, MD
Gynecology Service
Department of Surgery

Paul J Sabbatini, MD
Developmental Chemotherapy Service
Department of Medicine

Juan Santiago-Palma, MD
Pain and Palliative Care Service
Department of Neurology

Mark A Schattner, MD
GI/Nutrition Service
Department of Medicine

Moshe Shike, MD
*Director, MSK Cancer Prevention and
Wellness Program*

David R Spriggs, MD
*Chief, Developmental Chemotherapy
Service, Department of Medicine*

Steven L Soignet, MD
*Developmental Chemotherapy Service
Department of Medicine*

Ennapadam S Venkatraman, PhD
*Biostatistics Service
Department of Epidemiology and
Biostatistics*

Faculty of MD Anderson Cancer Center
1515 Holcombe Blvd, Houston, TX 77030

Michael W Bevers, MD
*Assistant Professor
Department of Gynecologic Oncology*

Charles Levenback, MD
*Associate Professor
Department of Gynecologic Oncology*

Diane C Bodurka, MD
*Assistant Professor
Department of Gynecologic Oncology*

Karen H Lu, MD
*Assistant Professor
Department of Gynecologic Oncology*

Thomas W Burke, MD
*Professor
Department of Gynecologic Oncology*

Anakara V Sukumaran, MD
*Professor
Department of Anesthesiology*

Patricia J Eifel, MD
*Professor
Department of Radiation Oncology*

VanAnh Trinh, PharmD
*Pharmacy Clinical Specialist
Pharmacy-PC Operations*

David M Gershenson, MD
*Professor & Chairman
Department of Gynecologic Oncology*

J Taylor Wharton, MD
*Professor, Special Assistant to the
President
Department of Gynecologic Oncology*

Anuja Jhingran, MD
*Assistant Professor
Department of Radiation Oncology*

Judith K Wolf, MD
*Assistant Professor
Department of Gynecologic Oncology*

Dedication

The editors wish to dedicate this book to all the MD Anderson and Memorial Sloan-Kettering fellows in gynecologic oncology, past, present and future; and to all women with gynecologic cancer.

The editors also wish to express their appreciation to our wives, Catherine D'Agostino, Diane Bodurka-Bevers, Michelle Gershenson, and Iffath Abbasi Hoskins, who have supported us during the development of this book.

1
Basic biostatistics

Ennapadam S Venkatraman

Statistics is the theory of the collection, analysis, and interpretation of data that are subject to random variation, and biostatistics is statistical theory applied to medical or biological data. The purpose of a statistical analysis is to numerically evaluate data and draw inferences on the population being studied. This chapter is aimed at providing the reader with the basic statistical concepts required to understand and interpret scientific reports in medical journals. It is divided into sections that will guide the reader through various aspects of statistical analysis. We use data from two studies to illustrate underlying statistical concepts. The first is a study on the relationship between preoperative CA-125 and the debulking status of Stage III ovarian cancer patients, and the second is a randomized trial comparing chemotherapy alone with chemotherapy and radiation in high-risk cervical cancer patients.

EXPLORATORY DATA ANALYSIS

Types of data

Data are defined as a collection of factual information used as a basis for inference. In statistics, individual categories of data are called *variables*. Variables from an experiment can be of two types: *independent* and *dependent*. Independent variables, or *covariates,* are those that can be controlled by the experimenter, whereas dependent variables are those that are measured as an outcome of the experiment. For example, data collected from a clinical trial might consist of independent variables such as the stage and grade of the disease, and of dependent variables such as tumor response and toxicity. Generally X or Y are used as notation for variables and x_i or y_i for the value of a variable for an individual subject i. The number of subjects in the data set is often denoted by n.

Data from a medical study can be classified into two types, called *quantitative* and *qualitative*. The values of a quantitative variable have numeric significance; hence, such a variable is also called *numeric*. Numeric variables can take values from either a continuum of numbers or from integers, and are, therefore, named *continuous* and *discrete*, respectively. The preoperative CA-125 level of an ovarian cancer patient is an example of a continuous variable, whereas the number of positive lymph nodes is discrete. The values of a qualitative variable, on the other hand, fall into categories, and thus such a variable is also called *categorical*. These categories can be numbered, but have no numeric significance. There are two types of categorical variables: *nominal* and *ordinal*. Nominal variables are those whose categories cannot be ordered in a meaningful way, whereas ordinal variables have categories that have some intrinsic order. For example, values for the histology of epithelial ovarian cancer consist of clear-cell, serous, mucinous, etc., which have no intrinsic order, and, therefore, histology is a nominal variable. The staging system, however, is designed so that Stage I refers to patients with the least extent of disease, followed by Stages II, III, and IV. Thus, stage is an ordinal variable.

Graphical techniques

The first step in a statistical analysis is to summarize and visually display the data. The simplest way of presenting data from a categorical variable is to use a table where the number (*frequency*) or the percentage or proportion (*relative frequency*) of observations in each category is reported. The table can also be graphically displayed using either *bar graphs,* where the heights of the bars represent the frequencies, or *pie charts,* where the angles of the wedges are proportional to the frequencies.

Numeric variables often take on too many values to construct meaningful summaries using the data as is. Frequency tables for numeric variables can, however, be constructed by grouping the values into categories. Categories can be obtained by breaking the set of possible values for the variable into groups, or *bins*, which are nonoverlapping and cover the entire range of values and are generally of the same width. For example, the age at diagnosis of ovarian cancer can be tabulated by grouping the patients as 20–29, 30–39, etc. The bar graph from such a frequency table is called a *histogram*. Another exploratory graph for numeric data is the *box and whisker* plot, a tool used to highlight the summary information in the quartiles. The center half of the data, from the first to the third quartile, is represented by a box, with the median (the middle value) indicated by a bar (the definitions of the median and the quartiles are given in the next section). One line or whisker extends from the third quartile to the maximum value and another one from the first quartile to the minimum value. The log(CA-125) values of the 100 patients in the CA-125 study are displayed using a histogram and a box and whisker plot in Figure 1.1(a) and 1.1(b), respectively.

Univariate summary measures

Once the data have been explored graphically, we need summary measures that are objective representations of the data. Since the values of a categorical variable have no numeric significance, they cannot be combined to provide a

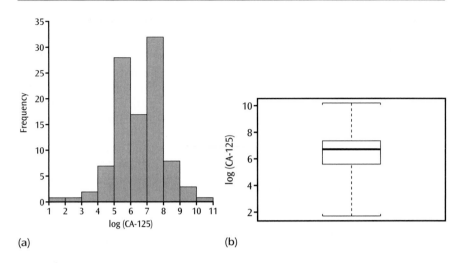

Figure 1.1

The logarithms of the preoperative CA-125 levels of the patients in the study are graphed as (a) a histogram and (b) a box and whisker plot.

single summary measure. Hence, the relative frequency table is the only summarization possible.

Often proportions are converted into *rates* by using a large multiplier (10,000 or 100,000) as in births, deaths, mortality, morbidity, etc. This makes the measure more understandable, especially when the proportion of subjects in a category is very small. For example, we could state that the proportion of women who are diagnosed with ovarian cancer is 0.00015. An equivalent way of saying this, however, is to state that the annual incidence rate of ovarian cancer is 15 per 100,000. When the rates are affected by the different compositions of the groups involved, they are *standardized* to account for these differences. For example, since the rates of ovarian cancer incidence in New York and Orlando can be affected by the differences in ages and ethnicity, they should be standardized.

We can summarize a numeric variable by measuring the center of the data and the amount of variability present, using measures of central tendency and measures of dispersion, respectively. A measure of central tendency is a value that represents the middle or the midpoint of the possible values of a variable. It provides a reference point to evaluate whether a particular observation is large or small. There are two commonly used measures of central tendency: the *mean* and the *median*. The mean is the average value of the data, and is denoted by $\bar{x}$. It is calculated by adding all the values in the data set and dividing by the number of observations: $\bar{x} = (x_1 + ... + x_n)/n$. The median is the middle value when the measurements are arranged from the smallest to the largest.

Let $x_{(1)} \leq x_{(2)} \leq \ldots \leq x_{(n)}$ be the data set in increasing order. The median is the observation that is at the halfway point, and is given by $x_{(m)}$, where $m = (n+1)/2$, for odd values of n, and by $(x_{(m)} + x_{(m+1)})/2$, where $m = n/2$, for even values of n. A generalization of the median is the *quantile*. For any number p between 0 and 1, the pth quantile is the value such that, after the observations have been ordered from the smallest to the largest, $100 \times p\%$ of the data are below this value and $100 \times (1-p)\%$ are above. The quantiles that correspond to $p = 0.25$ and $p = 0.75$ are called the *first and third quartiles*, and the median is the quantile that corresponds to $p = 0.5$.

A measure of dispersion describes the spread in the data (i.e., how variable the data are). The simplest measure of spread is the *range*, which is given by two numbers: the minimum and the maximum. The most commonly used measure of dispersion is the *variance*, which is defined as $s^2 = [(x_1 - \bar{x})^2 + \ldots + (x_n - \bar{x})^2]/n$. The difference $x_i - \bar{x}$ between an observation x_i and the mean of the data $\bar{x}$ is called the *deviation*. The variance of a data set is the mean of the squared deviations. The *standard deviation,* denoted by s, is defined as the square root of the variance. The standard deviation is reported more frequently because it has the same units of measurement as the mean, unlike the variance, which is in squared units.

Multivariate data

The previous section dealt with the summarization of data concerning a single variable. Observations on two or more variables are often recorded for a single individual. We can study the bivariate (2 variables) or multivariate (>2 variables) data to discover if any relationships exist between the variables and to determine how strong these relationships are. When values of two categorical variables are summarized in the form of a frequency table by cross-classifying them, the resulting frequency table is called a *contingency table*. In a contingency table, the row and column labels give us the categories of the two variables, and the cells represent the frequency of individuals who fall in those categories.

When values of two numeric variables are recorded on an individual, the resulting data can be thought of as a pair and displayed graphically in a bivariate plot called a *scatterplot*. In this plot, one variable is on the x-axis and the other is on the y-axis, and points represent the individuals. A scatterplot is a good way to graphically display how one variable is related to the other. Let us denote the two variables by X and Y. Since quantitative variables have numeric significance, we can ask the question: does the value of Y increase (or decrease) as the value of X increases? The *correlation coefficient* measures how well the relationship between X and Y can be explained using a straight line. The value of the correlation coefficient lies between -1 and 1, where 0 represents no association, 1 represents a perfect line that increases, and -1 represents a perfect line that decreases. The correlation coefficient ρ, is defined as $s_{xy}/(s_x \times s_y)$, where $s_{xy} = [(x_1 - \bar{x}) \times (y_1 - \bar{y}) + \ldots + (x_n - \bar{x}) \times (y_n - \bar{y})]/n$ is the covariance between X and Y and where s^2_x and s^2_y are the variances of the two variables.

Another form of the correlation coefficient that is applicable not only to numeric data but also to ordinal data is the *Spearman rank correlation*. This is calculated by replacing the real data with their ranks. It measures whether the variables have an increasing or a decreasing relationship and how strong it is, without specifying the relationship to be linear.

PROBABILITY

It is often of interest to study a particular characteristic of a population, such as the response rate of a new treatment for patients with ovarian cancer. While it may be theoretically possible to treat all patients in the population and obtain the response rate, it is not practical to do so. Thus, we select a subset of patients from the population, called a *sample,* on whom to conduct the study, where every subject in the population is equally likely to appear in the sample. Probability theory tells us the likelihood of observing a particular value of a variable for a randomly chosen subject. The *probability* or *chance* of observing a chosen value is defined as the relative frequency of that value in the population. If, for example, we were told that the relative frequency of response in the population is 25%, then the probability that a randomly chosen patient would respond to the new treatment is 0.25. The practice of statistics depends on the application of probability theory to real data.

In probability theory, the relative frequency table is called a *probability mass function* or a *density function*. It gives us the probability of individual values of a variable. An *event* is defined as a collection of values of the variable of interest, and the probability of an event can be calculated by summing the probabilities of individual values within it. For example, high-stage ovarian cancer can be considered an event whose values consist of Stages III and IV. The probability of being diagnosed with a high-stage ovarian cancer is the relative frequency of observing a Stage III or Stage IV ovarian cancer at diagnosis.

Another important concept is that of *conditional probability*, which is the probability of an event A occurring when it is known that another event B has occurred. The conditional probability of A given B, denoted by $P(A|B)$, is the proportion of subjects experiencing event A among those who experienced event B. Observe that this conditional probability is the ratio of two relative frequencies or probabilities. The numerator is the probability of a subject experiencing both events A and $B,$ and the denominator is that of a subject experiencing event B. Thus, the conditional probability is $P(A\&B)/P(B)$.

Events are called *independent* if the occurrence of one has no bearing on the occurrence of the other. When two events A and B are independent, the probability of observing them simultaneously is the same as the product of the probabilities of each individual one: $P(A\&B) = P(A) \times P(B)$.

Another important probability function for variables that can be ordered (i.e., numeric or ordinal) is the *cumulative distribution function*. If we define an event as all values that are smaller than a given number or level, the probability of that event is the cumulative distribution at that value. The cumulative distribution function is, then, these probabilities for the entire set of values of the variable.

Our goal in conducting a study is to answer some question about our population of interest. For example, we may be interested in the population response proportion of a novel drug or the mean of the age at diagnosis of the population of women who get ovarian cancer. These population quantities are referred to as *parameters*. As mentioned earlier, however, it is infeasible to use the entire population. Instead, we use a sample, and *estimate* the parameter of interest from this sample. We use the *sampling distribution* of the estimate to derive the probability of observing a given value of the estimate. In practice, there are two commonly used probability distributions: the *binomial* and the *normal*.

Binomial distribution

A categorical variable with two categories is called a *Bernoulli* or a *binary* variable. The two categories in a binary variable can be referred to as "success" and "failure." When we represent the success and the failure of a binary variable with a 1 and a 0, respectively, we can calculate its mean to be p and its variance to be $p \times (1-p)$, where p is the population proportion of a success. The sampling distribution of a binary variable is given by the binomial distribution. We can illustrate this with the following example.

Suppose we are interested in the population response proportion of a new treatment. We administer the treatment to a sample of 25 patients in order to estimate it. The two categories of the outcome are response and no response, which are the success and the failure of the binary variable. The number of responders among the 25 patients can be any value from 0 to 25. Earlier, we saw that a randomly chosen patient is likely to respond with a probability given by the population response proportion. Since the patients are independent, we can obtain how likely it is to observe 0, 1, . . ., or 25 responses using the population response rate and enumerating all ways of assigning a fixed number of responses to the 25 patients in the study. The probability distribution thus obtained is called the binomial distribution. It has two parameters: the total number of subjects studied, n, and the probability of success, p.

Normal distribution

The normal distribution is used for a continuous variable, such as the age at diagnosis of ovarian cancer. It is also called the *Gaussian distribution* or the *bell curve*. It is called the bell curve because the histogram of the population with small bins is shaped like a bell. We may often require a transformation, such as a logarithmic or square root transformation, to make the histogram have a bell shape. The normal distribution also has two parameters: the mean μ and the variance σ^2. The normal distribution with mean $\mu = 0$ and variance $\sigma^2 = 1$ is called the *standard normal,* and its cumulative distribution function is tabulated for a range of values. The standard normal tables are available in most statistics books. An important property of the normal distribution is that if a variable X has a normal distribution, then any rescaling of X by constants a and b given by $(X - a)/b$ also has a normal distribution. We get the standard normal distribution if we set a to be the mean and b to be the standard deviation.

One important theorem in probability theory is called the *central limit theorem,* which states that the distribution of the sample mean $\bar{x}$ can be approximated by a normal distribution with mean μ and variance σ^2/n, where μ is the population mean, σ^2 the population variance, and n the number of observations in the sample. The quantity $\sigma/\sqrt{n}$ is called the *standard error* of the mean; this is a measure of variability for the sample mean. In our example, we might also be interested in the distribution of the average CA-125 level of the patients in the sample. The central limit theorem could be applied to obtain the distribution of the sample mean.

More generally, the central limit theorem states that the estimate of a parameter from a sample has an approximate normal distribution with mean equal to the population parameter and the variance proportional to $1/n$. This approximation gets better as the sample size n gets larger. Note that the standard deviation of a population is fixed, whereas the standard error reduces with sample size.

STATISTICAL INFERENCE

We perform studies on a representative sample to estimate a population characteristic such as the response rate of a new treatment. In the section on probability, we showed the relationship between the population parameters of interest and their estimates from a sample. Since the population parameters are unknown, the problem becomes one of drawing conclusions about the population from the sample. This area of statistics is called *statistical inference.* The CA-125 study will be used to illustrate different aspects of statistical inference.

We collected data on preoperative serum CA-125 levels (continuous variable) and debulking status (categorical with levels optimal and suboptimal) from a series of 100 consecutive Stage III ovarian cancer patients. Among the 100 patients in our series, 45 had a complete resection or optimal debulking, giving us a sample proportion of 0.45. We can ask the following questions: (a) What is the true response rate? (b) Are the CA-125 levels comparable between the optimally and the suboptimally debulked patients? The two questions correspond to the two aims of statistical inference, called *confidence intervals* and *hypothesis testing,* respectively.

Confidence intervals

In the above example, the sample proportion is 0.45, which is only an estimate of the true population proportion and is therefore subject to uncertainty. In the section on probability theory, we saw that for any fixed true population proportion, the sample estimate can take a variety of values. The sampling distribution of the estimate enables us to give a range within which the estimate from a sample should fall with a high probability, say 95%. However, we obtain the estimate from a single sample, which could have come from a range of possible population proportions. Thus, the natural question is whether we can similarly give a range of values that we are confident contains the true population proportion. Confidence intervals provide an answer to this question.

Earlier we saw that the sampling distribution of a binary variable is given by the binomial distribution. Thus, the number of patients who were optimally debulked has a binomial distribution with parameters p, the population response rate, and sample size $n = 100$. Applying the central limit theorem allows us to conclude that the sample mean, which is the same as the sample proportion in the binomial case, has an approximate normal distribution with mean p and variance $p \times (1-p)/n$. Hence, if we denote the sample proportion by $\hat{p}$, then $(\hat{p} - p)/\sqrt{\hat{p} \times (1-\hat{p})/n}$ has a standard normal distribution. We substitute the sample variance in the formula, since the population variance is unknown. Now, suppose we want the central 95% region of a standard normal variable. From the standard normal probability tables, we ascertain that the lower and upper 2.5% quantiles are 21.96 and 1.96 respectively (i.e., 95% of the values of a standard normal variable lie between 21.96 and 1.96). That is, if we repeat this experiment many times, 95% of the values of $\hat{p}$ should satisfy $21.96 \leq (\hat{p} - p)/\sqrt{\hat{p} \times (1-\hat{p})/n} \leq 1.96$. However, for a given sample, the known value in this expression is the sample proportion $\hat{p}$ and not the population proportion p. If we now rearrange the expression by moving all the known terms from the middle, then we get $\hat{p} - 1.96\sqrt{\hat{p} \times (1-\hat{p})/n} \leq p \leq \hat{p} + 1.96\sqrt{\hat{p} \times (1-\hat{p})/n}$. This is called the *confidence interval*, and the probability value (0.95) used to obtain the interval is called the *confidence level*. In our example, the sample proportion is 0.45, and its standard error is 0.05 $(= \sqrt{0.45 \times (1-0.45)/100})$. Using these, we ascertain that $(0.45-p)/0.05$ should lie between 21.96 and 1.96 and that p should, therefore, lie within the interval (0.352, 0.548). We are, therefore, 95% confident that the true population proportion of patients who are optimally debulked is between 35% and 55%.

We get different intervals by replacing the probability used in the initial expression with larger confidence levels that lead to wider intervals. In general, we can obtain confidence intervals for any parameter by applying the central limit theorem to the sampling distribution of its estimate. The accuracy of the interval depends on how well the normal distribution, obtained by applying the central limit theorem, approximates the true sampling distribution.

Hypothesis testing

We shall now answer the second question, which asked whether the CA-125 levels of optimally and suboptimally debulked patients are similar. Since CA-125 levels are very skewed (most values are small to moderate, while a few are very large, making the histogram have a long tail), and since they do not have the bell shape, we shall transform them by taking the logarithms of the values. There are 45 patients who were optimally debulked, and the mean and variance of their log(CA-125) are 5.73 and 1.71, respectively. Similarly, there are 55 patients who were suboptimally debulked, and the mean and variance of their log(CA-125) are 7.11 and 1.43, respectively. Statistically, the question in which we are interested is whether the two means are different, or, phrased another way, whether there is enough variability in the data to prohibit ruling out the possibility that they are the same. The answer to this question leads us to hypothesis testing.

In the question posed above, we have two hypotheses. The first is that there is no reason to believe that the two means are different; this is called the *null hypothesis*. The other one is that there is a difference in the means; this is called the *alternative hypothesis*. The two true means could either be the same (i.e., the null hypothesis is true) or they could be different (i.e., the alternative hypothesis is true). Similarly, the data could lead us to claim either that the means are different (i.e., we can reject the null hypothesis) or that the means are the same (i.e., we cannot reject the null hypothesis). Thus, we can have two types of errors. A *type I error* occurs when we reject the null when it is actually true. A *type II error* occurs when we fail to reject the null when the alternative hypothesis is true. As there is uncertainty due to sampling, we can calculate the probability of a type I error when the null holds. This is called the *significance level,* or the *size* of the test, and is denoted by α. Similarly, we can calculate the probability of a type II error, which is denoted by β. The *power* of a test is defined as the probability that the test rejects the null hypothesis when the data are such that the alternative hypothesis is true. We can see that it is the same as the number of times it does not reject the null hypothesis subtracted from 1 (i.e., the power of the test is $1-\beta$).

In our example, the parameter in which we are interested is the difference between the two population means, which is estimated using the difference in the two sample means. We would like to determine whether this difference in means is different from 0. If we denote the true difference under the null hypothesis by θ, its estimate by $\hat{\theta}$, and its standard error by τ, then, by the central limit theorem, we can approximate $(\hat{\theta} - \theta)/\tau$, a *test statistic*, by a standard normal distribution. If we again use the fact that 95% of the values of a standard normal variable lie within 21.96 and 1.96, then a test with a 5% significance level is given by rejecting the null if $(\hat{\theta} - \theta)/\tau$ does not lie within 21.96 and 1.96. For our example, $\theta=0$, $\hat{\theta}=1.38$, and $\tau=0.253$, giving us the value of the test statistic to be 5.45, which does not lie within 21.96 and 1.96. Hence, we reject the null hypothesis (i.e., there is sufficient evidence in the data to suggest that the means of log(CA-125) are different between the two groups).

We can also use the normal distribution to answer the following question: If the means are not different, what is the probability of seeing a difference in the sample means greater than or equal to 5.46? This probability is called the *p-value* of the test; we usually quote this instead of simply reporting whether or not the test at a 5% significance level rejects the null hypothesis. Note that we can use the *p*-value to decide whether a test of any given size can reject the null hypothesis. Rejecting the null hypothesis by using a test of a smaller size provides stronger evidence against the null, which is an additional benefit of reporting the *p*-value. Since the probabilities are obtained through an approximation, however, we should refrain from reporting a *p*-value with more than two or three significant digits. In our example, the probability of a standard normal variable exceeding 5.46 is 2.38×10^{-8}; hence, we just report that the *p*-value is <0.01. This is interpreted as "the probability that this result occurred by chance is less than 0.01."

We tested whether the CA-125 levels are the same for the optimal and the suboptimal groups by comparing their means. The performance of the test used to compare them depends on how well the normal approximation works, which in turn depends on the data being nearly normal for small samples. An alternative test used to test the equality of the two samples is the *Wilcoxon rank sum* test, which is the name given to a procedure that does not make any assumptions on the underlying distributions. The Wilcoxon test is an example of a *nonparametric* procedure.

Sample size

Clinical trials are conducted in order to show that a novel treatment is efficacious. Thus, we have two parameters that correspond to the null hypothesis of no effect and the alternative hypothesis of a clinically relevant effect. In the preceding section, we defined the significance level and the power of a test, and described how they can be obtained from the sampling distribution and the null and alternative parameters. In addition to the true population parameter, the sampling distribution depends on the sample size. Since we do not want to reject the null when it is true and we want to do so when it is not, thresholds are used on the significance level, and the power of the test is used to prove efficacy. Traditionally, the significance level of the test is set at 5% and the power at 80%. Thus, the design of a clinical trial requires a sample size that would satisfy the size and power requirements. The central limit theorem tells us that the mean of the sampling distribution of an estimate is the population parameter and that the variance is proportional to $1/n$, that is, it decreases as the sample size n increases. Thus, with a high probability, the sample estimate gets very close to the true parameter as the sample size increases (i.e., for any test with a fixed significance level, the power increases as n increases). Hence, we can thereby obtain the minimum sample size required for a test to have a given size and power.

One nuance of the sample size calculation, however, is that the closer the null and the alternative parameters are, the harder it is to distinguish between them. Thus, the power decreases as the difference between the null and alternative parameters decreases, which implies that the sample size required increases as the difference between the null and the alternative becomes smaller. For example, a test of 5% significance level and power 80% requires a sample of 98 patients to compare a standard treatment with a 25% response proportion against a new treatment with a hypothesized response proportion of 45%. In contrast, it requires a sample size of 348 to compare treatments with response proportions of 25% and 35%.

ANALYSIS OF CATEGORICAL DATA

In the section on statistical inference, we described methods to evaluate an outcome variable and to compare them across two groups. It is, however, also of interest to explore the relationship between two variables. In this section, we shall describe methods for evaluating the association between categorical variables. If in the CA-125 study we categorize CA-125 levels above 500 as "high" and those below 500 as "low," we can obtain the contingency table given in Table 1.1 for the two categorical variables of interest: CA-125 level and debulking status.

The first question we would like to ask is whether optimal debulking is independent of CA-125 level. In other words, are patients with a high preoperative CA-125 level as likely to be optimally debulked as patients with a low preoperative CA-125? From the contingency table, we compute the probability of optimal debulking to be 0.45 (45/100) and the probability of low CA-125 to be 0.45 (also 45/100). If the two events, low CA-125 and optimal debulking, are independent, then the probability of observing both simultaneously is the product of the two probabilities, i.e., 0.2025. Thus, we would expect 20.25 out of the 100 patients studied to have low CA-125 and to be optimally debulked. We can fill out the other categories in a similar manner in order to get the expected frequencies, as in Table 1.2. The *chi-square test* of independence compares the observed (O) and the expected (E) numbers of subjects in each cell in order to test whether the data are consistent with the hypothesis of independence. The test statistic is given by $\chi^2 = \Sigma_i (O_i - E_i)^2 / E_i$, where the summation is

Table 1.1 Observed frequency table

	Optimal	Suboptimal	Total
Low CA-125	33	12	45
High CA-125	12	43	55
Total	45	55	100

Table 1.2 Expected frequency table			
	Optimal	Suboptimal	Total
Low CA-125	20.25	24.75	45
High CA-125	24.75	30.25	55
Total	45	55	100

over all cells, which are indexed by i. The statistic for our example is 24.5, with a p-value <0.001. Thus, we reject the null hypothesis and conclude that the preoperative CA-125 level impacts on a patient's chance of being optimally debulked.

We can similarly calculate this test statistic for a contingency table of any size – not just those from a binary variable. This test statistic has a distribution called the *chi-square distribution*, which depends on $(r-1) \times (c-1)$, where r is the number of rows and c is the number of columns in the contingency table. The approximation of the sampling distribution is not very good if the number of individuals in each cell is too small. In such cases, we use *Fisher's exact test,* which obtains the true sampling distribution rather than the normal approximation. Both the chi-square test and Fisher's exact test can also be used to compare two binomial proportions.

Now that we know that preoperative CA-125 levels and optimal debulking are not independent, we can explore further. We see from Table 1.1 that a higher proportion of patients with high CA-125 levels are suboptimally debulked compared with patients with low CA-125 levels. The question of interest, then, is how much more likely it is for a patient with a high CA-125 level to be suboptimally debulked than one with a low CA-125 level. There are two measures that quantify this.

We see from Table 1.1 that the probability (or risk) of suboptimal debulking in low CA-125 and high CA-125 patients is 0.267 (12/45) and 0.782 (43/55), respectively. The ratio of these two probabilities indicates to us the extent of greater probability of optimal debulking in low CA-125 patients compared with high CA-125 patients, and is called the *relative risk*. The term "risk" is used since suboptimal debulking is not a desirable outcome. If, instead of probability, we express the same measurement in odds, we conclude that the odds of optimal debulking are 12:33 and 43:12, respectively, in the low and high CA-125 groups. The ratio of these two odds is defined as the *odds ratio*. For our example, the relative risk and odds ratio are 2.93 and 9.85, respectively. In other words, the risk (odds) of a suboptimal debulking is 2.93 (9.85) times higher for a patient with a high CA-125 value than for a patient with a low one. The relative risk and the odds ratio are nearly equal when the probability of one category is very small. Very large or very small (close to 0) values of either denote a strong association. These can be generalized to variables with more than two categories.

EVALUATION OF DIAGNOSTIC TESTS

In clinical studies, diagnostic tools such as imaging and biomarkers are often used to noninvasively determine the value of a binary variable of interest, the levels of which are typically referred to as positive and negative. The true or error-free measurement of this outcome is the *gold standard* and a diagnostic tool is evaluated by being compared against it. Data from a diagnostic tool can be ordinal, as in imaging studies where the scans are scored using a ratings scale, or continuous, such as assay level of a biomarker. Subjects are classified as positive or negative using a threshold level for the diagnostic tool and they fall into one of the four bins as follows.

	Test-positive	Test-negative
True-positive	a	b
True-negative	c	d

True-positive and true-negative patients are those who are positive and negative, respectively, by the gold standard. The elements a and d are the subjects correctly classified and b and c are those misclassified by the diagnostic test. There are several measures of accuracy of a diagnostic tool, which are defined below.

The *sensitivity* or *true-positive rate* of a diagnostic test is the proportion, $a/(a+b)$, of true-positive patients classified as positive by the diagnostic test. Similarly the *specificity* or *true-negative rate* of a diagnostic test is the proportion, $d/(c+d)$, of true-negative patients classified as negative by the diagnostic test. The *positive* and *negative predictive values* are the proportion of true-positive and true-negative patients among those classified by the diagnostic test as positive and negative, respectively, or $a/(a+c)$ and $d/(b+d)$. A desirable diagnostic test should have a high sensitivity, specificity, and positive and negative predictive values. These measures depend on the choice of threshold level used to classify the subject. The optimal choice of the threshold depends on balancing the costs associated with the two types of misclassification.

A method used to evaluate the diagnostic test over the entire range of possible thresholds is the *receiver operating characteristic* (ROC) curve and the resultant analysis is called the ROC analysis. In this, the true-positive rate and the false-positive rate (1-specificity) are calculated for all choices of threshold values and plotted against each other. The area under the ROC curve (AUC) is a measure of accuracy of the diagnostic test. The value of AUC lies between 0 and 1, with larger values signifying better accuracy. An AUC of 1 corresponds to a perfect test and 0.5 to a coin toss. The AUCs can also be used to compare alternate diagnostic tests.

In the CA-125 study, the question of interest is whether preoperative CA-125 can be used to determine if a patient can be optimally (negative) or suboptimally (positive) debulked. The surgical result, which is the gold standard, was available for all patients. Large values of CA-125 correspond to a lower

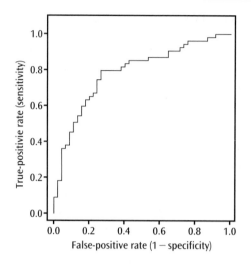

Figure 1.2

The receiver operating characteristic (ROC) curve for serum CA-125 as a predictor of debulking status.

chance of optimal debulking. If we classify patients with a CA-125 level above 500 as potentially suboptimal patients, then the sensitivity, specificity, and positive and negative predictive values are 0.782, 0.733, 0.782, and 0.733, respectively. If we move the threshold to 1,000, then they change to 0.655, 0.778, 0.783, and 0.648, respectively. The ROC curve for this problem of predicting debulking status is given in Figure 1.2 and its AUC is 0.79. These suggest that CA-125 is a good predictor of debulking status, but not a perfect one.

SURVIVAL ANALYSIS

In cancer studies, an important question is whether a new treatment prolongs the amount of time a person is alive or free of disease. In studies designed to address this question, the outcome is called a *failure time* variable, since it is the time taken for the treatment to fail (i.e., the time until the patient has a recurrence or dies). One approach to this question is to wait until all the subjects in the study fail and then analyze the failure times using methods discussed earlier. This process of analysis may be infeasible, however, since some of the patients may move and doctor–patient contact be lost. In addition, the time duration required to observe all of the failures might be too long for an experimenter to wait. Thus, for each subject, we have either the time of failure or the time duration observed during which the subject has not failed. In other words, we have two variables for each subject: the time of follow-up and a status indicator of whether an event occurred at the end of the time period. The subjects who are failure-free at the end of their follow-up times are called *censored*, since the true failure time has not been observed. The analysis of *censored data* is called *survival analysis*.

One key piece of information we would like to obtain from censored data is the proportion of subjects who are failure-free for any time interval of interest. For example, we may be interested in the proportion of people who are disease-free for 2 years after the completion of the treatment being studied, or the proportion who are alive for 5 years after the completion of treatment. Earlier, we defined the probability of a numeric variable not exceeding a given value as the *cumulative distribution*. Since we are interested in the probability of a variable being greater than a given value, we will look at the cumulative distribution subtracted from 1. This distribution is called the *survival distribution*. The goals of survival analysis are the estimation of the survival distribution and the test of equality of the survival distributions between two groups.

The most widely used method of estimating the survival distribution is a nonparametric procedure called the *Kaplan–Meier* or the *product–limit* method, which makes no assumptions about the underlying distribution of the survival times. This method works as follows: first, patients are ordered in increasing order according to their follow-up times. At any time-point *t* where a failure is observed, the probability of failing at *t* is calculated as the proportion of subjects who fail at *t* among those who are known to be failure-free. This probability of failure at a given time point is called the *hazard rate* at that time-point, and the set of subjects known to be failure-free is called the *risk set*. Note that if we are trying to obtain the hazard at 12 months, a subject who is censored at 8 months is not included in the risk set at 12 months, for even though we have not observed the subject there is a possibility that the subject failed between 8 and 12 months. A patient is failure-free beyond time *t* if and only if the patient is failure-free at all times prior to *t* and did not fail at *t*. This is known as *conditional probability*, and is used to calculate the survival probability at *t*. The variance of the survival probability estimate is obtained using *Greenwood's formula*, which gives us the uncertainty in the estimates. There is more uncertainty in the estimates for the larger time-points, since the tail of the distribution is unstable, because fewer subjects are at risk. Note that calculating the survival probability by either considering only the failures or by ignoring the status indicator would lead to incorrect results.

The *logrank test* is the most widely used test for comparing the survival distributions of two groups of patients. The null hypothesis for the logrank test maintains that the survival probabilities are equal for the two groups at all time-points. This implies that when a failure occurs, all the individuals who are failure-free at that time-point (i.e., those who belong to the risk set) are equally likely to fail. This gives us the expected number of failures in each group if the survival distributions are equal. We then form a chi-square statistic by comparing the expected number of failures in each group with the respective observed number of failures in order to test whether the data are consistent with equality of survival distributions.

A randomized trial was conducted at Memorial Sloan-Kettering Cancer Center to compare the survival rates of high-risk cervical cancer patients treated with adjuvant chemotherapy alone with those of similar patients treated with chemotherapy plus pelvic irradiation. A total of 89 patients (44 in chemo and

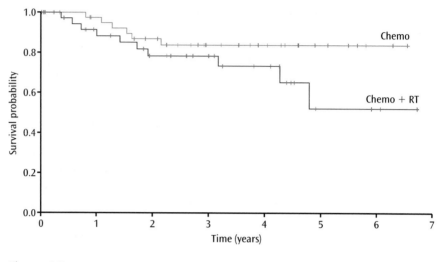

Figure 1.3
Kaplan–Meier survival curves.

45 in chemo + RT) were enrolled in the study. The Kaplan–Meier curves for the two groups are shown in Figure 1.3. The logrank test showed no statistically significant difference, with a p-value of 0.11.

REGRESSION MODELS

Earlier, we introduced the odds ratio and the correlation coefficient, which measure the association between two binary and two numeric variables, respectively. Regression models generalize the concept of association between one or more independent variables, which can be numeric or categorical, and a dependent variable, which can be numeric, binary, or a survival variable. Furthermore, these models give a mathematical expression for the relationship between the independent and the dependent variables.

Linear regression

Suppose we have data on independent variables $X_1, \ldots, X_k$, where $k \geq 1$, and the dependent variable is Y. We are interested in determining how Y is related to the Xs. Earlier, we defined the correlation coefficient, which is a measure of the linear relationship between two numeric variables; that is, it measures how well we can model the relationship between X and Y using a straight line of the form $Y = a_0 + a_1 X$, where a_0 is the intercept and a_1 is the slope of the line. This way of modeling a dependent variable by a single independent variable, both of which are numeric, is called *simple linear regression*. When we have more than one independent variable, we can use an equation of the form $Y = a_0 + a_1X_1 + \ldots + a_kX_k$ to generalize it. This extension of simple linear regression is called *multiple regression*, and together they are called *linear regression analysis*.

The above equation gives us the average value of the outcome, or dependent variable, for a fixed set of values of the independent variables. The outcome of an individual subject varies around this average, and this variation is called the *unexplained variation*. The remaining part of the overall variation in the outcome is called the *explained variation*. How well the model fits the data is given by R^2, which is the ratio of explained variation to overall variation. The intercept gives us the average value of the outcome when all independent variables are set to 0. The slope gives us the magnitude of change in the outcome variable resulting from a unit change in the independent variable. If the slope is zero, then the outcome does not change when the independent variable changes. Thus, a test of whether the slope is zero is conducted to evaluate the prognostic significance of the independent variable. The linear models can be extended to independent variables that are categorical. The resulting analysis is called an *analysis of variance*.

Logistic regression

Linear regression gives us a method to model a numeric outcome variable as a function of a collection of independent variables. The extension of the concepts of linear regression to a binary outcome variable is called *logistic regression*. In the section on the analysis of categorical data, we defined the concept of an odds ratio for a binary independent variable and binary outcome variable. In the example provided, we ascertained the odds ratio to be 9.85, which is interpreted to mean that the odds of suboptimal debulking for a patient with a high preoperative CA-125 level is 9.85 times higher than that for a patient with a low CA-125 level. Since CA-125 level is a numeric variable, we can also treat it as a continuous variable. We may then be interested in quantifying the increase in odds of suboptimal debulking as a patient's CA-125 level increases. Logistic regression provides a model for the odds ratio as a patient moves from one CA-125 level to the next. It uses a mathematical form similar to that in the linear regression analysis, and the parameters give us the logarithm of the odds ratio. Since an odds ratio of 1 means that the odds do not change, the prognostic significance of an independent variable can be evaluated by testing whether the odds ratio is 1.

Proportional hazards model

In the section on survival analysis, we introduced the concept of the hazard rate. Suppose we have two patients and the values of the independent variables given as A and B. The hazard ratio is defined as the ratio of the two hazard rates. The hazard ratio quantifies the greater likelihood of a patient with B failing at any given time-point than a patient with A. The proportional hazards model, also called the Cox model after the statistician who proposed it, models this hazard ratio as a function of independent variables. For example, with regard to the cervix data, we may be interested in the effect of the number of positive lymph nodes on overall survival. The Cox model would give us the hazard ratio. The proportional hazards model uses a mathematical form similar to the linear and the logistic-regression models. Since a hazard ratio of 1 means that the hazards are the same, the prognostic significance of an independent variable can be evaluated by testing whether the hazard ratio is 1.

CLINICAL TRIALS

Clinical drug trials are classified into three categories: Phase I, Phase II, and Phase III. A Phase I clinical trial is a dose-finding trial, a Phase II trial is a noncomparative efficacy trial, and a Phase III trial is a randomized, controlled trial designed to compare two competing treatment regimens.

The treatment of cancer involves cytotoxic drugs; therefore, patients experience toxic side effects. The goal of a Phase I trial is to find the *maximum tolerated dose,* which is defined as the dose level of the drug with acceptable *dose-limiting toxicity.* A small number of patients are treated in these trials following a dose-escalation scheme, and the escalation stops at the level at which unacceptable levels of toxicity are reached.

Phase II trials attempt to evaluate the potential efficacy of a treatment regimen. Typically, the major endpoint of interest is the tumor response. Usually between 20 and 50 patients are treated in such trials at the dose level established in the Phase I trial, and the endpoints are estimated, along with their confidence intervals. Often a *Gehan two-stage design* or a *Simon two-stage design* is employed to eliminate treatments that are potentially ineffective.

The Gehan design sets the number of patients at the first stage to be the minimum number of patients required for the 95% confidence limit of the response proportion to be smaller than the target response proportion. Suppose we are conducting a clinical trial of a new treatment regimen in order to evaluate its efficacy. If we need the target proportion to be 20% for the treatment to be considered effective, then the first stage requires 14 patients. If none of the 14 patients in the first stage has a response, the trial is stopped and the drug declared ineffective. If at least one responds, additional patients are treated and the response proportion estimated with the appropriate confidence interval.

The Simon design starts with an unacceptable response proportion p_0, a desirable response proportion p_1, and error rates α and β for the Type I and Type II errors, respectively. For specified values of p_0, p_1, α, and β, the optimal design is obtained by minimizing the average sample size. Suppose we consider a treatment with a 10% response rate to be ineffective and one with a

30% response rate to be effective, and we fix both the error rates at 10%; then the Simon design would treat 12 patients in the first stage. If, at most, one patient responds, then the trial is stopped and the drug declared ineffective. If two or more patients respond, then an additional 23 patients are treated, for a total of 35 patients. We declare that the drug warrants further study if at least six of the 35 patients in the study respond.

Phase II designs lack concurrent controls; results in Phase II trials are therefore compared against historical data. Since these trials are also subject to patient selection such that the sample is not always truly representative of the population of interest, results from these trials show variability over and above what can be expected due to random fluctuations. Thus, the results should be used as an indicator for further study of the treatment rather than as confirmatory proof of efficacy.

Phase III trials are aimed at comparing experimental treatments with their standard counterparts. These trials employ *randomization,* which is the process of allocating patients randomly to either of the two treatments in order to provide concurrent control and to balance any potential patient selection problems. The process of not informing the patient as to which treatment arm they belong is called *blinding,* or *double-blinding* in cases where treatment-arm information is also kept from the treating physician. Blinding and double-blinding are used to prevent alteration of the treatment's effect in a manner that may render the trial unbalanced. For example, if it is believed that the new treatment is better than the standard treatment, patients in the standard arm may seek alternate treatment prior to the end of study. This could lead to an alteration of the balance provided by randomization. In order to reduce variability, patients are *stratified* by major prognostic factors, and randomization is undertaken within each stratum. The randomization is done using a random permuted-block design in order that the numbers of patients within each stratum for the two treatment arms are nearly equal to one another and the balance thereby maintained.

Since Phase III clinical trials are aimed at proving that a new treatment offers an improvement over the standard, they are monitored periodically so that they may be stopped early if the new treatment proves effective. In this way, all patients can be offered the effective treatment. These analyses for monitoring are called *interim analyses,* and are implemented using *group sequential designs,* which adjust for inflation of size and loss of power that can result from multiple testing. Another issue seen in clinical trials is that of a randomized individual withdrawing from the trial or being administered a treatment different from the one assigned. In such cases, the data are collected from all patients, and the analysis includes each patient in the arm to which they were randomized. This is called an *intent-to-treat analysis.* The intent-to-treat analysis is conducted in order to minimize the potential bias, and any subsequent trial imbalance that may occur, due to patients' withdrawing or switching treatment arms.

SELECTED READING

Altman DG, *Practical Statistics for Medical Research*. New York: CRC Press, 1990.

Anderson JR, Crowley JJ, Propert KJ, Interpretation of survival data in clinical trials. *Oncology* 1991; **5**: 104.

Chatterjee S, Price B, *Regression Analysis by Example*. New York: Wiley, 1977.

Chi DS, Venkatraman ES, Masson V, Hoskins WJ, The ability of preoperative serum CA-125 to predict optimal primary tumor cytoreduction in stage III epithelial ovarian carcinoma. *Gynecol Oncol* 2000; **77**: 227.

Collett D, *Modelling Survival Data in Medical Research*. New York: CRC Press, 1994.

Curtin JP, Hoskins WJ, Venkatraman ES et al, Adjuvant chemotherapy versus chemotherapy plus pelvic irradiation for high-risk cervical cancer patients after radical hysterectomy and pelvic lymphadenectomy (RH-PLND): a randomized phase III trial. *Gynecol Oncol* 1996; **61**: 3.

Green S, Benedetti J, Crowley J, *Clinical Trials in Oncology*. New York: CRC Press, 1997.

Hosmer DW, Lemeshow S, *Applied Logistic Regression*. New York: Wiley, 1989.

Miller RG, *Survival Analysis*. New York: Wiley, 1998.

Pagano M, Gauvreau K, *Principles of Biostatistics*. Belmont, CA: Duxbury Press, 1993.

Tukey JW, *Exploratory Data Analysis*. Reading, MA: Addison-Wesley, 1977.

2
Pharmacology

VanAnh Trinh

PHARMACOLOGICAL MANAGEMENT OF PAIN

Pain causes unnecessary suffering; therefore, pain control demands appropriate medical attention. Effective management requires comprehensive assessment of pain and judicious individualization of therapy. Treatment planning should integrate multidisciplinary approaches to properly address the multifactorial aspect of pain.

Drug therapy remains the cornerstone of pain management, relying on three major classes of agents: (1) nonsteroidal anti-inflammatory drugs (NSAIDs) and acetaminophen; (2) opioids; (3) adjuvant analgesics. Drug selection should match pain intensity and can be facilitated by the WHO three-step analgesic ladder:

- **Step I:** Mild to moderate pain should be treated with acetaminophen or an NSAID.
- **Step II:** If pain persists or increases despite NSAID use, an opioid should be added.
- **Step III:** Moderate to severe pain or persistent pain despite the use of a Step II analgesic regimen should be managed with a more potent opioid.

The available dosage forms and usual dosing schedules of the commonly used analgesics are detailed in Table 2.1

NSAIDs and acetaminophen are effective in managing mild or moderate pain. They can be combined with opioids to relieve more severe pain. NSAIDs exhibit a "ceiling" analgesic effect and can produce serious adverse reactions such as platelet dysfunction, bleeding, gastric ulceration, and renal failure. Because of high protein binding, potential drug interaction exists with warfarin, methotrexate, cyclosporine, digoxin, and sulfa drugs. Selective cyclooxygenase-2 (COX-2) inhibitors with a potentially safer profile have recently been introduced. However, more data are required to confirm their efficacy and safety in the management of pain.

Opioid analgesics constitute the primary therapy for moderate to severe pain. They can be divided into three groups based on their interaction with different opioid receptors: full agonists, partial agonists, and mixed agonist–antagonists. Partial agonists and mixed agonist–antagonists (buprenorphine, pentazocine, butorphanol, dezocine, and nalbuphine) are not recommended, because of their ceiling effect and their risk of precipitating a withdrawal syndrome in patients receiving full agonists. Full opioid agonists can be further classified based on potency. Weak opioids (codeine, hydrocodone, propoxyphene) are usually formulated in fixed ratio with NSAID/acetaminophen to treat moderate pain. Potent opioids for severe pain include meperidine, morphine, hydromorphone, oxycodone, methadone, levorphanol, and fentanyl. Meperidine should not be used chronically or in the presence of renal dysfunction, because a toxic metabolite accumulates, causing dysphoria, agitation, and seizures. Methadone and levorphanol, with complex pharmacokinetics, are not recommended for initial therapy, and should be prescribed by pain specialists. Recently, methadone has become more popular in the management of cancer pain because of the following advantages: low cost, excellent oral bioavailability, lack of neuroactive metabolites, and extraopioid analgesic activity at the N-methyl-D-aspartate (NMDA) receptors. Common side effects of opioids include nausea, constipation, urinary retention, pruritus, sedation, and respiratory depression.

Adjuvant analgesics can be added to any level of pain management if indicated. Common agents are anticonvulsants, antidepressants, corticosteroids, local anesthetics, and bisphosphonates.

Analgesics can be delivered via different routes (available routes and modes of analgesic administration are detailed in Tables 2.2 and 2.3). Oral administration is preferred because of convenience and cost-effectiveness. When switching routes, dosage of analgesics must be adjusted to account for changes in systemic bioavailability. Conversion factors are given in Table 2.4.

Proper pain management also requires monitoring and handling of treatment-related side effects. Suggestions for the pharmacological management of adverse effects are given in Table 2.1. Concurrent use of misoprostol, famotidine, or omeprazole can reduce the risk of NSAID-induced gastric ulcers. Because constipation is a common problem associated with opioids, scheduled laxative must be ordered with opioids unless contraindicated. For opioid-induced nausea and vomiting, dopaminergic (metoclopramide, prochlorperazine) or cholinergic (scopolamine) antagonists can be used. Attempts to minimize persistent sedation should begin with administering opioid more frequently at a lower dose. If unsuccessful, central nervous system stimulants can be initiated. Switching to another opioid may reduce some adverse effects, such as sedation, hallucination, and myoclonus. When rotating opioids, clinicians need to consider the relative potency and the incomplete cross-tolerance of opioids. It is recommended to start the new opioid at 50% of the calculated equianalgesic dose and titrate up as clinically indicated. Conversion factors are given in Tables 2.4 and 2.5.

Table 2.1 Commonly used analgesics in adults and management of common side effects

Generic name	Usual dose for adults	Available dosage forms	Comments
Step I analgesics: NSAIDs and acetaminophen			
Acetaminophen (Tylenol®)	325–650 mg p.o./p.r. q 4–6 hrs Max 4,000 mg/day	Tablet: 325 mg, 500 mg, 650 mg Liquid: 160 mg/5 ml, 500 mg/5 ml Suppository: 325 mg, 650 mg	May mask fever No anti-inflammatory activity
Aspirin (Anacin®, Ecotrin®)	325–650 mg p.o./p.r. q 4–6 hrs Max 4,000 mg/day	Tablet: 325 mg, 500 mg, 650 mg Suppository: 325 mg, 650 mg	May mask fever Can cause platelet dysfunction, GI ulceration, renal impairment
Ibuprofen (Advil®, Motrin®)	200–800 mg p.o. q 4–6 hrs Max 2,400 mg/day	Tablet: 200 mg, 400 mg, 600 mg, 800 mg Suspension: 100 mg/5 ml	May mask fever Can cause dermatitis, platelet dysfunction, GI ulceration, renal impairment, and fluid retention
Naproxen (Naprosyn®)	250–500 mg p.o. q 8–12 hrs Max 1,500 mg/day	Tablet: 250 mg, 375 mg, 500 mg Suspension: 125 mg/5 ml	May mask fever Can cause dermatitis, platelet dysfunction, GI ulceration, renal impairment, and fluid retention
Ketorolac tromethamine (Toradol®)	10 mg p.o. q 6 hrs 30–60 mg i.v. × 1 then 15–30 mg i.v. q 6 hrs Max 40 mg/day (p.o.) 120 mg/day (i.v.)	Tablet: 10 mg Injection: 15 mg/ml, 30 mg/ml	Max duration 5 days ↓ dose by 50% in renal insufficiency or in elderly patients Cause headache, platelet dysfunction, GI ulcer, renal impairment, hyperkalemia, and fluid retention

Continued

Table 2.1 Continued

Generic name	Usual dose for adults	Available dosage forms	Comments
Celecoxib (Celebrex®)	100–200 mg b.i.d.	Capsule: 100 mg, 200 mg	Celecoxib and rofecoxib are selective COX-2 inhibitors Contraindicated in patients allergic to sulfa drugs or other NSAIDs
Rofecoxib (Vioxx®)	12.5–50 mg q day	Tablet: 12.5 mg, 25 mg Suspension: 12.5 mg/5 ml, 25 mg/5 ml	Less effect on platelet function compared with typical NSAIDs Effects on GIT, kidneys not yet established
Step II analgesics: opioid + NSAID/acetaminophen combinations			
Codeine	30–60 mg p.o./s.q. q 3–4 hrs	Tablet: 15 mg, 30 mg, 60 mg Liquid: 15 mg/5 ml Injection: 15 mg/ml, 30 mg/ml, 60 mg/ml	C-II
Codeine (C) + acetaminophen (T)	1–2 tablets p.o. q 4–6 hrs	Tablet: 30 mg(C)/300 mg(T) (Tylenol®3), 60 mg(C)/300 mg(T) (Tylenol®4) Suspension: 12 mg(C)/120 mg(T) per 5 ml	C-III Do not exceed 4 g (T)/day
Hydrocodone (H) + acetaminophen (T)	1–2 tablets p.o. q 4–6 hrs	Tablet: 5 mg(H)/500 mg(T) (Lortab 5/500®, Vicodin®) 7.5 mg(H)/500 mg(T) (Lortab 7.5/500®, Vicodin-ES®) 10 mg(H)/500 mg(T) (Lortab 10/500®)	C-III Do not exceed 4 g (T)/day

		Liquid: 2.5 mg(H)/167 mg(T) per 5 ml (Lortab®)	
Hydrocodone (H) + ibuprofen (I)	1 tablet p.o. q 4–6 hrs	Tablet: 7.5 mg(H)/200 mg(I) (Vicoprofen®)	C-III Do not exceed 4 tablets/day See previous comment on ibuprofen
Oxycodone (O) + acetaminophen (T)	1–2 tablets p.o. q 4–6 hrs	Tablet: 5 mg(O)/325 mg(T) (Percocet®) Capsule: 5 mg(O)/500 mg(T) (Tylox®) Liquid: 5 mg(O)/325 mg(T) per 5 ml	C-II Do not exceed 4 g (T)/day
Propoxyphene	1–2 capsules p.o. q 4–6 hrs	Capsule: 65 mg (propoxyphene HCl, Darvon®) Tablet: 100 mg (propoxyphene napsylate, Darvon-N®)	C-IV 100 mg napsylate = 65 mg HCl Toxic metabolite accumulates in renal insufficiency or with chronic use Not recommended for chronic use
Propoxyphene napsylate (P) + acetaminophen (T)	1–2 tablets p.o. q 4–6 hrs	Tablet: 50 mg(P)/325 mg(T) (Darvocet-N®) 100 mg(P)/650 mg(T) (Darvocet-N 100®)	C-IV Do not exceed 4 g (T)/day See comment on propoxyphene
Step III analgesics: opioids (C-II)			
Morphine sulfate immediate-release	30 mg p.o./p.r. q 3–4 hrs 10 mg i.v./s.q. q 3–4 hrs	Tablet: 15 mg, 30 mg Liquid: 10 mg/5 ml, 20 mg/5 ml Suppository: 5 mg, 10 mg, 20 mg, 30 mg Injection: From 1 mg/ml to 50 mg/ml	

Continued

Table 2.1 Continued

Generic name	Usual dose for adults	Available dosage forms	Comments
Morphine sulfate sustained-release	Dosage based on 24-hour requirement of short-acting narcotics	MS Contin® (tablet): 15 mg, 30 mg, 60 mg, 100 mg, 200 mg Oramorph SR® (tablet): 30 mg, 60 mg, 100 mg	Do not chew, crush, or break tablet q 8–12 hrs dosing interval
		Kadian® (capsule): 20 mg, 50 mg, 100 mg	May open capsule and sprinkle pellets on a small amount of apple sauce immediately before ingestion Do not chew, crush, or dissolve pellets q 12–24 hrs for Kadian®
Oxycodone immediate-release	30 mg p.o. q 3–4 hrs	Tablet: 5 mg, 10 mg, 30 mg Liquid: 5 mg/5 ml	
Oxycodone sustained-release tablets	Dosage based on 24-hour requirement of short-acting narcotics	Oxy Contin®: 10 mg, 20 mg, 40 mg, 80 mg, 160 mg	Do not chew, crush, or break tablet q 8–12 hrs dosing interval
Hydromorphone (Dilaudid®)	6 mg p.o./p.r. q 3–4 hrs 2 mg i.v./s.q. q 3–4 hrs	Tablet: 1 mg, 2 mg, 3 mg, 4 mg, 8 mg Liquid: 5 mg/5 ml Suppository: 3 mg Parenteral: from 1 mg/ml to 10 mg/ml	Sustained-release dosage form will soon be available
Meperidine (Demerol®)	200–300 mg p.o. q 3 hrs 100 mg i.v./s.q. q 3 hrs	Tablet: 50 mg, 100 mg Parenteral: 50 mg/ml, 100 mg/ml	Short duration of action: 2–3 hrs Toxic metabolite accumulates in renal insufficiency or with chronic use Not recommended for chronic use

Methadone (Dolophin®)	20 mg p.o. q 6–8 hrs 10 mg i.v./s.q. q 6–8 hrs	Tablet: 5 mg, 10 mg Liquid: 5 mg/5 ml, 10 mg/5 ml Parenteral: 10 mg/ml	Long half-life Accumulate with prolonged use Should only be used by pain specialists
Fentanyl transdermal patch (Duragesic®)	Dosage based on 24-hour requirement of short-acting narcotics	Patch: 25 µg, 50 µg, 75 µg, 100 µg	Contraindicated in postop analgesia or acute pain Take at least 24 hrs to reach steady state $\Rightarrow$ make sure to have available breakthrough pain medications Serum concentration $\downarrow$ by $\frac{1}{2}$ in about 17 hrs after patch removal q 72 hrs dosing interval
Oral transmucosal fentanyl citrate (OTFC) (Actiq®)	Start with 200-µg unit Gradual titration a must	OTFC: 200 µg, 400 µg, 600 µg, 800 µg, 1,200 µg, 1,600 µg	For breakthrough pain only in cancer patients who are opioid-tolerant Contraindicated in acute or postop analgesia Consume each unit in 15 minutes Should only be used by pain specialists

Adjuvant analgesics

Dexamethasone (Decadron®)	4–24 mg p.o./i.v. q.i.d.	Tablet: 4 mg Liquid: 0.5 mg/5 ml Parenteral: 4–24 mg/ml, 1 mg/ml	Dexamethasone and prednisone relieve nerve pain, bone pain, and pain associated with spinal-cord compression, brain and liver metastases If helpful, use lowest effective dose of dexamethasone or prednisone
Prednisone (Deltasone®)	20–50 mg p.o. b.i.d.	Tablet: 2.5 mg, 5 mg, 10 mg, 20 mg, 50 mg Liquid: 5 mg/5 ml	

Continued

Table 2.1 Continued			
Generic name	Usual dose for adults	Available dosage forms	Comments
Gabapentin (Neurontin®)	300–600 mg p.o. t.i.d.	Capsule: 100 mg, 300 mg, 400 mg, 600 mg, 800 mg	For neuropathic pain Slow titration to avoid sedation
Amitriptyline (Elavil®, Endep®)	10–150 mg p.o. q h.s.	Tablet: 10 mg, 25 mg, 50 mg, 100 mg, 150 mg	For neuropathic pain Start with 10–25 mg h.s. and titrate up Use cautiously in the elderly and patients at risk for arrhythmia
Mixelitine (Mexitil®)	150–200 mg p.o. q 8 hrs	Capsule: 150 mg, 200 mg, 250 mg	For neuropathic pain Start with 150 mg q day and titrate up Avoid if risk for arrhythmia presents
Pamidronate (Aredia®)	60–90 mg i.v. over 2–24 hrs q month		For pain associated with osteolytic bone lesions
Management of side-effects			
Misoprostol (Cytotec®)	100–200 μg p.o. q.i.d.	Tablet: 100 μg, 200 μg	Misoprostol, famotidine, and omepraxole prevent NSAID-induced gastric ulcers
Famotidine (Pepcid®)	20 mg p.o. b.i.d.	Tablet: 20 mg, 40 mg Suspension: 40 mg/5 ml Injection: 10 mg/ml	
Omeprazole (Prilosec®)	20 mg p.o. q day	Capsule: 10 mg, 20 mg, 40 mg	Do not chew, crush, or open omepraxole capsule

Drug	Dosing	Formulation	Comments
Psyllium (Metamucil®, Perdiem®)	1 packet p.o. q day b.i.d. Each dose must be mixed in a glass of water		Bulk-forming laxatives Avoid if poor p.o. intake or in bowel obstruction
Docusate (Colace®)	100–200 p.o. q day b.i.d.	Capsule: 50 mg, 100 mg Syrup: 50 mg/15 ml	Enhance water and fat incorporation in stool for stool softening Not used alone for opioid-induced constipation
Bisacodyl (Dulcolax®)	10 mg p.o./p.r. q day	Tablet: 5 mg Suppository: 10 mg	Peristalsis-stimulating laxatives Avoid in bowel obstruction, appendicitis, GI bleed
Senna + Docusate (Senokot-S®)	1–2 tablets p.o. q day t.i.d.		
Magnesium hydroxide (MOM®)	30–60 ml p.o. q day		Magnesium hydroxide and magnesium citrate cause osmotic retention of fluid and stimulation of peristalsis Avoid in severe renal insufficiency
Magnesium citrate	$\frac{1}{2}$–1 bottle p.o. × 1		Magnesium citrate is primarily used for bowel evacuation prior to surgery

Continued

Table 2.1 Continued

Generic name	Usual dose for adults	Available dosage forms	Comments
Lactulose (Enulose®)	15–60 ml p.o. q day		Causes osmotic retention of fluid and stimulation of peristalsis
Polyethylene glycol electrolyte (Golytely®)	4,000 ml p.o. × 1	Powder for oral solution: 2,000 ml, 4,000 ml, 6,000 ml	For bowel evacuation prior to surgery
Methylphenidate (Ritalin®)	5 mg p.o. q day b.i.d.	Tablet: 5 mg, 10 mg, 20 mg	Last dose should be given at noon to avoid insomnia

Table 2.2 Routes and modes of analgesic administration

Route	Comments
p.o.	Preferred owing to convenience and cost-effectiveness
p.r.	Avoid if having anal/rectal lesions, diarrhea, thrombocytopenia, or neutropenia
i.v., s.q.	More rapid onset
PCA	Allows patients to tailor analgesic dose based on their own needs Facilitates rapid pain control in patients with acute exacerbation
i.m.	Avoid because of pain and unreliable absorption
Transdermal	Delayed onset
Intraspinal	Reserved for patients whose pain cannot be controlled by other routes owing to unmanageable systemic toxicities Require professional experience and regular follow-up

Table 2.3 Commonly prescribed patient-controlled analgesia (PCA)

Generic name	Common starting dose		
	Basal	Demand	Nurse bolus
Morphine	1 mg/hr	1 mg q 15 min	3 mg q 3–4 hrs
Hydromorphone	0.2 mg/hr	0.2 mg q 15 min	1 mg q 3–4 hrs

Table 2.4 Conversion factors for opioid rotation (chronic dosing only)

Generic name	p.o.	Parenteral
Morphine	30 mg	10 mg
Hydromorphone	7.5 mg	1.5 mg
Oxycodone	20–30 mg	—
Methadone	Variable	Variable
Fentanyl	—	0.1 mg

Table 2.5 Conversion from p.o./parenteral morphine to fentanyl transdermal patch

Oral 24-hour morphine equivalent (mg/day)	Parenteral 24-hour morphine equivalent (mg/day)	Transdermal fentanyl dose (μg/hr)
45–134	8–22	25
135–224	23–37	50
225–314	38–52	75
315–404	53–67	100
405–494	68–82	125
495–584	83–97	150
585–674	98–112	175
675–764	113–127	200
765–854	128–142	225
855–944	143–157	250
945–1,034	158–172	275
1,035–1,124	173–187	300

Comments:
- Manufacturer's recommendations
- May result in dose underestimation when converting from oral morphine to fentanyl patch and overestimation when switching from patch to oral morphine
- Alternative dosing conversion: 60 mg oral morphine = 25 µg/hr fentanyl patch

THE HEMATOPOIETIC GROWTH FACTORS

Granulocyte colony-stimulating factor (G-CSF, filgrastim, Neupogen®) and granulocyte–macrophage colony-stimulating factor (GM-CSF, sargramostim, Leukine®, Prokine®)

The colony-stimulating factors (CSFs) present an additional supportive measure to patients at risk for neutropenic complications due to chemotherapy. Evidence-based practice guidelines for appropriate use of CSFs have been established by the American Society of Clinical Oncology. The following are the clinical situations in which CSF use is recommended:

- **Primary prophylaxis:** CSFs should be reserved for patients with a febrile neutropenic expectancy greater than 40%.
- **Secondary prophylaxis:** CSFs can be used in subsequent chemotherapy courses if febrile neutropenia occurred in the previous course and dose-intensity maintenance is desired. However, chemotherapy dose reduction after an episode of severe neutropenia should be considered as a primary therapeutic option.
- **Therapeutic use:** CSFs may be added to antibiotics to manage febrile neutropenia in selected high-risk patients: (1) those with neutrophil counts less than 100/mm^3 with a documented infection predictive of poor outcome (e.g., pneumonia, perirectal abscess, sepsis syndrome, or fungal infections); (2) those with neutrophil counts less than 500/mm^3 without evidence of clinical improvement after 48–72 hours of antibiotics.

Dosing schedules for G-CSF and GM-CSF are listed in Table 2.6.

EPO (recombinant human erythropoietin, Epogen®, Procrit®)

Anemia is common in cancer patients. Untreated anemia undermines patients' functional capacity and quality of life. There is also evidence suggesting the negative impact of anemia on the outcome of cancer therapy, particularly with therapeutic radiation. In fact, tumor response to radiation in the management of cervical cancer has been directly related to the patient's hemoglobin level during therapy. Thus, correction of anemia is important.

Since the cause of anemia can be multifactorial, careful workup is essential to determine treatment strategy. Anemia of chronic disease in cancer patients can respond favorably to EPO administration, providing an alternative to blood transfusion without the transfusion-related risks.

Dosing schedules for EPO are listed in Table 2.6.

Interleukin-11 (IL-11, oprelvekin, Neumega®)

Interleukin-11 stimulates megakaryocyte progenitor cell production and maturation. It is indicated to prevent severe thrombocytopenia and reduce the need of platelet transfusion after myelosuppressive chemotherapy for nonmyeloid malignancies. It is not indicated following myeloablative chemotherapy. Unfortunately, IL-11 can cause a number of serious adverse reactions (e.g., peripheral edema, dyspnea, pleural effusion, and atrial arrhythmia). See Table 2.6 for the dosing schedule for IL-11.

Table 2.6 Dosage and administration of growth factors		
Agent	Dosing	Comments
G-CSF	5 µg/kg s.q./i.v. q day Rounded to closest vial size	Vial size: 300 µg, 480 µg Begin 24–48 hrs after end of chemotherapy Stop when neutrophils $\geq$1,500/mm^3
GM-CSF	250 µg/m^2 s.q./i.v. q day Rounded to closest vial size	Vial size: 250 µg, 500 µg Start and stop date similar to G-CSF
EPO	Start at 150 units/kg s.q./i.v. t.i.w. If Hgb ↑ $\geq$1 gm/dl by week 4: same dose If Hgb ↑ <1 gm/dl: ↑ to 300 units/kg t.i.w. Stop if no change in Hgb after week 8	Alternate schedule: Start at 40,000 units s.q. q wk If Hgb ↑ $\geq$1 gm/dl by week 4: same dose If Hgb ↑ <1 gm/dl: ↑ to 60,000 units s.q. q wk Stop if no change in Hgb after week 8
IL-11	50 µg/kg s.q. q day	Start 24 hrs after end of chemotherapy Stop when platelets $\geq$50,000/mm^3

CHEMOTHERAPY-INDUCED NAUSEA/VOMITING

Uncontrolled chemotherapy-induced nausea/vomiting (CINV) can provoke medical complications, compromise quality of life, and cause refusal of chemotherapy. Risk factors for CINV include emetogenic potential of chemotherapeutic agents (Table 2.7) and patient's characteristics (female sex, young age, low alcohol intake, and poor control with prior chemotherapy). CINV is commonly classified as acute, delayed, anticipatory, and refractory.

Recommended antiemetic therapy for CINV is detailed in Table 2.8. The serotonin receptor (5-HT$_3$) antagonists are safe and effective against acute emesis induced by moderately to highly emetogenic chemotherapy. Their

Table 2.7 Emetogenic potential of single-agent chemotherapy

Level	Frequency of emesis (%)	Agent
5	>90	Cisplatin $\geq$50 mg/m^2 Cyclophosphamide >1,500 mg/m^2 Dacarbazine
4	60–90	Carboplatin Cisplatin <50 mg/m^2 Cyclophosphamide >750 mg/m^2, $\leq$1,500 mg/m^2 Dactinomycin Doxorubicin >60 mg/m^2 Ifosfamide Methotrexate >1,000 mg/m^2
3	30–60	Altretamine (oral) Cyclophosphamide $\leq$750 mg/m^2 Doxorubicin 20–60 mg/m^2 Gemcitabine Methotrexate 250–1,000 mg/m^2 Mitoxantrone Topotecan/irinotecan
2	10–30	Etoposide 5-Fluorouracil Methotrexate >50 mg/m^2, <250 mg/m^2 Mitomycin Paclitaxel/docetaxel
1	<10	Bleomycin Chlorambucil (oral) Hydroxyurea Methotrexate $\leq$50 mg/m^2 Melphalan (oral) Thiotepa Vinblastine/vincristine/vinorelbine

Table 2.8 Recommended antiemetic therapy

Emetogenic level	Antiemetics[a]	Comments
3–5	• Acute emesis (<24 hrs from chemotherapy): ondansetron 8–16 mg i.v. (16–24 mg p.o.) [granisetron 1 mg i.v. (2 mg p.o.)] [dolasetron 100 mg i.v./p.o.] + dexamethasone 20 mg i.v./p.o. ± lorazepam 0.5–2 mg i.v./p.o.	p.o. preferred if tolerated Combination chemotherapy: acute emesis based on agent with highest emetogenicity Multiday chemotherapy: acute emesis for each day based on emetic level of chemotherapy agent given on that specific day
	• Delayed (>24 hrs from chemotherapy): ondansetron 8 mg p.o. b.i.d. × 3 days [metoclopramide 30–40 mg p.o. q 6 hrs with diphenhydramine 25–50 mg p.o. q 6 hrs] + dexamethasone 8 mg p.o. b.i.d.	
	• Breakthrough emesis: Prochlorperazine 10 mg p.o./i.v. q 4–6 hrs [prochlorperazine 25 mg p.r. q 6 hrs] [haloperidol 1–2 mg p.o./i.v. q 4–6 hrs] [promethazine 25 mg i.v./p.o./ p.r. q 4–6 hrs] [metoclopramide 30–40 mg p.o. q 6 hrs with diphenhydramine 25–50 mg p.o. q 6 hrs] [ABH[b] 1 capsule p.o. q 4–6 hrs] [dronabinol 5 mg/m^2 p.o. q 4–6 hrs] [scopolamine 1 disc behind ear q 3 days]	p.o. preferred if tolerated
2	• Acute emesis: dexamethasone 4–8 mg p.o. • Delayed emesis: no routine antiemetics • Breakthrough: same as those for level 3–5	
1	• Acute or delayed: no routine antiemetics	

[a] [ ] represents an alternative antiemetic regimen.
[b] ABH is a compounded combination of Ativan®, Benadryl®, and Haldol®.

PROPHYLACTIC AND THERAPEUTIC ANTIBIOTICS FOR COMMON INFECTIONS

Gynecologic surgery can be classified as clean-contaminated, contaminated, or dirty (Table 2.10). Antimicrobial prophylaxis is recommended for clean-contaminated procedures. For contaminated or dirty procedures, antibiotics should be instituted with therapeutic intent.

Antibiotic selection should be directed towards commonly encountered organisms (e.g., enteric aerobes and anaerobes, staphylococci, group B streptococci, and enterococci). First-generation cephalosporins (cefazolin) are still prophylactic agents of choice for most gynecologic procedures. Second-generation cephalosporins (cefotetan, cefoxitin) should be reserved for procedures requiring anaerobic coverage, such as those involving the colorectal area. Recommended antibiotics for surgical prophylaxis are listed in Table 2.11.

Proper timing of antibiotics is critical. Intravenous antibiotics should be given within 30 minutes of incision. A single-dose regimen is as effective as a multidose regimen for procedures that are 2 hours or less in length. For longer operations, antibiotics should be redosed based on their half-lives.

For elective surgeries involving the colorectum, complete bowel preparation should be performed, with mechanical cleansing and antibacterial decontamination. Oral antibiotics should be given in divided doses within 19 hours preoperatively. Most surgeons advocate the use of parenteral prophylaxis in conjunction with mechanical and antibiotic decontamination.

Recommended antibiotic therapy for commonly encountered infections in patients with gynecologic problems is detailed in Table 2.13.

Table 2.10 Classification of gynecologic procedures

Procedures	Criteria	Antibiotics
Clean-contaminated	Entrance of genitourinary (GU)/biliary tract in absence of infected urine/bile Entrance of gastrointestinal (GI) tract with minimal spillage Entrance of vagina Appendectomy	Prophylactic
Contaminated	Entrance of GU/biliary tract in presence of infected urine/bile Entrance of GI with gross spillage Encounter of acute, nonpurulent inflammation	Therapeutic
Dirty	Presence of perforated viscus Encounter of acute, purulent inflammation	Therapeutic

Table 2.11 Recommended antibiotics for surgical prophylaxis

Procedures	Antibiotics	Comments
Gynecologic	Cefazolin/cefotetan/cefoxitin 1–2 g i.v. (dose q 4–6 hrs if prolonged)	30 min prior to incision Cefazolin as effective as cefoxitin/cefotetan
	Clindamycin 600–900 mg i.v. [or metronidazole 1 g i.v.] + gentamicin 1.5 mg/kg i.v.	If allergic to penicillin
Gastroduodenal/ Biliary	As above	
Colorectal	Cefotetan/cefoxitin 1–2 g i.v. 30 min prior to incision (Dose q 4–6 hrs if prolonged)	For elective surgery, 1 day preop: Golytely: 1.5 liters/hr till clear diarrheal effluent Neomycin + erythromycin base 1 g each p.o. × 3 doses 19, 18, and 9 hrs preop Clear liquid diet Remember to provide antiemetics with preop bowel preparation
If at risk for endocarditis (Table 2.12)	Ampicillin 2 g i.v. + gentamicin 1.5 mg/kg i.v.	30 min prior to procedures Repeat ampicillin 6 hrs later
	Vancomycin 1 g i.v. + gentamicin 1.5 mg/kg i.v.	For patients allergic to penicillin

Table 2.12 Conditions in which endocarditis prophylaxis is recommended

Cardiac conditions	Procedures
High-risk: Prosthetic valves Previous bacterial endocarditis Congenital heart disease (e.g., transposition of great arteries, tetralogy of Fallot, single ventricle) Surgically constructed systemic pulmonic shunts **Moderate risk:** Other congenital heart disease Hypertrophic cardiomyopathy Mitral valve prolapse + regurgitation/ thickened leaflet	**Respiratory:** Bronchoscopy with rigid bronchoscope Bronchoscopy with flexible bronchoscope[a] **Gastrointestinal:** Dilatation of esophageal stricture ERCP with biliary obstruction Biliary-tract surgery Surgery involving intestinal/biliary tract **Genitourinary:** Urethral dilatation/cystoscopy Vaginal delivery/hysterectomy[a]

[a]Prophylaxis is optional for high-risk patients.

Table 2.13 Recommended antibiotics for commonly encountered infections[a]

Conditions	Antibiotics	Comments
Gastrointestinal-tract infections		
C. difficile colitis	Metronidazole 250 mg p.o. q 6 hrs	• × 7–10 days • Can be used i.v. if needed
	Vancomycin 125 mg p.o. q 6 hrs	• × 7–10 days • i.v. not effective
Diverticulitis	Ciprofloxacin 500 mg p.o. q 12 hrs + metronidazole 500 mg p.o. q 6 hrs	• If no signs of perforation
	Gentamicin[b] 1.5 mg/kg i.v. q 8 hrs + metronidazole 500 mg p.o. q 6 hrs Piperacillin/tazobactam 3.375 g i.v. q 6 hrs Imipenem 500 mg i.v. q 6 hrs	• If perforated • Must cover enteric aerobes and anaerobes
Urinary-tract infections		
Cystitis	Sulfamethoxazole/trimethoprim DS 1 tablet p.o. b.i.d.	• × 3 days
	Ciprofloxacin 500 mg p.o. q 12 hrs	• × 3 days
Pyelonephritis	Ciprofloxacin 400 mg i.v. q 12 hrs	• i.v. until afebrile → p.o. ciprofloxacin
	Ampicillin 2 g i.v. q 6 hrs + gentamicin[b] 1.5 mg/kg i.v. q 8 hrs	• Total antibiotics × 2 weeks
Genital infections/sexually transmitted diseases		
Chlamydia trachomatis	Doxycycline 100 p.o. b.i.d.	• × 7 days
	Azithromycin 1 g p.o.	• × 1 dose only
Gonorrhea	Ceftriaxone 125 mg i.m. Ciprofloxacin 500 mg p.o.	• × 1 dose • With empiric therapy for C. trachomatis as above
Disseminated gonococcal disease	Ceftriaxone 1 g i.v./i.m. q day	• i.v. until afebrile → p.o. ciprofloxacin • Total antibiotics × 7 days
Chancroid	Ceftriaxone 250 mg i.m. Azithromycin 1 g p.o.	• × 1 dose only
Syphillis, early (<1 year)	PenG benzathine 2.4 million units i.m.	• × 1 dose only
Syphillis, late (>1 year)	PenG benzathine 2.4 million units i.m. q wk	• × 3 weeks
Neurosyphillis	PenG 3–4 million units i.v. q 4 hrs Ceftriaxone 1 g i.v./i.m. q day	• × 2 weeks • Very difficult to treat

Table 2.13 Continued

Conditions	Antibiotics	Comments
Trichomoniasis	Metronidazole 2 g p.o.	• × 1 dose only • Same dose for sex partner
Herpes simplex, primary genital	Acyclovir 400 mg p.o. t.i.d. Valacyclovir 1 g p.o. b.i.d.	• Immunocompetent • × 10 days
Herpes simplex, recurrent genital	Acyclovir 400 mg p.o. t.i.d. Valacyclovir 1 g, p.o. b.i.d.	• Immunocompetent • × 5 days
Herpes simplex, suppression	Acyclovir 400 mg p.o. b.i.d. Valacyclovir 500 mg p.o. q.d.	• If >10 recurrences/year
Herpes simplex, mucocutaneous	Acyclovir 5 mg/kg i.v. q 8 hrs Famciclovir 500 mg p.o. b.i.d.	• Immunocompromised only • × 7 days
Herpes zoster	Acyclovir 800 mg p.o. 5 × day Famciclovir 500 mg p.o. t.i.d. Valacyclovir 1 g p.o. t.i.d.	• Immunocompetent • × 7 days
Herpes zoster	Acyclovir 10–12 mg/kg i.v. q 8 hrs begin within 3 days of onset	• Immunocompromised • × 14 days
Pelvic inflammatory disease	Ofloxacin 400 mg p.o. b.i.d. + metronidazole 500 mg p.o. b.i.d.	• p.o. for less severe cases only
	Cefoxitin 2 g i.v. q 6 hrs + doxycycline 100 mg i.v. q 12 hrs Piperacillin/tazobactam 3.375 g i.v. q 6 hrs Clindamycin 900 mg i.v. q 8 hrs + gentamicin[b] 1.5 mg/kg i.v. q 8 hrs	• i.v. for severe cases • Clindamycin + gentamicin if patient is allergic to penicillin
Vaginal candidiasis	Fluconazole 200 mg p.o.	• × 1 dose
	Miconazole 200 mg q.h.s. (vaginal suppository)	• × 3 days
Bacterial vaginosis	Metronidazole 500 mg p.o. b.i.d. Metronidazole 1 applicator b.i.d. Clindamycin 300 mg p.o. b.i.d.	• × 7 days • Intravaginally × 5 days • × 7 days
Respiratory-tract infections		
Pneumonia, community-acquired, mild	Azithromycin 1 g p.o. × 1 then 250 mg p.o. q day × 5 days	
	Amoxillin/clavulanate 875 mg p.o. b.i.d. Levofloxacin 500 mg p.o. q day	• × 7–10 days
Pneumonia, community-acquired, hospitalized	Azithromycin 500 mg i.v. q day + cefotaxime 2 g i.v. q 8 hrs	• Any second- or third-generation cephalosporin
	Levofloxacin 500 mg i.v. q day	• Enhanced activity against pneumococci

Continued

Table 2.13 Continued

Conditions	Antibiotics	Comments
Pneumonia, nosocomial	Imipenem 500 mg i.v. q 6 hrs Ceftazidime 2 g i.v. q 8 hrs + levofloxacin 500 mg i.v. q day Ceftazidime 2 g i.v. q 8 hrs + gentamicin[b] 1.5 mg/kg i.v. q 8 hrs Piperacillin/tazobactam 4.5 g i.v. q 6 hrs Imipenem 500 mg i.v. q 6 hrs	• Use aztreonam + gentamicin[b] or levofloxacin if patient is allergic to penicillin
Skin and soft-tissue infections		
Wound cellulitis without sepsis	Nafcillin 2 g i.v. q 4 hrs Cefazolin 1–2 g i.v. q 8 hrs	• Need draining/debridement
	Cefoxitin 2 g i.v. q 6–8 hrs	• In patients with diabetes
Wound cellulitis with sepsis	Piperacillin/tazobactam 3.375 g i.v. q 6 hrs Imipenem 500 mg i.v. q 6 hrs	
Sepsis syndrome		
Sepsis	Piperacillin/tazobactam 3.375 g i.v. q 6 hrs Imipenem 500 mg i.v. q 6 hrs ceftazidime 2 g i.v. q 8 hrs + gentamicin[b] 1.5 mg/kg i.v. q 8 hrs	
Catheter-related sepsis	Vancomycin 1 g i.v. q 12 hrs (single agent in normal host)	• Add to above regimen if immunocompromised

[a]Adjust dose in renal insufficiency.
[b]Once-daily aminoglycosides can also be used.

Table 2.14 Distribution of fluid in the body

	Total body water = 0.6 × total body weight		Intracellular 2/3
	Extracellular 1/3		
i.v. fluid (1 L)	Intravascular 1/4	Interstitial 3/4	
NS	250 ml	750 ml	—
D5W	83 ml	250 ml	667 ml
½ NS	167 ml	500 ml	333 ml

Table 2.15 Composition of various fluids (mEq/L)

Fluid	Na	Cl	K	HCO₃	Ca	Glucose	Osmolarity (mOsm/L)
Body fluid							
Gastric	60	100	10	0			
Duodenal	110	105	5	10–30			
Ileal	120	100	5	10–30			
Bile	150	100	5	40			
Pancreas	140	80	5	120			
Extracellular	140	102	4	28	5		
Intravenous replacement fluid							
Normal saline(NS)	154	154					308
3% saline	513	513					1,026
2 NS	77	77					154
Lactated Ringer's	130	109	4	28	3		273
5% dextrose (D5W)						50 g	253
D5NS	154	154				50 g	561
D51/2NS	77	77				50 g	407
D51/4NS	34	34				50 g	330

FLUID AND ELECTROLYTES

In many diseases, patients are unable to maintain sufficient oral intake to offset daily water and electrolyte losses. Thus, correction of fluid and electrolyte imbalance is important.

Proper handling of fluid/electrolytes requires knowledge of normal body water/solute physiology (Tables 2.14 and 2.15) and the underlying pathophysiology of a specific disorder. One must attempt to correct the etiology if possible. Therapy (agent, rate, and route of administration) should be modified based on the severity of the problem, which can be determined by the acute onset (<48 hours), the presence of symptoms, and the magnitude of laboratory abnormality. Function of major organs, especially heart and kidneys, should also be factored into treatment decision.

Replacement therapy consists of providing maintenance requirement and replacing ongoing abnormal losses. On the other hand, removal of excess fluid/electrolyte requires a different approach, including physiologic antagonists, agents that reduce intestinal or renal absorption, resin exchangers, or dialysis. Suggested management of fluid and electrolyte abnormalities is detailed in Tables 2.16 and 2.17. Volume loss secondary to trauma, surgery, or coagulopathy should also be corrected with appropriate blood products (Table 2.18).

Table 2.16 Fluid replacement

Requirement	Volume
Maintenance	1,000–1,500 ml/m^2 of body surface area
Fever	↑ insensible loss by 20% for each °C above normal *Note:* normal insensible loss ≈ 900 ml/day (1/2 via skin + 1/2 via lungs)
Hyperventilation	Doubling ventilatory rate ↑ insensible loss from lung by 50%
Gastric suctioning	Measure loss
Diarrhea	Measure loss

Table 2.17 Electrolytes

Electrolyte	Treatment decision
Na	Abnormalities generally reflective of body water imbalance Assess symptoms, volume status, serum + urine Na, serum + urine osmolarity Slow correction a must

K	1 mEq/L ↓ in serum K indicates a K deficit of 100–200 mEq (normal condition)
	Assess symptoms, EKG changes, pH, HCO_3, Mg, renal function, ongoing losses, drugs, lab error (blood sample hemolysed/drawn from line)
	
	Hypokalemia (serum K < 3.5 mEq/L):
	Serum K: 3.6–3.9 mEq/L → 20 mEq i.v./p.o.
	Serum K: 3.0–3.5 mEq/L → 40–60 mEq i.v.
	Use 1/2 dose in renal dysfunction
	i.v. infusion rate ≤10 mEq/hr unless monitored by telemetry
	Maximal concentration for peripheral line: 80 mEq/L
	
	Hyperkalemia (serum K > 5 mEq/L):
	Serum K < 6 mEq/L and no EKG change → Na polystyrene sulfonate (Kayexelate)
	    15–30 g p.o./p.r. as enema; repeat q 4–6 hrs if needed
	Serum K ≥ 6 mEq/L + EKG change →
	    Ca gluconate 1–2 g i.v. over 10–15 minutes
	    Dextrose 50% 50–100 ml + insulin 1 unit per 3–5 g dextrose i.v.
	    $NaHCO_3$ 50–100 mEq i.v. over 2–5 minutes, especially if acidotic
	    Kayexelate as above
	    Hemodialysis, especially if renal insufficiency

Mg	Assess symptoms, renal function, ongoing losses, drugs
	1 g $MgSO_4$ = 8 mEq elemental Mg
	
	Hypomagnesemia (serum Mg < 1.8 mg/dl):
	Serum Mg > 1.2 mg/L →
	    Mg oxide 500 mg p.o. q.i.d. or $MgSO_4$ 0.5 mEq/kg i.v. over 24 hrs
	Serum Mg < 1.2 mg/L →
	    $MgSO_4$ 1 mEq/kg i.v. over 24 hrs
	Use 1/2 dose in renal dysfunction
	Prolonged infusion more effective than bolus
	
	Hypermagnesemia (serum Mg > 3 mg/dl): Rare
	Ca gluconate 1–2 g i.v. over 10–15 min

Table 2.17 Continued

Electrolyte	Treatment decision
Ca	Assess symptoms, ionized calcium, PO$_4$, renal function, ongoing losses, drugs
	Hypocalcemia (serum Ca $<$ 8.5 mg/dl) and symptomatic: Ca gluconate 1–2 g i.v. over 10–15 minutes; repeat if symptoms recur, then daily supplement: calcium carbonate 1–2 g p.o. t.i.d. with meals
	Hypercalcemia (serum Ca $>$ 10.5 mg/dl): NS 150–200 ml/hr i.v. Furosemide 40 mg i.v. after intravascular volume repleted; repeat as needed Pamidronate 60–90 mg i.v. over 2–24 hrs If refractory: calcitonin 4–8 units/kg s.q. q 12 hrs
PO$_4$	Assess symptoms, Ca, renal function, ongoing losses, drugs Select KPO$_4$ if serum K $<$ 4 mEq/L; 10 mmol PO$_4$ $\rightarrow$ 15 mEq K Select NaPO$_4$ if serum K $>$ 4 mEq/L

	Hypophosphatemia (serum PO$_4$ $<$ 2.4):
	Serum PO$_4$: 2.0–2.3 mg/dl $\rightarrow$
	  Neutra-Phos powder 2 packets p.o. t.i.d. or
	  i.v. PO$_4$: 0.15–0.25 mmol/kg i.v. at rate $\leq$3 mmol PO$_4$/hr
	Serum PO$_4$: 1.0–2.0 mg/dl $\rightarrow$
	  i.v. PO$_4$: 0.15–0.25 mmol/kg i.v. at rate $\leq$3 mmol PO$_4$/hr
	Serum PO$_4$ $<$ 1.0 mg/dl $\rightarrow$
	  i.v. PO$_4$: 0.3–0.5 mmol/kg i.v. at rate $\leq$3 mmol PO$_4$/hr

	Hyperphosphatemia (serum PO$_4$ $>$ 4.5 mg/dl): Calcium carbonate 1–2 g p.o. t.i.d. with meals Alternagel 30 ml (600 mg/5 ml) p.o. q.i.d. with meals

Table 2.18 Blood products

Product	Content	Indication	Comment
Packed red cells	Red blood cells (hematocrit: 70%; 250 ml)	Anemia Blood loss	Transfusion-related risk 1 unit $\uparrow$ Hgb by 1 g/dl
Fresh-frozen plasma	All clotting factors 400 mg fibrinogen; 220 ml	Coagulopathy	1 unit $\uparrow$ fibrinogen by 10 mg/dl
Cryo-precipitate	Factor VIII 250 mg fibrinogen; 10 ml	Deficiency of factor VIII or fibrinogen	1 unit $\uparrow$ fibrinogen by 5 mg/dl
Platelets	Random-donor platelets; 50 ml	Bleeding + platelet $<$50,000 Nonbleeding + platelet $<$10,000	1 unit $\uparrow$ platelet by 6,000/mm^3

SELECTED READING

Pharmacological management of pain

Agency for Health Care Policy and Research – Cancer Management Panel: Management of Cancer Pain – Clinical Practice Guideline #9, 1994.

Brietbart W, Chandler S, An alternative algorithm for dosing transdermal fentanyl of cancer-related pain. Oncology 2000; 14: 695.

Bruera E, Neumann CM, Role of methadone in the management of pain in cancer patients. Oncology 1999; 13: 1275.

Cherny N, Ripamonti C, Strategies to manage the adverse effects of oral morphine: an evidence-based report. J Clin Oncol 2001; 19: 2542.

Hawkey CJ, COX-2 inhibitors. Lancet 1999; 353: 307.

Hematopoietic growth factors

Groopman JE, Itri LM, Chemotherapy-induced anemia in adults: incidence and treatment. J Natl Cancer Inst 1999; 91: 1616.

Ozer H, Armitage JO, 2000 update of recommendations for the use of hematopoietic colony-stimulating factors: evidence-based, clinical practice guidelines. J Clin Oncol 2000; 18: 3558.

Rubenstein EB, Elting L, Incorporating new modalities into practice guidelines: platelet growth factors. Oncology 1998; 12: 381.

Chemotherapy-induced nausea/vomiting

American Society of Clinical Oncology, Recommendations for the use of antiemetics: evidence-based, clinical practice guidelines. J Clin Oncol 1999; 17: 2971.

National Comprehensive Cancer Network, NCCN antiemesis practice guidelines. Oncology 1997; 11: 57.

Initial antimicrobial therapy for neutropenic fever

Infectious Diseases Society of America, 1997 guidelines for the use of antimicrobial agents in neutropenic patients with unexplained fever. Clin Infect Dis 1997; 25: 551.

National Comprehensive Cancer Network, NCCN practice guidelines for fever and neutropenia. Oncology 1999; 13: 197.

Prophylactic and therapeutic antimicrobials for common infections

Nichols RL, Surgical antibiotic prophylaxis. Med Clin North Am 1995; 79: 509.

Price SA, Polk HC, Prophylactic and therapeutic use of antibiotics in pelvic surgery. J Surg Oncol 1999; 71: 261.

Fluid and electrolytes

Lindeman RD, Papper S, Therapy of fluid and electrolyte disorders. Ann Intern Med 1975; 82: 64.

Wagner BK, D'Amelio LF, Pharmacologic and clinical considerations in selecting crystalloid, colloidal, and oxygen-carrying resuscitation fluids. Clin Pharm 1993; 12: 335.

3
General principles of chemotherapy

Jakob Dupont, Steven L Soignet, David R Spriggs

Chemotherapy agents are among the most toxic medications prescribed by physicians. Medication errors in dose, schedule, or route of administration are always serious, and may be fatal. Even in the appropriate dose and schedule, 1–3% of patients die during chemotherapy for gynecologic cancers. Extreme care must be utilized during the prescription, reconstitution, and administration of these drugs, and attentive follow-up is essential for patient safety. No patient should receive chemotherapy without histologic confirmation of malignancy, preferably at the institution's own pathology department. The decision to prescribe chemotherapy should be predicated on several decisions. First, is this patient potentially curable? If so, aggressive combination therapy can be justified, and the moderate toxicity will be acceptable to both patient and physician. In contrast, if palliation is the goal, quality-of-life issues become paramount. Noncurative therapy is primarily directed at the palliation or prevention of symptoms and the maintenance of a normal lifestyle. An explicit discussion of therapeutic goals should be held with the patient and involved family. Second, an informal risk/benefit analysis is required. Patients with poor performance status, poor nutrition, or multiple prior therapies will generally have a higher risk of toxicity and a lower rate of response than more vigorous patients. For some patients, the risk of serious complications may clearly outweigh the potential for benefit, and supportive care may be the best alternative. A modest delay (one to two weeks) in therapy will often distinguish recovering patients from those whose disease is progressing quickly. With the exception of the treatment of gestational trophoblastic disease and the initial chemotherapy for ovarian cancers, chemotherapy is not urgent. Optimal chemotherapy administered to a stable patient is far superior to ill-considered haste.

DOSE INTENSITY

The practice of chemotherapy is an exercise in brinksmanship, since the effective dose of most chemotherapy agents is uncomfortably close to the toxic dose. During much of the last decade, the dictum that "more is better" was unquestioned. "Dose intensity" is an artificial estimate of chemotherapy administered, expressed as mg/wk therapy. However, it is increasingly clear with platinum, taxanes, and perhaps other agents that the dose–response curves are neither steep nor monotonic. Retrospective analysis of clinical-trial data supports the importance of dose, although most analyses are based on data near or below the conventional dose level. Carboplatin dosing is a good example. While low doses are clearly less effective, results of randomized trials suggest that the effective dose of carboplatin may be as low as an AUC (area under the curve) of 4–5, and there are no data to support pushing the dose beyond an AUC of 6. In general, a high priority should be given to the timely administration of *effective* doses of chemotherapy, maintaining a "density" of dose that relies on minimum intertreatment intervals while avoiding unnecessary toxicity associated with excessive doses. The use of dose-intensive chemotherapy requiring stem-cell or bone-marrow support for gynecologic malignancy is unjustified by randomized data outside of well-designed clinical trials.

APPROACH TO THE CHEMOTHERAPY PATIENT

The approach to the chemotherapy patient is outlined in Table 3.1. There are a handful of key questions that will form the core of the chemotherapy visit:

1. **Does the patient have *proven* cancer?**
   Histologic proof of malignancy is required.
2. **Is the patient curable by chemotherapy or other modality?**
   Referral for chemotherapy does not preclude more appropriate therapy by either surgery or radiation for local disease.
3. **Was the prior therapy associated with severe toxicity?**
   For patients with severe toxicity, dose modification or treatment delay may be necessary. Some general rules for dose modification are presented in Table 3.2. More extensive dose modification may be required, depending on the overall health of the patient. If the patient is on a clinical trial, the protocol should be consulted for dose modification.
4. **Has all acute toxicity resolved?**
   Treatment should be delayed for a neutrophil count of less than 1,000/dl or a platelet count of less than 100,000/dl. Nausea, mucositis, and diarrhea should resolve prior to additional therapy. Renal and hepatic function should return to baseline values. Skin toxicity should also resolve. Chronic toxicities such as neuropathy should be assessed and documented with every course of therapy.
5. **Is the patient responding to current therapy?**
   Regular assessment of therapeutic effect is an essential part of chemotherapy management. Treatment should not be continued in the face of progressive disease. Table 3.3 presents the most common definitions of response to therapy.

Table 3.1 Approach to the chemotherapy patient

Chart review
(1) Establish diagnosis
(2) Review pathology report
(3) Review recent radiographic information
(4) Review other medications for potential interactions

History and physical exam
(1) Verify patient identity
 • Beware of common names and unfamiliar patients
(2) Collect height and weight information to calculate doses
 • Weight changes of more than 5% require recalculation
(3) Review toxicity from previous cycle (both myeloid and nonmyeloid)
 • Document worst grade and duration
 • Consider dose modification for toxicity ≥ grade 3 (see Table 3.2)
 • Verify recovery from all toxicity
 ? Treatment delay or dose modification
(4) Assess for progression or response
 • Measure and document clinical lesions

Data review
(1) Review blood counts (WBC > 3,500/dl, ANC > 1,500/dl, plts > 125,000/dl)
(2) • Review critical organ function (within 24 hrs)
 • Normal renal function for drugs via the kidney
 • Normal bilirubin, AST/ALT (SGOT/SGPT) drugs excreted via the liver
 • Cardiac function for anthracyclines
 • Pulmonary function for bleomycin
(3) Assess objective measures of response or progression
 • Review tumor markers (hCG, AFP, CA-125)
 • Consider/review radiographic assessment

Chemotherapy treatment plan
(1) Choose agent or combination to be used
(2) Calculate actual doses of treatment
 • Use only generic names *without abbreviations*
 • Specify both dose/square meter and actual dose
 • Use milligrams for all doses, and include leading zero (0.5 mg: not 500 μg, not .5 mg)
 • Clearly specify route of administration
 • Identify both frequency of treatment and duration
 • State the actual total daily dose
(3) All doses should be recalculated by another medical professional
(4) Specify parameters for therapy (e.g., hold drug for WBC < 1,000/dl)
(5) Prescribe hydration and premedications
(6) Specify the antiemetic regimen (both acute and delayed)
(7) Patient education regarding potential side effects

Follow-up plan
(1) Order interval laboratory studies (e.g., weekly blood counts)
(2) Consider response assessment
(3) Designate follow-up appointment with bloodwork/radiographs

Table 3.2 Minimum dose modification for toxicity[a]

	No change in dose	25% dose reduction	50% dose reduction
Absolute neutrophil count	Nadir ≥ 500 PMN/dl		
Platelet count	Nadir ≥ 50,000/dl	Nadir 10,000–50,000/dl (CTC Gr 3)	Nadir ≤ 10,000/dl or bleeding (CTC Gr 4)
Diarrhea	CTC Gr 1–2	≥ 7 stools/day or requires i.v. fluids for dehydration	Cardiovascular collapse ICU care (CTC Gr 4)
Mucositis	Ulcers or erythema, able to eat (CTC Gr 1–2)	Unable to eat, requires i.v. fluids (CTC Gr 3)	Requires parenteral nutrition (CTC Gr 4)
Liver function (*reversible*)	Peak values ≤ 4 × upper limit of normal	Peak values 5–10 × upper limit of normal (CTC Gr 3)	Peak value > 10 × upper limit of normal (CTC Gr 3–4)
Renal function (creatinine) (*reversible*)	Peak values ≤ 3 × upper limit of normal	Peak value 3–6 × upper limit of normal	Peak value > 6 × upper limit of normal

[a]These guidelines represent aggressive chemotherapy dosing and are based on quantitative values that correspond to the Common Toxicity Criteria (CTC), Version 2.0. For patients receiving noncurative therapy, more extensive dose modification or a change of agent may be more appropriate than the criteria listed above. *Consultation with an experienced chemotherapist is always required before selecting additional treatment for patients with grade 3/4 toxicity.*

The Common Toxicity Criteria, Version 2.0 contain grade-specific definitions for a variety of more qualitative toxicities such as fatigue, nausea, or neuropathy. In general, grade 3 and 4 toxicities will require dose modification.

6. **Is the patient fit enough for additional therapy?**
   This includes resolution of all toxicity and normal excretory function as well as other medical conditions. Patients with active infections, bowel obstructions, or poor performance status are at high risk for complications, and should be delayed or switched to best supportive care.

If one can answer these questions, the approach outlined in Table 3.1 should be safe and appropriate.

Table 3.3 Criteria for objective response/progression

Response category	Bidimensional disease	Unidimensional disease
Complete response	Complete disappearance of all disease without the appearance of any site of new disease	Complete disappearance of all disease without the appearance of any site of new disease
Partial response	50% decrease in the sum of all individual lesion diameter products of all disease without the appearance of any site of new disease	30% decrease in the sum of all lesion diameters
Stable disease	Effect meeting neither the response nor the progression criteria without new lesions	Effect meeting neither the response nor the progression criteria without new lesions
Progressive disease	25% increase in the sum of the cross-products (for maximum perpendicular diameters) for all lesions or any new lesions	30% increase in the sum of all unidimensional diameters or any new lesions

CHOICE OF CHEMOTHERAPY AGENTS

The choice of chemotherapy agent is generally empiric, based on published disease-specific efficacy data. For chemotherapy with curative intent, combination chemotherapy is generally the standard of care. The preferred combination regimens for specific disease states are described in the disease-oriented chapters and summarized in Appendix 4. However, there are some general principles that apply. Optimal combinations usually draw agents from different classes of chemotherapeutics. Single-agent activity is required for each agent in the combination. Ideally, the combined agents should have different dose-limiting toxicities and compatible schedules for convenient combinations. Combinations that require major reduction in administered dose are unlikely to be superior to sequential treatment. In the palliative setting, combination therapy generally has a higher response rate, a higher rate of toxicity, and little impact on survival. As a result, most chemotherapy in the relapsed-disease setting utilizes sequential single agents.

Selection of single agents depends on many factors. The goal of in vitro chemotherapy screening has proven to be elusive, and most authorities remain skeptical about the utility of such in vitro assays. There are few randomized comparisons of single agents or combinations in the relapsed-disease setting.

Lacking level 1 clinical evidence, the choice among "salvage" agents is made based on schedule, expected toxicity, cost, and patient preference.

CHEMOTHERAPY AGENTS USED IN GYNECOLOGIC ONCOLOGY

Platinum complexes

Cisplatin

Cisplatin (Platinol®, Platinol-AQ®, cis-diamminedichloroplatinum(II), CDDP) is one of the most important agents in the chemotherapy of gynecologic cancer. It is among the most active agents in the treatment of nearly all gynecologic cancers (except certain sarcomas), but it also has significant potential toxicities.

Mechanism of action
Cisplatin functions as a bifunctional electrophile, cross-linking DNA to form both interstrand (dG–dG) and intrastrand DNA (dGpdG) cross-links. These DNA cross-links cross conformational "kinks" in DNA and lead to DNA damage repair and apoptosis.

Elimination
Cisplatin and its active species are filtered and excreted by the kidney. However, the active aquated species of cisplatin is an avid electrophile that binds with proteins and nucleic acids with a very short half-life to form inactive complexes. The protein-bound cisplatin is eventually metabolized and excreted over a period of months. No modifications are required for hepatic disease.

Dosing and schedules
The common dose schedules for cisplatin are shown in Table 3.4. For most purposes, cisplatin is generally administered as an intermittent short infusion given every 1–3 weeks. The other schedules are used for chemoradiation combinations and for germ-cell tumors.

Administration
Cisplatin is highly emetogeneic. Serum creatinine should be assessed on the day of therapy, and cisplatin should generally not be administered to a patient with a rising serum creatinine or serum creatinine greater than 2.0 mg/dl. Adequate white blood cell (WBC) and platelet counts are also required. All patients should receive at least 1–2 liters of hydration (1 liter pretreatment and 1 liter post-treatment) with cisplatin, and particular attention to the serum K^+ and Mg^{2-} is necessary, since the toxicity of cisplatin can lead to electrolyte wasting.

Table 3.4 Cisplatin dosing

Schedule of administration	Dose	Indications
Every 3 weeks	50–100 mg/m^2 as single agent or in combination	Cervical cancer Ovarian cancer Endometrial cancer
Weekly	20–40 mg/m^2	Radiation sensitization
Daily × 5	20 mg/m^2/day (in combination)	Germ-cell tumors Stromal tumors Gestational trophoblastic disease

Expected side effects
Alopecia is rare. Both acute and delayed nausea and vomiting are very common. The most common other toxicity is renal damage, with decreased glomerular filtration rate (GFR) as well as magnesium and potassium wasting. Sensory neuropathy, tinnitus, and high-frequency hearing loss are also frequent. Myelosuppression from cisplatin is generally modest and reversible. Some of the cisplatin toxicities may be prevented by co-administration of amifostine.

Drug interactions
Synergistic renal toxicity may be observed in patients receiving aminoglycosides, intravenous contrast agents, or other nephrotoxins. Cisplatin administration may injure the kidney and potentiate other drugs excreted by renal mechanisms, such as bleomycin and methotrexate.

Carboplatin
Carboplatin (Paraplatin®, CBDCA) is a closely related platinum complex with an improved therapeutic index and a similar anticancer profile.

Mechanism of action
The mechanism of action of carboplatin is identical to that of cisplatin. Its principal distinguishing property is slower activation. Nearly 75% of carboplatin is excreted unchanged in the urine. It appears to be cross-resistant with cisplatin, and has little value in cisplatin-resistant disease.

Elimination
Carboplatin is excreted in the urine, and must be dosed according to renal function (see below). The half-life of carboplatin is approximately 2.5–3 hours.

Dosing and schedule
Carboplatin is generally administered on an every 3- to 4-week basis. The

delayed platelet nadir associated with carboplatin may require longer intervals. The safe dosing of carboplatin requires an accurate assessment of glomerular filtration, either by nuclear-medicine study or estimate by serum creatinine or 24-hour urine collection. The dose of carboplatin is then calculated by the Calvert formula (Dose = AUC × [GFR + 25]), where the AUC is a clinically derived target area under the curve. An AUC of 4–7 is generally recommended, depending on the other drugs administered, while the GFR is usually estimated by using creatinine clearance and the Jellife or Crockcroft/Gault equations. The Gynecologic Oncology Group (GOG) protocols generally use the formula GFR = 0.9 × (98 − 0.8 × [age − 20])/serum creatinine.

Administration
Carboplatin is highly emetogenic, although less so than cisplatin. It is not nephrotoxic and does not require pre- or posthydration, and can generally be given as a short outpatient infusion. While ototoxicity and neurotoxicity are observed, these toxicities are also less common than with cisplatin. Unfortunately, carboplatin is much more myelosuppressive than cisplatin. Prior to administration, the serum creatinine must be assessed and adequate WBC counts, neutrophil counts, and platelet counts should be documented.

Expected side effects
Alopecia is rare. Nausea and vomiting are common and a good antiemetic regimen is required, but other gastrointestinal effects are minimal. Both leukopenia and thrombocytopenia are frequently observed after carboplatin, and may occur 14–21 days after treatment. Neurotoxicity and ototoxicity are generally mild. Of note, true allergic reactions are common after multiple carboplatin exposures and may require discontinuation of this treatment.

Drug interactions
Prior administration of paclitaxel appears to attenuate the thrombocytopenia associated with carboplatin administration.

Oxaliplatin

Oxaliplatin (oxaliplatinum, Eloxatin®, Transplatine®), a platinum-containing antineoplastic, has recently been designated an orphan product for use in the treatment of ovarian cancer.

Mechanism of action
Oxaliplatin is a cisplatin analogue. It is the first available diaminocyclohexane platinum derivative. Its mechanism of action is thought to be similar to that of cisplatin. Cisplatin cross-resistance is less likely with oxaliplatin than with carboplatin because oxaliplatin adducts are not substrates for the mismatch repair system.

Elimination
Oxaliplatin is primarily eliminated in the urine. Renal clearance of platinum significantly correlates with GFR. The elimination half-life of oxaliplatin is about 70 hours.

Dosing and schedule
Oxaliplatin has been administered as single-agent therapy to heavily pretreated ovarian cancer patients on an every 3-week basis. In general, 59–130 mg/m^2 of oxaliplatin is administered as a 20-minute or 2-hour infusion. Oxaliplatin (130 mg/m^2) has also been administered sequentially with cisplatin (100 mg/m^2) to platinum-pretreated ovarian cancer patients. Two-hour infusions of each are given, separated by 2 hours; oxaliplatin is given first.

Administration
Oxaliplatin, like the other platinum agents, is highly emetogenic. Clearance of platinum is lower in patients with moderate renal impairment; however, no marked increase in drug toxicity was noted. The effect of severe renal impairment on platinum clearance and toxicity is currently unknown. Oxaliplatin should not be given to patients with significant renal or hepatic dysfunction.

Expected side effects
Alopecia is uncommon. The main cumulative dose-limiting toxicity of oxaliplatin is peripheral sensory neuropathy. The drug can also produce diarrhea, vomiting, mucositis, transaminase elevation, and myelosuppression. Unlike cisplatin, oxaliplatin has not been reported to cause renal failure or peripheral motor neuropathy, and the sensory neuropathy is partially reversible. Unlike carboplatin, oxaliplatin produces only mild to moderate myelosuppression.

Drug interactions
Oxaliplatin given in combination with irinotecan (Camptosar®, CPT-11) can cause an increased risk of cholinergic syndrome (abdominal pain, hypersalivation). Oxaliplatin should also be administered cautiously in combination with other drugs that can cause renal, hepatic, or sensory toxicities.

Alkylating agents

A variety of alkylating agents have been used in the treatment of gynecologic malignancy. They are summarized in Table 3.5.

Table 3.5   Alkylating agents

Drug	Metabolism and elimination	Dose and schedule	Common side effects	Drug–drug interactions
Altretamine	Efficient absorption Extensive first-pass metabolism	260 mg/m² daily In 4 divided doses for 14–21 days	Nausea and vomiting Neuropathy Myelosuppression	Pyridoxine may decrease activity Does not increase cisplatin neuropathy
Melphalan	Active uptake into cells Poor and uneven absorption Absorption increased by fasting	1 mg/kg orally, usually as 0.25 mg/kg/d × 4 days every 4–6 weeks	Myelosuppression (occurs late and may be cumulative) Late leukemogenesis	Degraded by alkaline pH
Chlorambucil	Efficiently absorbed Hepatic metabolism	0.1–0.2 mg/kg/d for 5–14 days	Myelosuppression Nausea and vomiting Secondary leukemia	
Ifosfamide (requires MESNA; see below)	Requires hepatic activation by hepatic mixed oxidases	1,200–2,000 mg/m² daily × 5 days as short infusion 5,000 mg/m² as 24-hr infusion Requires hydration	Confusion/lethargy Hemorrhagic cystitis Renal damage Myelosuppression Alopecia	CNS toxicity increased by other sedating drugs
Cyclophosphamide	Requires hepatic activation by hepatic mixed oxidases	600–1,000 mg/m² Requires hydration	Nausea and vomiting Myelosuppression Hemorrhagic cystitis Alopecia	Increased activation by barbiturates, phenytoin Cimetidine increases myelotoxicity
MESNA	Renal clearance 50% oral bioavailability	25–30% of ifosfamide dose administered in 3 divided doses prior to ifosfamide and then 4 and 8 hrs after treatment		Mild nausea

Taxanes

Paclitaxel

Paclitaxel (Taxol®) has become an important part of gynecologic cancer chemotherapy for ovarian, endometrial, and some cervical cancers. It is a diterpene compound originally isolated from the bark of the Pacific Yew, *Taxus brevifolia*.

Mechanism of action

Paclitaxel appears to act as a mitotic spindle poison, promoting the disordered polymerization of tubulin monomers and preventing their subsequent depolymerization. The result is cell-cycle arrest and cell death.

Elimination

Paclitaxel is hepatically excreted after metabolism by members of the P450 enzyme class. The pharmacokinetics of paclitaxel are complex, with a long terminal half-life (21–65 hours), and may lead to some schedule dependence. Patients with hepatic function abnormalities should not receive standard doses of paclitaxel.

Dosing and schedule

The typical schedule of paclitaxel has been an every 3-week schedule administered as a 3-hour infusion ($175 \, \text{mg/m}^2$) or a 24-hour infusion ($135 \, \text{mg/m}^2$). The 3-hour schedule is less myelosuppressive but more neurotoxic than the 24-hour infusion schedule. Several studies have suggested that there is no increase in response rate above $175 \, \text{mg/m}^2$. Of note, a weekly 1-hour infusion schedule ($80 \, \text{mg/m}^2$) has also been shown to be active, with very little myelosuppression. Long infusions are associated with more diarrhea and myelosuppression.

Administration

The first administration of paclitaxel can be associated with life-threatening hypersensitivity reaction. All patients should receive 20 mg of dexamethasone 6 hours and 12 hours before treatment, as well as 50 mg of diphenhydramine and 300 mg of cimetidine 30 minutes before the first dose of paclitaxel. While premedication has decreased the incidence of acute hypersensitivity reactions to approximately 2%, it is still essential that a physician be present for the first paclitaxel administration. The hypersensitivity reactions to paclitaxel will occur within the first 15 minutes of therapy. The majority of paclitaxel reactions will be histamine-release reactions, with flushing, urticaria, and chest tightness. These reactions are usually treated by discontinuation of the infusion and readministration of dexamethasone 20 mg i.v. and diphenhydramine 50 mg. In 15–20 minutes, the infusions can be slowly restarted (in the presence of a physician) without further complications. *However, patients with severe bronchospastic reactions, hypotension, or laryngeal edema should not be rechallenged.* Acute hypersensitivity to paclitaxel is rare after the initial two exposures. After an uneventful first therapy, most authorities will use a single intravenous dose of dexamethasone (10–20 mg) prior to each subsequent paclitaxel treatment.

Expected side effects
In addition to the hypersensitivity reactions described above, other side effects of paclitaxel include alopecia, myelosuppression, and neuropathy. Alopecia is universal after paclitaxel treatment. Leukopenia is common but generally short in duration and not often associated with the complications of neutropenia. Thrombocytopenia is rare. Nausea is uncommon and antiemetics are not usually required. As with the platinum complexes, a sensory neuropathy appears after extended treatment with paclitaxel, and can be debilitating. However, unlike platinum neuropathy, the sensory changes from paclitaxel are generally reversible. A separate syndrome of myalgia/arthralgia is sometimes seen 3–4 days after short paclitaxel infusions, and may require narcotic analgesics. Asymptomatic arrhythmias and bradycardia are sometimes observed during paclitaxel treatment, but do not require specific changes in therapy.

Docetaxel
Docetaxel (Taxotere®) is another taxane with antitumor activity against ovarian cancer. Its mechanism of action is similar to that of paclitaxel. It has been reported to have activity in paclitaxel-treated patients.

Elimination
Docetaxel is excreted through the liver via the P450 CYP 3A4 enzyme system with a terminal half-life of approximately 12 hours. Patients with abnormal liver function tests should receive modified doses of docetaxel, and patients receiving other drugs cleared by the P450 CYP 3A4 system (e.g., ketoconazole and erythromycin) should be treated with caution.

Dosing and schedules
The optimal dose and schedule for docetaxel is not known. Generally, it is administered as a 1-hour infusion at a dose of 75–100 mg/m^2.

Administration
As with paclitaxel, acute hypersensitivity reactions can occur with docetaxel therapy, and premedication with dexamethasone, diphenhydramine, and cimetidine is recommended (see paclitaxel). The incidence of hypersensitivity reactions may be less than with paclitaxel. However, a more extended dexamethasone treatment is required to prevent fluid retention. A regimen of dexamethasone 8 mg b.i.d. for 3 days beginning the day before therapy appears to be effective in preventing this side effect. Antiemetics are not always required.

Expected side effects
Docetaxel probably has more myelosuppression than paclitaxel. Alopecia and diarrhea are also common. It is also notable for fluid retention, including anasarca and pleural effusions, which can be prevented by dexamethasone pretreatment.

Drug interactions
Agents eliminated by P450 CYP 3A4 may interfere with clearance of the taxanes, particularly docetaxel. Such agents include many common drugs, such as vinorelbine, ketoconazole, erythromycin, lovastatin, and some calcium-channel blockers. Agents such as phenobarbital may induce P450 enzyme levels and promote excretion.

Vinca alkaloids

Vincristine, vinblastine, and vinorelbine
Three different vinca alkaloids have found their place in modern chemotherapy: vincristine, vinblastine, and vinorelbine. All three inhibit tubulin polymerization at a site distinct from the taxane-binding site. All three are neurotoxic and myelosuppressive.

Elimination
All three agents are hepatically cleared by a biliary mechanism, which may be inhibited by inhibitors of the *MDR1* gene mechanism. Patients with abnormal liver function tests should not receive vinca-derived drugs.

Dosing: vincristine
The dose of vincristine is $1–1.4\,mg/m^2$, with a maximum dose of 2 mg. The drug is usually given as part of combination regimen every 2–3 weeks.

Dosing: vinblastine
The usual dose of vinblastine is $6\,mg/m^2$ or 0.1–0.2 mg/kg. The drug is usually given as part of a combination regimen every 2–3 weeks.

Dosing: vinorelbine
The usual dose of vinorelbine is $20–30\,mg/m^2$ every 1–2 weeks as a single agent.

Administration
The vinca alkaloids are all potent vesicants. Extravasation is likely to lead to severe tissue damage, which may may require skin grafting. These drugs should never be administered subcutaneously, intramuscularly, intraperitoneally, or intrathecally. The vinca alkaloids should be administered by experienced personnel via a recently placed intravenous catheter or a central venous catheter.

Expected side effects
In addition to being potent vesicants, the vinca alkaloids are all neurotoxic and myelosuppressive. They are all moderately emetogenic. As a generalization, vincristine is more neurotoxic and less myelosuppressive than either vinblastine or vinorelbine. The vinca neurotoxicity is characterized by a sensory peripheral neuropathy and loss of deep tendon reflexes, which occurs in an exposure-dependent manner. Both high doses and long exposures are risk factors. A unique neurotoxicity is the abdominal pain, severe obstipation, and ileus observed after vinblastine administration, paticularly with cisplatin combinations. Particular attention to laxatives is needed for vinblastine-treated patients. The myelosuppression associated with vinca-alkaloid exposure is early (approximately 7 days) and brief. Neutrophils are generally more affected than platelets and red cells. Alopecia is common.

Drug interactions
The vinca alkaloids are all substrates for the MDR1 extrusion pump and may be affected by MDR1 inhibitors.

Topoisomerase I/II inhibitors

Topotecan
Topotecan (Hycamptin®) is a semisynthetic derivative of camptothecin, which targets the topoisomerase I enzyme. It is active in ovarian cancer and small-cell cancers.

Mechanism of action
Topotecan stabilizes the DNA–topoisomerase complex, resulting in single-strand DNA breaks and cell death.

Elimination
Topotecan is excreted primarily via the kidney. Glomerular filtration rates below 40 ml/min are associated with a marked increased risk for neutropenia. In patients with normal renal function, the terminal half-life is approximately 3 hours. Hepatic dysfunction appears to have no impact on topotecan toxicity.

Dosing and schedules
The standard schedule for topotecan is a daily × 5 days schedule. In this schedule, a dose of 1–1.5 mg/m² is recommended, depending on the amount of prior therapy and renal function. While oral dosing, a daily × 3 schedule and a 21-day infusion have been explored. No comparative data exist to support the superiority of alternatives to the daily × 5 schedule.

Administration
Topotecan is generally administered as a 30-minute infusion daily for 5 days. It is moderately emetogenic, but does not require hydration or premedication for hypersensitivity reactions, which are very rare.

Expected side effects
The principal side effect of topotecan is myelosuppression, affecting all three cell lineages. Neutropenia is very common, although brief in duration and not cumulative in nature. Thrombocytopenia is less common. Anemia is a common side effect with topotecan, and patients may require either transfusion or erythropoietin support. Alopecia, fatigue, and rash can also be seen.

Irinotecan

Irinotecan (Camptosar®, CPT-11) is another camptothecin derivative, approved for the treatment of colorectal cancer in the USA. It has been reported to be active in both ovarian cancer and cervical cancer.

Elimination
The inactive parent form of irinotecan is metabolized in the liver to its active metabolite, SN38. Excretion of both irinotecan and SN38 is via the liver and bile, with some evidence for hepatic recirculation. The half-life of SN38 may be as long as 12–15 hours.

Dosing and schedules
The initial schedule of irinotecan as a single agent was 80–110 mg/m^2 weekly for 4 out of 6 weeks. This schedule is the current preferred schedule for colorectal cancer treatment. Other schedules, including a bolus treatment once every 3 weeks, have been piloted.

Administration
Irinotecan is generally given as a 90-minute infusion. It is moderately emetogenic and premedication with antiemetics is required. Hydration is not required.

Expected side effects
Life-threatening diarrhea has been reported with irinotecan, and the earliest signs of diarrhea require aggressive management. The diarrhea occurs in two forms. The immediate diarrhea follows within the first few hours of irinotecan administration and is accompanied by flushing and cramps. It is generally controlled with loperamide. The late diarrhea, occurring after 2–3 weeks of therapy, is more ominous. Up to 20% of patients may experience grade 4 diarrhea. These patients should receive 4 mg of loperamide immediately and then 4 mg every 2 hours until the diarrhea has resolved for at least 12 hours. Leukopenia, thrombocytopenia, alopecia, nausea, vomiting, and rare pulmonary toxicity have also been observed.

Etoposide

Etoposide (VP-16) is the only current epipodophyllotoxin derivative (produced from the mandrake plant, *Podophyllum peltatum*) incorporated in the armamentarium for gynecologic malignancies. It is used as a single agent or in combination for the treatment of gestational trophoblastic disease, ovarian cancer, germ-cell tumors, and uterine sarcomas.

Mechanism of action
The cytotoxic effects of etoposide likely occur from its interaction with topo-isomerase II, resulting in a stable topoisomerase–DNA complex. This allows multiple single- and double-strand DNA breaks that lead ultimately to cell death.

Elimination
Etoposide is well absorbed in the gastrointestinal tract, with a bioavailability of 50%. It is highly protein-bound and undergoes hepatic metabolism to form hydroxy acids, which rapidly distribute into body water. However, this agent is excreted predominantly in the urine unmetabolized. It has a terminal half-life of between 3 and 19 hours, which is significantly prolonged in patients with hepatic insufficiency.

Dosing and schedules
The following are several of the doses and schedules used for the treatment of gynecologic malignancies:

- Epithelial ovarian cancer: 50–100 mg **p.o.** daily for 21 days of a 28-day cycle.
- Ovarian germ-cell tumor as part of the BEP regimen: 100 mg/m^2 **i.v.** over 30 minutes on days 1–5, repeated on a 3-week cycle.
- High-risk gestational trophoblastic disease as part of the EMA/CO (see Appendix 4) regimen: 100 mg/m^2 **i.v.** over 30 minutes on days 1 and 2, repeated every 21 days.

Administration
When given intravenously, this agent should be diluted to a concentration not exceeding 0.4 mg/ml and infused over 30–60 minutes. Premedication with an antiemetic is required, since it has moderate emetogenic potential.

Expected side effects
Myelosuppression (leukopenia > thrombocytopenia) is dose-limiting, with the nadir occurring approximately 14 days after initiation of therapy. Nausea and vomiting occurs in one-third of patients, and is usually controlled with antiemetics. Alopecia is dose-related and seen in approximately 60% of patients. Hypersensitivity reactions, chemical phlebitis, and peripheral neuropathy are uncommon. Secondary malignancies, including acute leukemia, have been reported.

Anthracyclines

Doxorubicin HCl

Doxorubicin HCl (Adriamycin®, Rubex®, hydroxydaunorubicin) is an anthracycline antibiotic obtained from *Streptomyces peucetius* var *caesius*. It is one of the most commonly used anticancer agents in both solid and hematologic malignancies. This agent has no known antagonistic interaction and is therefore commonly used in combination with other cytotoxic agents.

Mechanism of action
Doxorubicin appears to have multiple mechanisms by which it induces its cytotoxic effects. In general, it intercalates between base pairs in the DNA double helix and inhibits DNA topoisomerase I and II, resulting in DNA fragmentation and cell death.

Elimination
This agent is approximately 75% protein-bound and is rapidly distributed in body tissues. Doxorubicin undergoes extensive hepatic metabolism to glucuronide conjugates and the hydroxylated metabolite doxorubicinol, and then is excreted primarily in bile and feces. Approximately 5–10% is also excreted in the urine. A 50–75% dose reduction is required in the setting of hepatic insufficiency. The elimination half-life is about 30 hours.

Dosing and schedules
The dose ranges of this agent given alone or in combination with other cytotoxic agents on a 3-week cycle are 60–90 mg/m^2 and 45–60 mg/m^2, respectively. A weekly i.v. bolus dose of 20 mg/m^2 or a 96-hour continuous infusion of 60–90 mg/m^2 is also employed. Because of the dose-dependent cardiotoxicity of this agent, the *maximum lifetime cumulative dose is approximately 500 mg/m^2*. Dexrazoxane (Zinecard®) is a cardioprotectant that is occasionally used with doxorubicin after significant cumulative doses.

Administration
Doxorubicin, like all anthracyclines, is a vesicant and should be administered carefully in a free-flowing i.v. line as a bolus injection over a 5- to 10-minute period. It is incompatible with heparin and should not be given via a heparin lock. If the agent is diluted in NS or D5W, it should be used within 8 hours of mixing. When administered as a continuous infusion, the mixture should be protected from light.

Expected side effects
Myelosuppression is the dose-limiting toxicity. Leukopenia occurs approximately on days 10–12 and resolves by day 21. Thrombocytopenia is usually not as severe. There are two patterns of cardiac toxicity. The first occurs within 24 hours of administration of the drug and is not dose-related. It is manifested

as electrocardiographic changes that have rare clinical significance. The second pattern, and the one of most concern, is a dose-related cardiomyopathy (frequently irreversible) that presents as congestive heart failure. A baseline echocardiogram or MUGA scan should be obtained to evaluate cardiac function before the initiation of therapy. Other expected side effects include alopecia and mucositis. This agent is highly emetogenic and requires prophylactic management.

Drug interactions
Doxorubicin is mostly incompatible with antiviral agents and with most drugs when it is given at concentrations of 2 mg/ml.

Liposomal doxorubicin HCl
Liposomal doxorubicin HCl (Doxil®) has a small volume of distribution and has a much longer half-life compared with doxorubicin HCl.

Mechanism of action
Liposomal doxorubicin binds DNA and inhibits nucleic-acid synthesis.

Elimination
The percentage of this agent that is protein-bound is unknown. The metabolite doxorubicinol is found in small concentration after the administration of liposomal doxorubicin in comparison with conventional doxorubicin.

Dose and schedule
This agent is commonly used as second-line therapy for advanced ovarian cancer. An initial starting dose is 50 mg/m^2 given every 4 weeks. Dose reduction is required for hepatic insufficiency.

Administration
Liposomal doxorubicin is mixed in at least 250 ml D5W and administered intravenously over 30 minutes. In-line filters should *not* be used, since this may alter the characteristics of this agent.

Expected side effects
The side-effect profile is similar to that for doxorubicin. However, this agent has been associated with *palmar–plantar erythrodysethesia* (hand and foot syndrome – characterized by painful erythema and edema), which can be a dose-limiting toxicity. Another unique feature when compared with doxorubicin is an *acute infusion-related reaction* that has been reported in approximately 7% of patients. It is characterized by flushing, chills, back pain, shortness of breath, and hypotension. This reaction generally resolves within hours by either slowing down or discontinuing the infusion. This agent is mildly emetogenic.

Epirubicin

Epirubicin (Pharmorubicin®) is an anthracycline derivative of doxorubicin developed in an attempt to reduce the cardiotoxicity that is observed with doxorubicin. Epirubicin is currently under investigation in the USA. However, in Phase I and II trials, this agent appears to be promising in the treatment of ovarian cancer.

Mechanism of action
Similar to doxorubicin, epirubicin exerts its antitumor effects via interference with DNA synthesis and function. Maximal activity appears to occur during the S-phase of the cell cycle.

Elimination
Epirubicin is rapidly distributed into body tissues following i.v. administration. It undergoes extensive hepatic metabolism. The terminal half-life of the parent compound and its metabolites ranges between 20 and 38 hours. A minimum of 50% reduction in dose is required in the presence of moderate hepatic dysfunction. Less than 15% of this agent is renally excreted.

Dosing and schedules
In clinical trials, epirubicin has been given as a single agent and in combination at doses ranging between 70 and 90 mg/m^2 every 3–4 weeks. For equivalent degrees of myelosuppression seen with doxorubicin, a 20% higher dose of epirubicin is needed.

Administration
Epirubicin has been administered by a variety of techniques, including bolus injection and continuous infusion.

Expected side effects
Myelosuppression, particularly leukopenia, is dose-limiting, with the nadir occurring by day 14 and full recovery by day 21. Common nonhematologic toxicities observed are nausea and vomiting, stomatitis, and alopecia. Congestive heart failure occurred in 35% of patients treated with cumulative doses in excess of 1,000 mg.

Antimetabolites

This class of agents includes structural and chemical analogs of naturally occurring substrates in the metabolic pathways directed toward the synthesis of purines, pyrimidines, and nucleic acids. Antimetabolites are generally S-phase-specific and are most active against rapidly dividing cells. This group of compounds can be subclassified into purine analogs, fluorinated pyrimidines (5-FU), ribonucleotide reductase inhibitors, and folic-acid antagonists (methotrexate).

Methotrexate

Methotrexate (Folex®, Mexate®, MTX) is an analog of folic acid and is the principal folate antagonist used clinically.

Mechanism of action

This agent causes an arrest in DNA, RNA, and protein synthesis by blocking the reduction of dihydrofolate to tetrahydrofolic acid, the active form of folic acid required for purine synthesis.

Elimination

Approximately 50% of methotrexate is bound to plasma proteins, and has a triphasic half-life pattern with $t_{1/2\alpha}$, $t_{1/2\beta}$, and $t_{1/2\gamma}$ of 45 minutes, 2–4 hours, and 8–10 hours, respectively. The majority of the drug is filtered and secreted unchanged in the urine. Methotrexate readily distributes into body water and has a volume of distribution of approximately 0.6 L/kg. *Caution must be taken when used in patients with effusions, since this agent accumulates in the fluid collection, resulting in delayed drug clearance and increased toxicity.* Methotrexate is also available in an oral formulation with a bioavailability of 30–40%.

Dosing and schedules

There are multiple doses and schedules used for this agent, ranging from doses of 30–50 mg p.o. or i.v. weekly to 1–12 g/m² given as a continuous infusion over a period of 24 hours or longer. The oral preparation is available in 2.5 mg tablets.

Administration

Methotrexate can be administered intravenously, intramuscularly, orally, or intrathecally. When given intravenously, it is usually administered as a rapid infusion over 15–30 minutes. Prior to treatment with high doses, sodium bicarbonate should be used to *alkalinize the patient's urine* to maintain a pH greater than 6.5. To minimize toxicity, *leucovorin rescue* is mandatory when methotrexate is given in doses of 240 mg/m² or greater. Methotrexate levels should be monitored at least once or twice per 24 hours after administering doses of 1 g or greater until the levels fall below 0.1 micromolar. If levels remain above 1 micromolar 48 hours after dosing, leucovorin rescue should be initiated using a dose of 100 mg/m² and repeated q 6–12 hours until the levels fall below 1 micromolar. Both liver and kidney function should be monitored before each dose.

Expected side effects

Myelosuppression is common, and involves the leukocytes, platelets, and hemoglobin. The nadir occurs in two phases: the first between days 4 and 8 (mild) and the second between days 14 and 21, with recovery by day 24. Nausea and vomiting is common (moderate emetogenic potential), and is usually prevented with standard antiemetics. Renal failure can occur with high doses of therapy, but is easily prevented by alkalinizing the urine and giving generous i.v. hydration. Diarrhea is frequently reported. Photosensitivity is common; therefore, patients should be advised to wear sunscreen and avoid significant sun exposure. Severe mucositis can also occur with high-dose therapy.

5-Fluorouracil
5-Fluorouracil (Efudex®, Fluoroplex®, Adrucil®, 5-FU) is a fluoropyrimidine used in the treatment of a variety of malignancies as a single agent or concurrently with radiation therapy as a radiosensitizer.

Mechanism of action
5-Fluorouracil is initially metabolized to the nucleotide 5-FUTP, which is incorporated into RNA and inhibits its metabolism. 5-FUTP is further metabolized to 5-FdUMP. This metabolite covalently binds and inhibits thymidylate synthase, which prevents the production of dTMP and thereby alters DNA synthesis. Leucovorin potentiates the antitumor activity of this agent by enhancing the formation of the ternary complex consisting of thymidylate-synthase–FdUMP–reduced-folate.

Elimination
5-Fluorouracil is catabolized in the liver by dihydrouracil dehydrogenase to DHFU, which is further metabolized and excreted in the urine. There are several nonhepatic sites of metabolism; therefore, altered liver function does *not* require dose reduction.

Dosing and schedules
This agent is usually given at a dose of 500–1,000 mg/m²/day as a continuous infusion for 4–5 days, and repeated every 3 weeks. This dose and schedule is frequently employed in the treatment of recurrent cervical cancer.

Administration
5-Fluorouracil can be given as a bolus injection over a period of 2–5 minutes. If administered as a continuous infusion, it should be diluted in 500–1,000 ml of D5W or NS.

Expected side effects
The dose-limiting toxicities of 5-FU involve the bone marrow and gastrointestinal tract. Myelosuppression peaks around days 10–12 and recovers by days 25–30. Diarrhea is common and can be life-threatening. This toxicity is most pronounced when 5-FU is given as a continuous infusion. This agent has mild to moderate emetogenic potential.

Capecitabine
Capecitabine (Xeloda®) is an oral prodrug that is ultimately converted in

tumor tissue to the active cytotoxic agent 5-FU. Capecitabine is used primarily in the treatment of metastatic breast cancer and colorectal cancer. It can also be used in the treatment of ovarian cancer.

Mechanism of action
The mechanism of action of capecitabine is the same as that of 5-FU, within cancer cells.

Elimination
Capecitabine is primarily eliminated in the urine. The elimination half-life is about 45 minutes. Food reduces the rate and extent of absorption of capecitabine.

Dosing and schedule
The pharmacokinetics of capecitabine and its metabolite are dose-dependent over a dosage range of 500–3,500 mg/m^2/day. Standard dosing is 1,500–2,000 mg/m^2 daily in two divided doses for 2 weeks with a 1-week rest period. Capecitabine dosing is modified in the presence of mild to moderate renal insufficiency (creatinine clearance 30–50 ml/minute). Patients with severe renal insufficiency (creatinine clearance < 30) should not receive capecitabine.

Administration
Capecitabine is an *oral* chemotherapeutic agent. It should be taken in divided doses, 12 hours apart. It should be administered, with water, 30 minutes after a meal. Serum creatinine and complete blood counts should be assessed prior to starting a cycle of capecitabine. Liver function should also be monitored while a patient is receiving capecitabine therapy.

Expected side effects
As noted above, the final step in the conversion of capecitabine to its active metabolite occurs preferentially in tumor cells. Consequently, capecitabine treatment results in less systemic toxicity than direct administration of fluorouracil. The most common side effects are hematologic (i.e., neutropenia, anemia, and thrombocytopenia) and gastrointestinal (i.e., diarrhea, vomiting, nausea, stomatitis, abdominal pain, constipation, and dyspepsia). Usually, these events are mild to moderate. Other events less frequently seen include palmar plantar erythrodysesthesia (hand and foot syndrome) and hyperbilirubinemia. Significant alopecia is not associated with capecitabine.

Drug interactions
Antacids (containing aluminum hydroxide and magnesium hydroxide) can increase circulating drug levels of capecitabine. Oral anticoagulants such as Coumadin® (warfarin) can be affected by capecitabine. Patients receiving an oral anticoagulant and capecitabine simultaneously might have an increased

risk of bleeding. Thus, coagulation parameters must be followed closely in patients receiving both agents.

Gemcitabine

Gemcitabine (Gemzar®) is a deoxycytidine analogue that is structurally related to cytosine arabinoside, which is an important antileukemic agent. Although best known for its use in the treatment of adenocarcinoma of the pancreas, gemcitabine has activity against several other tumors, including ovarian cancer.

Mechanism of action

Gemcitabine is a prodrug that is di- and triphosphorylated in tumor cells by nucleoside kinases. The diphosphate inhibits ribonucleotide reductase, which would block the conversion of ribonucleotides to deoxyribonucleotides and thereby alter DNA synthesis.

Elimination

This agent has a high volume of distribution. The terminal half-life of the parent compound is approximately 1 hour. However, the metabolite difluorodeoxyuridine is detected in the plasma 24 hours after dosing. Renal clearance is rapid, with nearly 75% of the dose excreted in the urine (<5% parent compound).

Dosing and schedules

The dose and schedule commonly used is 800–1,000 mg/m^2 given weekly × 3 and repeated on a 4-week schedule. Dose adjustments are made based on the absolute neutrophil count (ANC) and platelet count (plt): ANC > 1,000 and plt > 100,000, give full dose; ANC 500–999 or plt 50,000–99,000, give 75% of scheduled dose; and ANC < 500 or plt < 50,000, hold treatment.

Administration

Once reconstituted, this agent should not be refrigerated, since it may form crystals. The rate of administration should be no faster than 20 mg/minute (a usual dose is generally given over 90 minutes) to optimize its cytotoxic effect. An *acute infusion-associated reaction* characterized by dyspnea, flushing, chills, headache, back pain, and hypotension is reported to occur in approximately 5% of patients treated. Symptoms generally resolve within 24 hours of stopping the infusion.

Expected side effects

Myelosuppression is the dose-limiting toxicity. Leukopenia occurs approximately at days 10–14 and resolves by day 21. Less than 10% of the patients develop a nadir neutrophil count < 500. Thrombocytopenia is usually not as severe, and rarely falls below 50,000. Nonhematologic side effects include a macular papular rash, cellulitis, peripheral edema, and dyspnea. A *flu-like illness*, including fever, has been reported to occur in 15–20% of patients. This agent has moderate emetogenic potential.

Antitumor antibiotics

Dactinomycin
Dactinomycin (actinomycin-D, Cosmegen®) is a *Streptomyces* fermentation product that appears to function as a DNA intercalator, preventing the transcription of RNA species.

Elimination
Dactinomycin is rapidly taken up by tissue, but is eventually cleared unchanged in both bile and urine. The need to adjust dosing for renal and hepatic impairment is not well understood.

Dosing and schedules
As a single agent, dactinomycin is given as 0.04 mg/kg (40 mg/kg) once every 2 weeks or as a divided dose of 0.008–0.015 mg/kg/day for 5 consecutive days. It is also given as part of combination regimens, including EMA-CO, for gestational trophoblastic disease.

Administration
Dactinomycin is generally given as a bolus or short infusion.

Expected side effects
Dactinomycin is highly emetogenic. Alopecia is common. Myelosuppression and stomatitis are common. *Dactinomycin is a vesicant.*

Drug interactions
Dactinomycin is an MDR1 substrate.

Bleomycin
Bleomycin (Blenoxane®) is a complex mixture of glycopeptides derived from *Streptomyces verticullis.* It is quantitated in units, not milligrams.

Mechanism of action
Bleomycin acts in the presence of metal ions, including cobalt, copper, and iron, to cause single-stranded DNA breaks. It has little effect on either RNA or protein species.

Elimination
Bleomycin is principally excreted unchanged in the urine. Dose reduction is required for renal insufficiency, and caution is required when bleomycin is co-administered with nephrotoxins such as cisplatin.

Dosing and schedules
For germ-cell tumors of the ovary, bleomycin is given as a weekly bolus of 30 units. A subcutaneous test dose of one unit is favored by some authorities to

screen for acute hypersensitivity reactions prior to the first dose. As a single agent, doses of 10–20 mg/m² are given weekly. *Cumulative doses of greater than 360 units should be avoided to prevent fatal pulmonary toxicity.*

Administration
Bleomycin is usually given intravenously.

Expected side effects
The most important toxicity of bleomycin is irreversible pulmonary fibrosis, exacerbated by exposure to high oxygen tension. The total dose of bleomycin should be capped at 360 units. Patients treated with bleomycin should be monitored for changes in D_{LCO} by serial pulmonary function testing, and patients with decrements in pulmonary function should receive alternative therapy. Bleomycin also causes fever (usually within 24 hours), mucositis, alopecia, skin hyperpigmentation, anorexia, and myelosuppression.

Epidermal growth factor receptor (EGFR) inhibitors

ZD-1839

ZD-1839 (Iressa®) is a small-molecule inhibitor of the epidermal growth factor receptor (EGFR) tyrosine kinase domain. ZD-1839 is under clinical development in cancer patients. In vitro and in vivo studies suggest that this agent has activity against ovarian cancer. Experimental models also suggest that ZD-1839 has synergy with other chemotherapeutic agents, including paclitaxel, and also with radiation therapy. Phase III trials are underway combining ZD-1839 with gemcitabine, cisplatin, carboplatin, or paclitaxel.

Mechanism of action
ZD-1839 is an orally active quinazolone derivative that selectively inhibits the EGFR tyrosine kinase domain. EGFR expression is increased on a number of human cancers, and inhibition of the EGFR signaling pathway is thought to prevent an important growth signal in cancer cells.

Elimination
It is unclear at present how ZD-1839 is metabolized. Urinary recovery of the drug is minimal, suggesting that this is not the major route of elimination. The elimination half-life is 28 hours.

Dosing and schedule
ZD-1839 has been administered at a dosing schedule of 100 mg once daily for 3 days in early clinical trials. In the lung cancer trials, daily doses of 250–500 mg were administered with carboplatin and paclitaxel. However, dose-limiting toxicity has not been reached with this dosing schedule.

Administration
ZD-1839 is an *oral* chemotherapeutic agent. A food-effect study showed that food intake with ZD-1839 did not affect the elimination half-life.

Expected side effects
The most common side effects noted were dematologic and gastrointestinal. Patients receiving ZD-1839 developed an acneform rash, which was self-limiting. Diarrhea was also seen.

Drug interactions
No significant drug interactions of ZD-1839 are known at present.

Cetuximab
Cetuximab (IMC-C225) is a chimeric monoclonal antibody that binds selectively to the EGFR. This agent is also under clinical development in cancer patients. Recent studies have shown that cetuximab is active in combination with irinotecan in patients with irinotecan-refractory colorectal cancer. Cetuximab has also been used in combination with radiation therapy for the treatment of head and neck cancer. Surprisingly, cetuximab appears to be equally effective in EGFR-overexpressing tumors and tumors that do not overexpress EGFR.

Mechanism of action
Cetuximab is directed against the extracellular domain of the EGFR. This agent also selectively inhibits activation of the EGFR tyrosine kinase. This interaction is thought to prevent EGFR-mediated growth signaling in cancer cells.

Elimination
The elimination of cetuximab is not well established.

Dosing and schedule
Cetuximab is administered intravenously at 200–250 mg/m^2 on a weekly basis.

Administration
Cetuximab is administered intravenously.

Expected side effects
Cetuximab is very well tolerated, with minimal adverse effects. The most common side effects are allergic reactions, fever, chills, asthenia, transaminase elevation, nausea, and skin toxicities. Skin toxicity was an acne-like skin rash.

Drug interactions
No significant drug interactions of cetuximab are known at present.

OSI-774
OSI-774 is an orally active small-molecule inhibitor of the EGFR tyrosine kinase domain. This agent is currently in Phase II trials in ovarian cancer.

Mechanism of action
OSI-774 is a selective small molecule inhibitor of the EGFR tyrosine kinase domain (similar to ZD-1839). The interaction of OSI-774 with the tyrosine

kinase domain is thought to prevent EGFR-mediated growth signaling in cancer cells. Preliminary activity in ovarian cancer has been observed.

Elimination
The elimination of OSI-774 is not well established. The elimination half-life is 24 hours.

Dosing and schedule
OSI-774 is an *oral* antineoplastic agent. It is administered at $150\,mg/m^2$ on a daily basis.

Administration
OSI-774 is administered orally and continuously.

Expected side effects
The most common side effects associated with OSI-774 are dermatologic and gastrointestinal. Acne-like rash and diarrhea are most frequently seen in patients taking this drug. Fatigue and headache are also common.

Drug interactions
No significant drug interactions of OSI-774 are known at present.

SUPPORTIVE CARE IN CHEMOTHERAPY

Antiemetic therapy

Recent advances in antiemetic therapy have made chemotherapy much less difficult for the patient with cancer. Attention to the efficacy of antiemetic therapy will make a major impact on patient quality of life. In Table 3.6, three classes of antiemetic therapy are listed, based on the emetogenic potential of the agents to be used. Patients with refractory nausea may also receive anti-anxiety agents. Patients with anticipatory nausea prior to chemotherapy may benefit from pretreatment the night prior to therapy.

Hematopoietic growth factors/cytokine support

A frequent compromising toxicity of chemotherapy is myelosuppression. Supportive-care measures such as the administration of antibiotics, blood and platelet transfusions, and dose reduction and/or delaying the administration of the cytotoxic agents are often required. A relatively recent advance in cancer medicine has been the discovery and clinical development of the hematopoietic growth factors, which are now commonly used to reduce and limit the hematopoietic toxicity of chemotherapy. These cytokines are polypeptide hormones that support the survival and differentiation of one or more lineages of mature blood cells from progenitor cells. The production of these physiologic regulators occurs in three sites. Granulocyte colony-stimulating factor

Table 3.6 Summary of antiemetic recommendations[a]

Degree	Chemotherapy agents	Acute emesis	Delayed emesis
Highly emetogenic	Cisplatin Dactinomycin Carboplatin Cyclophosphamide Ifosfamide Doxorubicin Epirubicin Hexamethylmelamine Oxaliplatin	**Dexamethasone 20 mg** with a 5-HT$_3$ antagonist dolasetron 100 mg i.v. or p.o. or granisetron 1 mg i.v. 2 mg p.o. or ondansetron 8 mg i.v. 12–24 mg/d p.o. tropisetron 5 mg i.v. or p.o. **May add antianxiety agent** **for breakthrough**	**Dexamethasone 8 mg p.o. b.i.d. × 3 d** with either **metoclopramide 30 mg p.o. q 6 hrs** or **a 5-HT$_3$ antagonist** dolasetron 100 mg p.o. or granisetron 2 mg p.o. or ondansetron 12–24 mg/d p.o. tropisetron 5 mg p.o.
Intermediate emetic risk	Irinotecan Paclitaxel Docetaxel Topotecan Capecitabine Gemcitabine Etoposide High-dose methotrexate	**Dexamethasone 4–8 mg × 1 p.o.**	None usually required
Low emetic risk	Vinorelbine Vincristine Methotrexate 5-Fluorouracil Bleomycin Vinblastine Melphalan Chlorambucil	None routinely required Some patients may require therapy similar to intermediate-risk patients	None routinely required

[a]Adapted from ASCO Guidelines

Table 3.7 Growth factors

Growth factors	Generic name (Trade name)	Supplied	Possible indications	Dosing	Side effects
EPO	Epoetin alfa (Epogen®, Procrit®)	In vials of 10,000, 20,000, and 40,000 units/ml	Anemia in patients: (1) receiving chemotherapy (2) scheduled for elective surgery with chronic renal failure (3) HIV-infected	150 g/kg t.i.w. (approx. 10,000 units) Given s.q. or 40,000 units weekly	Hypertension Thrombosis Allergic reactions
G-CSF	Filgrastim (Neupogen®)	300 g/ml 480 g/ml	(1) Primary prophylaxis of febrile neutropenia when expected incidence is > 40% (2) Secondary prophylaxis (3) Possible for neutropenia fever (4) Mobilization of stem cells	300–480 g s.q. daily (not to be given during chemo- or radiotherapy)	Bone pain ↑ LDH, uric acid, and alkaline phosphatase
GM-CSF	Sargramostim (Leukine®, Prokine®)	250 and 500 g/ml vials	(1) Post autologous transplant (2) Mobilization of stem cells (3) Possible role in fungal-infected patients	250 g/m²/d	Bone pain Myalgias Fever Capillary leak syndrome Allergic reaction ↑ LDH, uric acid, and alkaline phosphatase
IL-11	Oprelvekin (Neumega®)		Thrombocytopenia: (1) Patients at high risk for severe thrombocytopenia following myelosuppressive therapy (2) Drug-induced (3) Associated with liver disease (4) HIV-associated (5) Aplastic anemia		Thrombocytosis Thrombosis Bone-marrow fibrosis Antibody formation

material. This variation accounts for the poor contrast of radiation portal verification films.

(3) *Pair-production* absorption is related to Z^2. Because it only begins to dominate at photon energies of more than about 30 MeV, pair production is of limited importance in current radiation therapy.

Electrons and other particles

Electrons

The dose from an electron beam is relatively homogenous up to a depth that is related to the beam's energy. Beyond this depth, the dose decreases very rapidly to nearly zero. Electrons are used to treat relatively superficial targets, without delivering a significant dose to underlying tissues. The approximate depth at which the rapid falloff in dose occurs can be estimated by dividing the electron energy by 3.

Protons

These charged particles are much more massive than electrons. Protons scatter minimally as they interact with matter, depositing increasing amounts of energy as they slow down and then stop at a depth related to their initial energy. This results in rapid deposition of most of their energy at depth (called the *Bragg peak*), with a steep falloff in dose to near zero shortly after the peak. Modulating the energy can spread this peak out. The absence of an exit dose makes proton beams ideal for conformal therapy, and interest in their use has increased as the cost of producing proton generators has become somewhat more reasonable.

Neutrons

Neutrons are neutral particles that tend to deposit most of their energy in a single intranuclear event. The falloff of a neutron dose is similar to that of a photon beam of 4–6 MeV, but these densely ionizing beams have a high RBE that has been of interest to clinical investigators. Clinical studies of neutron treatments in cervical cancer patients were plagued by high complication rates, however, and today neutrons are rarely, if ever, used to treat gynecologic tumors.

Measurement of absorbed dose

Absorbed dose is a measure of the energy deposited by the radiation source in the target material. The unit currently used to measure radiation dose is the gray (Gy), which is equal to 1 joule per kilogram of absorbing material. Before the early 1980s, absorbed doses of radiation were measured in "rad," where 1 rad=1 cGy, and 1 gray=100 rad.

DELIVERY METHODS IN RADIATION THERAPY

Teletherapy

Teletherapy refers to x-rays delivered at a distance from the body (external-beam therapy). This is usually delivered using a linear accelerator that produces high-energy photons and electrons. Most treatment plans combine two or more beams to create a dose distribution designed to:

(1) maximize the dose of radiation delivered to the target;
(2) produce a relatively homogeneous dose within the volume of interest to minimize hot or cold spots that would increase the risks of complications or recurrence, respectively;
(3) minimize the dose delivered to uninvolved tissues, taking into account the different tolerances of various normal tissues.

The resulting treatment plan must include the primary-target volume (gross tumor or tumor bed), any areas at risk for microscopic spread of disease, and a margin of tissue to account for uncertainties in the location of the target, reproducibility of the set-up, and organ motion. The overall plan is often designed to deliver different doses to areas of greater or lesser risk (e.g., gross versus microscopic residual disease) by boosting areas at greater risk with smaller treatment fields after initial treatment to a relatively large volume.

Brachytherapy

The inverse square law
The inverse square law pertains to methods of radiation therapy delivery, such as brachytherapy, that use a radioactive isotope placed within or near tissue. This law states that the dose of radiation at a given point from the source is inversely proportional to the square of the distance from the center of radiation. This law implies that a large dose of radiation can be delivered to the tumor and immediately surrounding tissues with a rapid falloff that is proportional to the square of the distance from the source.

Intracavitary treatment
Any treatment that involves placement of radioactive sources within an existing body cavity is termed *intracavitary treatment*. The most common gynecologic applications involve placement of intrauterine or intravaginal applicators that are loaded with encapsulated radioactive sources (e.g., ^{137}Cs, ^{226}Ra, or ^{192}Ir). Conventionally, brachytherapy has been delivered at a low dose rate, usually 0.4–0.6 Gy/hour. Low-dose-rate (LDR) brachytherapy permits recovery of sublethal radiation injury, differentially sparing late-responding normal tissue versus tumor cells. With the advent of computer-controlled remote afterloading, it became possible to deliver brachytherapy treatments at high dose rates (in minutes rather than hours). High-dose-rate (HDR) treatment may

offer practical advantages because it is typically performed on an outpatient basis, although treatment must usually be divided into five or more fractions to achieve acceptable normal tissue effects.

Interstitial implants

Interstitial brachytherapy refers to the placement of radioactive sources within tissues. Various sources of radiation, such as ^{192}Ir and ^{125}I, may be obtained as radioactive wires or seeds. Sources may be positioned in the tumor or tumor bed in a variety of ways:

(1) Permanent implants of seeds (usually ^{125}I or ^{198}Au), inserted using a specialized seed inserter, are sometimes used to implant pelvic or aortic lymph nodes, particularly in recurrences after irradiation.

(2) Temporary implants of Teflon catheters can be intraoperatively placed and subsequently loaded with radioactive sources (usually ^{192}Ir). These are sometimes used to treat tumor beds. Transperineal needle implants can be placed with guidance using a Lucite template with regularly spaced holes and a central obturator that can hold a tandem or additional needles. Most gynecologic interstitial implants are temporary, low-dose-rate implants. Like intracavitary therapy, interstitial therapy delivers a relatively high dose of radiation to a small volume, potentially sparing surrounding normal tissues.

Intraperitoneal radioisotopes

Intraperitoneal radioisotopes (usually ^{32}P) have been used to treat epithelial ovarian cancer in an effort to address the transperitoneal spread pattern characteristic of the disease. If distribution of a radioisotope within the peritoneum is even, it is theoretically possible to irradiate the entire peritoneal surface. However, the pattern of energy deposition within the abdomen and the dose delivered beneath the peritoneal surfaces depend on many factors, including the physical characteristics of the isotope used, the energies of its decay products, and the distribution of the isotope within the peritoneal cavity.

CLINICAL USES OF RADIATION

Cervical cancer

Although specific radiation therapy techniques may vary, the curative treatment of cervical cancer usually includes a combination of external pelvic irradiation and brachytherapy. The goal of radiation therapy is to eliminate cancer in the cervix, paracervical tissues, and regional lymph nodes. All of these regions can be encompassed in a pelvic irradiation field. The dose that can be delivered to the pelvis is limited, however, by the tolerance of intrapelvic normal tissues, most importantly the rectosigmoid, bladder, and small bowel.

Because the bulkiest tumor is usually in the cervix, this region typically requires higher doses than the rest of the pelvis to achieve local regional control. It is usually possible to deliver these high doses with intracavitary therapy.

Treatment volume

Typical external-beam fields are designed to include the primary tumor, paracervical tissues, and the iliac and presacral lymph nodes, all with 1.5–2 cm margins. If the common iliac or aortic nodes are involved, the treatment fields are usually extended to include at least the lower paraaortic region. Vaginal disease must be covered with a margin of at least 3–4 cm. If lateral fields are used, care must be taken to cover the entire tumor as well as the iliac and presacral nodes and the uterosacral ligaments.

Radiation dose

For FIGO Stage IB or greater, the pelvis is usually treated with an initial course of external-beam therapy to a dose of 40–45 Gy to sterilize possible microscopic regional disease and decrease endocervical disease to facilitate optimal intracavitary therapy. The dose to the central tumor is then supplemented with one or two LDR intracavitary treatments or with a variable number of HDR treatments. Some practitioners block central structures during part of the external-beam treatment and increase the dose of intracavitary treatment. The total dose to point A (external-beam and LDR intracavitary therapy) believed to be adequate to achieve central disease control is usually between 75 Gy (for Stage IA) and 90 Gy (for locally advanced disease). Point A is described as 2 cm lateral and 2 cm superior to the external cervical os in the plane of the implant.

Results of treatment

Radiation as primary treatment

Radiation therapy is extremely effective for Stage IB1 cervical cancer: 5-year disease-specific survival rates and pelvic control rates are approximately 90% and 98%, respectively. Pelvic control rates gradually decrease as tumor size and FIGO stage increase, although large single-institution experiences report 5-year pelvic control rates of 60–70% and disease-specific survival rates of 40–50% even for bulky Stage IIIB cancers.

Recent studies have demonstrated a marked improvement in pelvic disease control and survival when cisplatin-containing chemotherapy is given concurrently with irradiation for patients with local-regionally advanced disease.

Adjuvant pelvic radiation therapy after radical hysterectomy

Lymph-node involvement is probably the strongest predictor of local recurrence and death. Therefore, most clinicians recommend postoperative radiation therapy of patients with positive lymph nodes. Parametrial involvement and involvement of surgical margins are also indications for postoperative therapy. A Gynecologic Oncology Group (GOG) study demonstrated a 50%

reduction in the risk of recurrence when cisplatin and 5-FU were added to pelvic irradiation for patients with these risk factors.

For patients with negative nodes, large tumor size (e.g., ≥4 cm), deep stromal invasion (e.g., ≥2/3), or involvement of lymph-vascular spaces predict an increased risk of pelvic recurrence after radical hysterectomy and pelvic lymphadenectomy. In another GOG study, 277 patients with at least two of these risk factors and negative pelvic lymph nodes were randomized to receive adjuvant pelvic irradiation or no further treatment. The recurrence rate was significantly lower for patients who had postoperative radiation therapy.

Complications

Late complications of radical irradiation for cervical cancer occur in 5–15% of patients, and are related to the dose per fraction, the total dose, the volume irradiated, and the extent of initial disease. Patient factors such as previous abdominal surgery, pelvic infection, and diabetes mellitus may also play a role. Late effects in the bladder may include hematuria, fibrosis, contraction, or fistula. Late effects in the rectosigmoid or terminal ileum may involve bleeding, stricture, obstruction, or perforation. Agglutination of the apex of the vagina is common. Severe vaginal shortening is less frequent, and is probably correlated with the patient's age, menopausal status, and sexual activity, and with the initial extent of disease. Although late effects may occur many years after treatment, most gastrointestinal complications occur within 30 months of radiation therapy.

Endometrial cancer

The role of radiation therapy in the treatment of endometrial carcinoma can be briefly summarized as follows:

(1) Adjuvant treatment to prevent pelvic recurrence after total abdominal hysterectomy with bilateral salpingo-oophorectomy (TAH-BSO).
(2) Preoperative treatment for patients with very extensive cervical stromal involvement.
(3) Curative treatment for some patients with medical problems that preclude surgery and for occasional patients with Stage III disease involving the vagina.
(4) Curative treatment for patients with isolated vaginal or pelvic recurrence, usually using a combination of external-beam and intracavitary or interstitial irradiation.
(5) Palliative treatment of massive pelvic or metastatic disease.
(6) Uterine papillary serous cancers, which have a particularly poor prognosis and tend to spread intraperitoneally, may be effectively treated with whole-abdominal irradiation (WAR) if there is minimal residual disease after hysterectomy.

Table 4.1 shows a possible schema used for FIGO Stage I patients.

Table 4.1 Possible schema for staging FIGO Stage I patients[a]

| | Myometrial invasion | | |
	None	<50%	≥50%
Grade 1	No RT	V	P ± V
Grade 2	V	V	P ± V
Grade 3	V	V ± P	P + V

[a]V, vaginal vault RT (ICRT); P, pelvic RT.

Fields and doses

The fields used in the treatment of endometrial cancer are very similar to those used to treat cervical cancer. Four fields (AP, PA, and laterals) are often used to avoid the small bowel. For postoperative adjuvant treatment, the pelvis is usually treated to 45–50 Gy. The vaginal cuff may be boosted or treated entirely with intracavitary therapy.

Results of treatment

Adjuvant irradiation reduces the risk of pelvic recurrence but has never been proven to improve survival. Unfortunately, no randomized study of this question has had enough power to detect or rule out moderate survival improvements. Two randomized trials addressing this question in intermediate-risk FIGO Stage I patients showed an improvement in local control but no improvement in overall survival with the addition of radiation therapy. However, in both of these trials, the majority of the patients were in the low-risk category where radiation therapy was probably not needed at all, and the follow-up for both trials was very short. Irradiation alone for medically inoperable patients results in survival rates of 50–60%.

Ovarian cancer

The primary treatment for ovarian cancer is usually surgery followed by chemotherapy. Selected patients with Stage I–III disease with minimal (<0.5 cm) tumor remaining after surgery may, however, be effectively treated with WAR.

Fields and doses

In WAR, the whole abdomen receives 1–1.5 Gy each day with a single pair of AP/PA fields, with posterior kidney blocks placed to limit the dose to the kidney to less than 18 Gy and AP/PA liver blocks to limit the dose to the liver to

25 Gy. Doses to whole abdominopelvic fields are 22.5–30 Gy, usually followed by a boost to the pelvis to bring the total dose to 45–50 Gy.

Toxicity

Acute toxic side effects of abdominopelvic irradiation include nausea, anorexia, general fatigue, and diarrhea in most patients. These symptoms are usually fairly well controlled with appropriate medications. About 10% of patients develop significant myelotoxicity (platelet count < 100,000 or neutrophil count <1,500). The risk, however, is much higher in patients who have this treatment after chemotherapy, the extent of risk depending on the drugs and duration of previous treatment. Transient, asymptomatic pneumonitis in the base of the lungs develops in about 15% of patients, and up to 40% of patients have transiently elevated levels of alkaline phosphatase. Symptomatic hepatitis is rare if the dose of radiation to the liver does not exceed 27 Gy. In the absence of tumor recurrence, late bowel complications are rare, but the risk tends to increase with the extent and number of previous abdominal operations (particularly lymphadenectomy).

Vulvar cancer

The role of radiation therapy in the treatment of vulvar cancer has increased dramatically during the past two decades. Improved radiation therapy equipment and techniques have reduced the toxicity that discouraged early attempts to treat the vulva with radiation, and prospective studies have increased interest in this effective modality. In particular, the landmark randomized study published by Homesley et al in 1986 demonstrated a marked improvement in survival when patients with positive lymph nodes were treated with pelvic and inguinal irradiation after vulvectomy and lymphadenectomy. The use of concurrent "sensitizing" chemotherapy (e.g., with continuous-infusion 5-FU or cisplatin) to improve control rates has been explored in a number of uncontrolled studies. The encouraging response rates and long-term control of gross disease reported in these trials and the successful use of chemoradiation in cervical and anal cancer are contributing to interest in this approach.

Radiation can be used:

(1) to reduce regional recurrence and improve survival in patients with inguinal node metastases;
(2) to reduce the risk of vulvar recurrence in patients with positive surgical margins, multiple local recurrences, or other high-risk features;
(3) to avoid exenterative surgery in patients whose disease involves the anus or urethra;
(4) as a possible alternative to inguinal lymphadenectomy in selected patients with clinically negative groins.

Vaginal cancer

Radiation therapy plays a major role in the treatment of vaginal cancer. Patients with FIGO Stage II–IVA are primarily treated with radiation therapy, either with a combination of external-beam radiation and brachytherapy or with external beam alone. Patients with FIGO Stage I disease can be treated either with radiation alone or with surgery; however, surgery usually involves either a total vaginectomy or even exenteration to get negative margins.

Treatment volume

External-beam fields must include the primary lesion and the regional lymph nodes. Fields should be individualized according to the primary site. When tumors involve the lower third of the vagina, pelvic fields should be enlarged to include at least the medial inguinal lymph nodes. When four fields are used to treat the pelvis, care must be taken to cover all the draining lymph nodes, especially the posterior perirectal nodes. Intracavitary is of little value in the treatment of locally advanced vaginal cancers because the dose falls off very rapidly from the surface of a vaginal cylinder. Interstitial brachytherapy can provide better coverage of thick vaginal tumors.

Radiation dose

When good brachytherapy coverage of the tumor can be accomplished, an effort should be made to treat the tumor to a dose of 75-85 Gy with a combination of external-beam radiation and brachytherapy. However, when brachytherapy is not possible, some patients may be cured with external-beam irradiation alone, using shrinking pelvic fields to deliver a tumor dose of 60–66 Gy. Treatment should be completed within 6–7 weeks. Lee and colleagues reported a significantly lower pelvic recurrence in patients whose entire treatment course was completed in 9 weeks or less.

Results of treatment

Radiation therapy is extremely effective in patients with vaginal cancer. Disease-specific survival is in the range of 75–95% in patients with FIGO Stage I disease treated with definitive radiation. As in cervical cancer, survival decreases with advancing tumor size and FIGO staging; however, even in patients with FIGO Stage III disease, definitive radiation therapy yields disease-specific survival in the range of 30–50%.

Because primary vaginal carcinomas are rare, few reports have specifically addressed the role of chemotherapy in the treatment of this disease. However, vaginal carcinoma resembles cervical carcinoma in its location, pattern of spread, histologic appearance, relationship to HPV infection, and response to radiation therapy. It may therefore be reasonable to extrapolate from randomized trials demonstrating a benefit from concurrent chemoradiation in patients with locally advanced cervical cancer to justify a similar approach in selected patients with high-risk invasive vaginal cancer.

SELECTED READING

Creutzberg CL, van Putten WL, Koper PC et al, Surgery and postoperative radiotherapy versus surgery alone for patients with stage-1 endometrial carcinoma: multicentre randomised trial. PORTEC Study Group. Post Operative Radiation Therapy in Endometrial Carcinoma. *Lancet* 2000, **355**: 1404.

Dembo AJ, Radiotherapeutic management of ovarian cancer. *Semin Oncol* 1984; **11**: 238.

Hall EJ, *Radiobiology for the Radiologist*, 5th edn. Philadelphia: JB Lippincott, 2000.

Homesley HD, Bundy BN, Sedlis A, Adcock L, Radiation therapy versus pelvic node resection for carcinoma of the vulva with positive groin nodes. *Obstet Gynecol* 1986; **68**: 733.

Johns HE, Cunningham JR, *The Physics of Radiology*. Springfield, IL: Charles C Thomas, 1978.

Morris M, Eifel PJ, Lu J et al, Pelvic radiation with concurrent chemotherapy compared with pelvic and paraaortic radiation for high-risk cervical cancer. *N Engl J Med* 1999; **340**: 1137.

Morrow CP, Is pelvic radiation beneficial in the postoperative management of Stage IB squamous cell carcinoma of the cervix with pelvic node metastases treated by radical hysterectomy and pelvic lymphadenectomy? *Gynecol Oncol* 1980; **10**: 105.

Morrow CP, Bundy BN, Kurman RJ et al, Relationship between surgical–pathological risk factors in outcome of clinical stage I and II carcinoma of the endometrium. A Gynecologic Oncology Group study. *Gynecol Oncol* 1991; **40**: 55.

Rose PG, Bundy BN, Watkins J et al, Concurrent cisplatin-based chemotherapy and radiotherapy for locally advanced cervical cancer. *N Engl J Med* 1999; **340**: 1144.

5
Critical care

Diane C Bodurka, Michael W Bevers,
Anakara Sukumaran

Care of the critically ill patient requires a thorough knowledge of pathophysiology and pharmacology, as well as an understanding of the numerous diagnostic and imaging tools available. This overview of critical care is meant to serve as an aid to the organization of a diagnostic and therapeutic approach, as well as a springboard for further investigation. For simplicity, the outline is organized into three broad topics: organ failure, shock, and endocrine and metabolic conditions. Although presented by organ system, the reader should have the understanding that all of the systems are fully interactive.

ORGAN FAILURE

Mechanical ventilation

Supplemental oxygen support is used to facilitate adequate oxygen uptake and delivery to the vital organs. Many methods are available to enhance oxygen delivery (Table 5.1).

Maintaining adequate oxygenation and elimination of CO_2 cannot always be accomplished with these conservative methods. The decision to begin mechanical ventilation is primarily a clinical judgement following conservative respiratory support. In addition to clinical judgement, there are parameters that may help guide the decision to proceed with intubation (Table 5.2).

Once the decision for mechanical ventilation has been made, the patient is properly positioned, sedation and neuromuscular blocking agents are administered, if clinically indicated, and endotracheal intubation is performed. The initial ventilator settings (Table 5.3), as well as the mode of ventilation, are then selected.

There are currently several possible modes for the delivery of mechanical ventilation (Table 5.4). The assist/controlled mechanical ventilation (A/C) and intermittent mandatory ventilation (IMV) modes are the most commonly used in the intensive care unit setting. There are also adjuncts to the modes of mechanical ventilation, including positive end-expiratory pressure (PEEP) and pressure support ventilation (PSV).

Table 5.1 Methods of supplemental oxygen support

Method	Oxygen delivery (FI_{O_2})
Nasal canula	24–44%
Venturi mask	24%, 28%, 31%, 35%, 40%, 50%
Nonrebreathing mask	90%
Continuous positive airway pressure (CPAP)	Variable

Table 5.2 Parameters suggesting necessity of mechanical ventilation

Variable	Criteria
Pa_{O_2}	<60 mmHg with $FI_{O_2} > 60\%$
Pa_{CO_2}	>50 mmHg with pH < 7.35
Vital capacity	<10 cc/kg
Negative inspiratory force	More positive than -20 cmH$_2$O
Respiratory rate	>35 breaths/min

Table 5.3 Initial ventilator management

Mode	Assist/controlled (A/C)
Respiratory rate	8–12 breaths/min
Tidal volume	10–12 cc/kg
FI_{O_2}	80–100%
I:E ratio	1:3

PEEP is the maintenance of positive airway pressure at the end of expiration. This allows the small alveoli to remain open, thereby decreasing the shunt fraction and allowing gas exchange to continue between breaths. Clinically, PEEP allows better oxygenation at lower levels of FI_{O_2}. Acute respiratory-distress syndrome and pulmonary edema are examples of clinical situations in which PEEP may be beneficial. As a consequence of increasing PEEP, intrathoracic pressure increases, and barotrauma and cardiovascular compromise may occur.

PSV is an adjunct to modes of ventilation that allow the patient to breathe spontaneously: IMV, synchronized intermittent mandatory ventilation (SIMV), and continuous positive airway pressure (CPAP). Pressure support ventilation is the delivery of gas flow (during a spontaneous breath) with a defined posi-

Table 5.4 Common modes of mechanical ventilation

Mode	Characteristics
Assist/controlled mechanical ventilation (A/C)	• Ventilator-delivered breath for every patient-initiated breath • Controlled ventilator-delivered breath when patient's spontaneous rate falls below the back-up rate
Intermittent mandatory ventilation (IMV)	• Patient may breathe at a spontaneous rate and tidal volume between preset ventilator-delivered rate and tidal volume
Synchronized intermittent mandatory ventilation (SIMV)	• Same as IMV except that the ventilator coordinates preset ventilator-driven breath with the patient's spontaneous breath
Continuous positive airway pressure (CPAP)	• Ventilator provides only PEEP, FI_{O_2}, and humidification, and does not deliver any mechanical breaths

tive pressure that is selected on the ventilator. This positive pressure is summated with the negative pressure generated by the patient's effort. The net result is enhancement of the positive pressure gradient across the lungs, and, as a result, enhancement of the spontaneous tidal volume. Clinically, PSV allows the respiratory muscles to perform a manageable amount of work with less fatigue. Like PEEP, PSV may result in cardiovascular alterations due to decreased venous return. These alterations are less pronounced with commonly used PSV settings. PSV is often utilized as a weaning tool.

Following the initial ventilator settings, subsequent changes are based on the arterial blood gas values and the overall clinical setting. Certain principles may be followed to reach desired endpoints for the P_{CO_2} (=35–45 with pH 7.35–7.45) and P_{O_2} (>60). First, adjustments in P_{CO_2} are accomplished by adjustments in the respiratory rate or tidal volume. Second, P_{O_2} changes are accomplished by adjusting the FI_{O_2} or the PEEP. Third, ventilator settings that affect the same parameter (P_{CO_2} or P_{O_2}) should not be adjusted at the same time, especially during the weaning phase.

Once the underlying disease process necessitating mechanical ventilation has been addressed and resolved, a trial of weaning can then be attempted. During weaning, the PEEP or PSV should be decreased slowly to prevent decompensation. Commonly used weaning techniques are IMV mode, PSV, and the T-tube. Once certain ventilatory or "weaning" parameters are satisfactory (Table 5.5), extubation is performed and supplemental oxygen supplied.

Table 5.5 Weaning parameters

Weaning variable	Acceptable value for extubation
Mental status	Alert and cooperative
Pa_{O_2}	>60 mmHg with FI_{O_2} < 50%
Pa_{CO_2} and pH	Acceptable range for individual patient
Respiratory rate	<30 breaths/minute
Vital capacity	>10 cc/kg
Minute ventilation	<10 L/min
Tidal volume	4–7 cc/kg
Negative inspiratory force	More negative than −20 cmH$_2$O
Positive end-expiratory pressure (PEEP)	<5 cmH$_2$O

Acute respiratory failure

Acute respiratory failure is a clinical condition in which the pulmonary system fails to maintain adequate gas exchange. There is an alteration in the respiratory drive, airway patency, or pulmonary function that results in hypercapnia, acidemia, or hypoxia.

Etiology

There are many causes of acute respiratory failure, including intrapulmonary and extrapulmonary etiologies. The differential diagnoses of airway obstruction yielding acute respiratory failure include mechanical obstruction (foreign body), mucus plugging, anaphylactic shock, displaced airway, and cancer. Intrapulmonary etiologies include parenchymal dysfunction secondary to pneumonia, pulmonary edema, congestive heart failure, acute respiratory-distress syndrome, chronic obstructive pulmonary disease (COPD), aspiration pneumonitis, and atelectasis. Destructive disease (abscess, cancer, and tuberculosis) and restrictive disease (pleural effusion, pneumothorax, and hemothorax) may also contribute. Extrapulmonary causes include embolism, cardiac failure or anemia yielding inadequate perfusion, cardiovascular accident, neuromuscular blocking antibiotics, metabolic abnormalities, and spinal cord trauma or lesion.

Diagnosis

The clinical manifestations of acute respiratory failure depend upon the underlying cause and the extent of tissue hypoxia. After obtaining the medical history and performing a physical examination, a chest x-ray and arterial blood gas (ABG) analysis should be obtained. A complete blood count, sputum studies, pulmonary function testing, ventilation/perfusion scan, and bronchoscopy should be performed as clinically indicated. Acute respiratory failure is present when Pa_{O_2} is less than 50 mmHg and/or Pa_{CO_2} is greater than 50 mmHg. These criteria include a pH level of less than 7.35 in patients with a chronically elevated Pa_{CO_2}.

Management

The goals of management are to treat the underlying cause, to promote gas exchange, to correct the acidosis, and to prevent complications. The airway must be maintained. Any form of obstruction should be cleared, and the head tilt and jaw thrust maneuver performed. Note that an oropharyngeal airway (correct size measured from tragus to corner of mouth) may cause gagging in an alert patient; a nasopharyngeal airway is frequently better tolerated in this situation. Oxygen should be administered to keep Pa_{O_2} greater than 90 mmHg. Intubation and mechanical ventilation may be required. Positive airway pressure should be administered in the form of either constant positive airway pressure or PEEP. Medications should be used as clinically indicated. Mucolytics, brochodilators, β_2 agonists or anticholinergic agents may be appropriate. Steroids, analgesics, sedation, or neuromuscular paralysis may be required – again depending upon the clinical scenario. The use of bicarbonate for severe acidosis (pH < 7.2) is controversial. Antibiotics and stress ulcer prophylaxis with an H_2-receptor antagonist should be considered. Complications such as cardiac dysrhythmias or pulmonary embolism should be treated in the conventional manner. Nutritional support should not be overlooked.

Acute respiratory-distress syndrome

Acute respiratory-distress syndrome (ARDS) is an inflammatory syndrome marked by a disruption of the alveolar capillary membrane. This syndrome is part of and originates in the same inflammatory–immune-mediated response as the multiple-organ dysfunction syndrome (MODS). ARDS is a pulmonary injury that is the result of an accumulation of protein-rich fluid in the alveoli secondary to increased microvascular permeability of the plasma proteins.

Etiology

ARDS is associated with a variety of clinical conditions, including aspiration, trauma, pneumonia, and sepsis. Severe pancreatitis, pulmonary embolism, disseminated intravascular coagulation, and shock states may also contribute.

Diagnosis

The clinical manifestations of ARDS include a variety of signs and symptoms related to the precipitating event. Patients may present with tachypnea, restlessness, apprehension, or agitation. They may also experience dyspnea or fatigue. The physical examination may reveal use of accessory muscles or fine crackles upon auscultation. The arterial blood gas analysis demonstrates a low Pa_{O_2}. Although the chest x-ray may be normal for the first 24 hours after the process begins, diffuse interstitial and alveolar infiltrates resulting in consolidation of the lungs soon appear, yielding the classic "white out" associated with ARDS. Criteria for diagnosis according to the American–European Consensus Committee on ARDS include acute onset, a Pa_{O_2}/FI_{O_2} ratio of 200 mmHg or less, bilateral infiltrates on chest x-ray, and pulmonary capillary wedge pressure (PCWP) of 18 mmHg or less with no clinical evidence of left atrial hypertension.

Management
The goals of management are to treat the underlying cause, to promote gas exchange, to support tissue oxygenation, and to monitor and treat complications. Supplemental oxygen should be provided at the lowest level to support tissue oxygenation. While A/C or SIMV ventilator modes are initially chosen, sedation or neuromuscular paralysis may require other ventilator modes. PEEP is added to help decrease FI_{O_2}. Both cautious fluid management and maintenance of cardiac output are essential in order to decrease the amount of fluid leaking into the lungs. A low intravascular volume (PCWP 5–8 mmHg) is maintained with fluid restriction and diuretics, while vasoactive drugs and inotropic agents are utilized to support the cardiac output. Stress ulcer prophylaxis and nutritional support should be provided. Arterial blood gas analysis and hemodynamic monitoring are used to monitor changes and guide therapy. The use of nonsteroidal anti-inflammatory agents (NSAIDs), thromboxane synthetase inhibitors, surfactant replacement, and other substances to block or neutralize mediators released as part of the inflammatory–immune response and to improve gas exchange by reducing intrapulmonary shunt is currently under investigation.

Acute renal failure

Acute renal failure is a clinical syndrome that is characterized by an abrupt decline in the glomerular filtration rate, with resultant retention of metabolic waste products from protein catabolism, an inability to maintain electrolyte and acid–base homeostasis, and disturbance in fluid volume regulation. Acute renal failure is reversible if treated promptly, but may progress to chronic renal failure if left untreated or if the patient fails to respond to appropriate care.

Etiology
Acute renal failure is divided into three basic etiologies: prerenal, intrarenal, and postrenal. Prerenal acute renal failure is a physiologic response to an insult that occurs before the blood reaches the kidney, resulting in renal hypoperfusion; the integrity of the kidney structure and kidney function are preserved. Events associated with hypovolemia, such as hemorrhage, shock, severe gastrointestinal losses, renal trauma, volume depletion ("third-spacing"), or renal losses from diuretics, diabetes insipidus or osmotic diuresis, result in renal hypoperfusion with subsequent oliguria.

Intrarenal acute renal failure is a physiologic response to an insult that occurs at the site of the nephrons and involves the glomeruli and/or tubular epithelium (acute tubular necrosis). This disease is caused by processes that damage the intrinsic renal unit, such as glomerulonephritis, hypertension, thrombus, diabetes mellitus, nephrotoxic drugs, poisons, and renal stenosis.

Postrenal acute renal failure is a physiologic response to disruption of the normal flow of urine within the urinary tract. It may be caused by obstructive disorders and tumors.

Diagnosis

The purpose of the assessment and diagnosis is to determine whether the acute renal failure is the result of a prerenal, intrarenal, or postrenal event. It is important to examine the mucous membranes and assess skin turgor, since this provides information regarding hydration status. The patient's chart should be consulted for fluid intake and output; insensible losses should be accounted for. Serum analyses should include electrolytes, blood urea nitrogen (BUN), creatinine, calcium, glucose, magnesium, bicarbonate, phosphorus, albumin, and liver function studies. Urine should be sent to assess electrolytes, creatinine, glucose, osmolality, specific gravity, and culture and sensitivity. The results from the above studies can then be utilized to ascertain the type of acute renal failure present (Table 5.6).

In addition to laboratory tests, radiologic studies should be ordered as clinically indicated. For suspected obstruction, cystoscopy, retrograde pyelogram, radionuclide excretion studies, and intravenous pyelogram may be useful. For suspected parenchymal disease, the sedimentation rate, a complete blood count, and autoantibodies should be checked. An ultrasound-guided renal biopsy or contrast computed tomography (CT) of the abdomen may be indicated.

Management

The goals of management are to prevent chronic renal failure, correct the acute problem, and promote regeneration of remaining renal capacity. In high-risk patients, the use of nephrotoxic drugs and NSAIDs should be avoided; the use of intravascular x-ray contrast media should be delayed. Fluid administration should be carefully monitored, with ongoing evaluation and frequent adjustment through hemodynamic monitoring, careful assessment of fluid intake and output, and daily weights. BUN and creatinine should be checked daily, along with applicable electrolytes. Hyperkalemia causes dysrhythmias. Treatment consists of immediate discontinuation of potassium; intravenous diuretics, insulin, and glucose may also be required. Bicarbonate and Kayexalate may be administered; dialysis remains an option as well. Dilutional hyponatremia is treated first by fluid restriction, then by hypertonic saline. Calcium supplements and aluminum hydroxide preparations may be administered for hypocalcemia and hyperphosphatemia. Diuretics and/or dopamine may be required to maintain adequate urine output. For patients who are taking nutrition orally, a

Table 5.6 Diagnosis of renal failure

Diagnosis	Serum BUN:creatinine ratio	Urinalysis[a]	Urine sodium (mEq/L)	FENa (%)	Urine osmolality (mOsm/kg H$_2$O)	Comments
Prerenal						
Prerenal azotemia	>20:1	Hyaline casts; may be normal	<20	<1	>600	Clinical signs of volume depletion
Intrinsic renal disease						
Acute glomerulonephritis	>20:1	RBCs, RBC casts, proteinuria	<20	<1	>600	History of sore throat, pyoderma or other infection
Acute interstitial nephritis	<20:1	WBCs, WBC casts, eosinophils	Variable	Variable	Variable	Drug exposure, eosinophilia
Acute renal failure	<20:1	Granular casts, proteinuria, ± RBCs, ± WBCs	>20	>1	~250–300	Exposure to nephrotoxic drug or radiocontrast; volume depletion or decreased blood pressure
Intratubular obstruction						
Intratubular obstruction	>20:1	Variable	Variable	Variable	Variable	Hyperuricemia; rhabdomyolysis; multiple myeloma
Obstructive uropathy						
Obstruction of collecting system	>20:1	Variable, may be normal	Variable (<20)	Variable (<1)	Variable	History of fluctuating urine volume; bilateral hydronephrosis

[a]RBC, red blood cell; WBC, white blood cell

renal diet should be provided. Protein, potassium, sodium, and phosphorus are restricted, while carbohydrates are increased. Fluid removal may be accomplished through administration of diuretics, hemodialysis, peritoneal dialysis, hemofiltration, or continuous renal-replacement therapy.

Acute pancreatitis

Acute pancreatitis is described as the acute onset of mild or severe abdominal pain accompanied by a rise in pancreatic enzymes. It is usually edematous or hemorrhagic in form.

Etiology

The most common causes of acute pancreatitis are alcoholism and gallstones. Other etiologies include peptic ulcer disease, surgical trauma, vascular disease, and the use of certain drugs (furosemide, oral contraceptives, sulfonamides, and thiazides).

Diagnosis

The signs and symptoms of pancreatitis frequently mimic those of other disorders. Patients may present with mild to severe abdominal pain, nausea and vomiting, and abdominal distention. On exam, the patient may be hypertensive, appear jaundiced, and exhibit abdominal guarding. The Grey Turner sign (gray–blue discoloration of the flank) and Cullen sign (discoloration of the umbilical region) may be present, and bowel sounds may be hypoactive or absent.

The Ranson criteria provide useful prognostic information. Severe illness and increased mortality are associated with patient age greater than 55 years, a white-blood-cell (WBC) count greater than 16,000/mm^3, serum aspartate aminotransferase (AST) (glutamic–oxaloacetic transaminase, SGOT) greater than 250 IU/L, glucose greater than 200 mg/dl, or serum lactate dehydrogenase (LDH) greater than 350 IU/L on admission. Other criteria include a rise in BUN greater than 5 mg/dl, a drop in hematocrit of greater than 10%, arterial oxygen tension less than 60 mmHg, serum calcium less than 8.0 mg/dl, a base deficit greater than 5 mg/dl, or estimated fluid sequestration greater than 6 L during the first 48 hours after admission.

Abdominal CT is the imaging method of choice. Typical findings include extensive pancreatic and retroperitoneal inflammation with superimposed patchy or generalized areas of necrosis and hemorrhage in the pancreas and surrounding tissues.

Management

The goals of management are to ensure adequate circulatory volume, to minimize pancreatic function, to correct metabolic abnormalities, and to manage local and systemic complications. Therapy is largely supportive.

Aggressive volume replacement with intravenous fluids must be performed,

Management

Since there is no specific treatment for individual organ failure, the management of multisystem organ failure focuses on supportive treatment for each affected organ. Appropriate diagnostic tests should be performed for continued assessment of each involved system.

Broad-spectrum antibiotics, including antifungals, antivirals, and agents for specific opportunistic or mycobacterial infections, should be administered. Although invasive procedures should be limited, surgery may ultimately be required. Experimental agents currently used in the treatment of sepsis include NSAIDs, prostaglandins, and anti-tumor necrosis factor (anti-TNF) antibodies.

A second goal of management is the improvement of tissue perfusion. Hemodynamic monitoring is essential. Fluids and blood should be given; vasoactive substances may be required. Experimental agents currently used to improve tissue perfusion include hyperosmolar saline, prostaglandins, naloxone, and calcium-channel blockers.

Oxygen requirements should be met; intubation and mechanical ventilation may be required. Arterial blood gas analyses and blood lactate levels should be monitored as a guide to adequate oxygen delivery. Blood products should be transfused to keep the hemoglobin level above 10.

Metabolic abnormalities should be appropriately corrected, and nutritional requirements met through enteral feedings or TPN. Stress ulcer prophylaxis should be administered; nasogastric tube suction may be required. Experimental pharmacologic agents currently under evaluation for repair of specific organ damage include O_2-free-radical scavengers (mannitol, vitamin C, furosemide), pentoxifylline, fibronectin, and adenosine 5′-triphosphate complexes.

SHOCK

Shock is defined as a state of inadequate tissue perfusion that, unless reversed, results in progressive organ dysfunction, damage, and death. Patients who develop shock typically pass through three stages. Stage I corresponds to a ≤10% reduction in effective intravascular volume, and patients may be asymptomatic. Compensatory mechanisms include sympathetic discharge that results in tachycardia and mild peripheral vasoconstriction, with blood pressure normal to slightly depressed. Stage II corresponds to a 15–25% reduction in effective intravascular volume. Despite intense activity of compensatory mechanisms, blood pressure declines and organ hypoperfusion begins. Tachycardia may be prominent, orthostatic signs may be present, and the patient may be restless or agitated. Stage III represents a >25% reduction in effective intravascular volume. Compensatory mechanisms begin to fail, blood pressure declines, and end-organ hypoperfusion becomes more evident. Clinically, this stage presents as decreased urine production, altered mental status, and cool clammy skin.

Etiology

Shock states can be classified into four broad categories (Table 5.7).

Diagnosis

A systematic and problem-focused history and physical exam should be performed, with particular attention paid to the possible underlying etiology of the shock state. Clinical findings will depend on the etiology and severity of the shock state (Table 5.8).

Initial diagnostic tests performed should include arterial blood gas analysis, complete blood count, electrolytes, BUN, creatinine, glucose, calcium, liver functions, and coagulation profile. If sepsis is suspected, additional laboratory tests include serum lactate level, blood, urine, and sputum culture tests. In addition, Foley, arterial-line, and central-venous catheters are placed. Each of the shock states has a characteristic hemodynamic pattern that can be identified by placing a Swan–Ganz catheter (Table 5.9).

Treatment

In addition to maintaining an airway, breathing, and oxygenation, the main goal of therapy of any form of shock state is to re-establish tissue perfusion. Fluid therapy with crystalloids or colloids and vasoactive drugs in the form of vasopressors and inotropes are used to accomplish this goal. Examples of these

Table 5.7 Shock classifications	
Type of shock	Etiologies
Hypovolemic	• Relative: internal shifting of fluid from the intravascular to extravascular space • Absolute: external fluid loss from the body (hemorrhage)
Cardiogenic	• Acute myocardial infarction, cardiopulmonary arrest, structural problem (septal rupture, cardiomyopathies, tumor, valve dysfunction, tamponade), dysrhythmias
Distributive	• Septic: combination of endotoxin effects from a variety of micro-organisms and immune mediators • Anaphylactic: IgE-mediated mast-cell release of mediators, rapidly developing, systemic allergic reaction as a result of beta-lactam antibiotics, chemotherapy drugs • Anaphylactoid: direct mast-cell-mediated release as a result of radiocontrast dye
Obstructive	• Massive pulmonary embolus, amniotic fluid embolism, tumor embolism

Diagnosis

The clinical features of SIADH are primarily neurologic, and are due to an osmotic water shift leading to increased intracellular fluid volume and brain-cell swelling. The severity of the symptoms depends upon the rapidity of onset and the decrease in plasma [Na$^+$]. Initially, patients may experience nausea and malaise. These symptoms progress to headache, lethargy, confusion, and an obtunded state. If the plasma [Na$^+$] acutely falls below 120 mEq/L, stupor, seizures, and coma may occur.

The underlying cause of hyponatremia can often be established from an accurate history and physical examination. The serum sodium and osmolality, urine sodium, osmolality, and specific gravity should be checked. In patients with SIADH, the serum osmolality and serum sodium are decreased, while the urine sodium, urine osmolality, and specific gravity are increased. Other diagnoses, such as congestive heart failure, renal failure, liver failure, adrenal insufficiency, and hypothyroidism, should be excluded. A chest x-ray or CT scan may establish malignancy as the etiology of this syndrome.

Management

SIADH may be corrected by limiting the intake of water or by promoting water excretion. Standard first-line therapy is water restriction. If this is not successful, or if the patient is symptomatic, agents that enhance water excretion may be administered. The combination of loop diuretics and salt tablets can enhance free water excretion, as can administration of urea. Drugs that decrease the effectiveness of ADH on renal tubules should only be considered in situations unresponsive to more conservative management; these drugs include demeclocycline, lithium carbonate, and phenytoin. No drug is available to prevent the secretion of ADH from the pituitary or from tumor.

Diabetic ketoacidosis

Diabetic ketoacidosis (DKA) is the most common form of diabetic emergency in which there is an absolute or relative lack of insulin within the systemic circulation and an excess of counterregulatory hormones (e.g., glucagon). Patients with type I diabetes are predisposed to DKA; however, DKA may occur in any diabetic patient who is sufficiently stressed.

Etiology

Diabetic ketoacidosis occurs essentially due to a lack of insulin. This may be due to increased endogenous glucose caused by stressful events with concurrent decreased exogenous insulin, as well as an excess of counterregulatory hormones. Precipitating events include infection, stress, trauma, and MI. An imbalance between food intake and amount of exogenous estrogen received and medications that affect carbohydrate metabolism and insulin secretion may also cause patients to develop DKA.

Diagnosis

Patients with DKA commonly present with nausea, vomiting, and vague abdominal pain without localizing signs. They may complain of polydipsia or polyuria. The skin may be flushed and dry; tachycardia, hyperventilation, and hypothermia may be present. The patient may rapidly become unstable. Confusion, shock, or coma may follow.

Laboratory evaluation reveals an elevated serum glucose in the majority of cases, as well as the presence of serum ketones, and metabolic acidosis with an elevated anion gap. Other laboratory abnormalities may include hyperkalemia, hyponatremia, increased BUN and creatinine, hyperosmolarity, decreased magnesium and phosphorus, and an elevated serum amylase unrelated to abdominal pathology.

DKA requires a precipitating event. Since an occult infection may exist, close examination of the hands and feet, blood and urine cultures, and a chest x-ray are required. Since MI may be a precipitating event, an electrocardiogram (ECG) should be obtained for cardiac evaluation. If the patient has not been previously diagnosed with diabetes, it is important to remember that DKA may be a presenting manifestation of type I diabetes. Other causes of metabolic acidosis, including starvation, alcoholism, toxic chemicals, lactic acidosis, and uremia, should also be considered.

Management

The therapy for DKA should include reversal of dehydration, treatment and prevention of circulatory collapse, restoration of the appropriate insulin-to-glucagon ratio, and identification of the precipitating cause. For patients in shock or coma, resuscitative measures should be promptly initiated.

The fluid deficit is often significant, and requires aggressive restoration of intravascular volume. This should be guided by the patient's cardiac and renal function. Initial fluid resuscitation consists of rapid infusion of isotonic (0.9%) saline or lactated Ringer's solution in patients with normal cardiac function. Volume replacement should then be administered at a rate of 1 L/hr (or greater) until the intravascular deficit has been corrected. Fluid replacement should be guided by careful monitoring of vital signs, urine output, and precipitating signs of secondary illness (e.g., cardiac failure) that may require central monitoring. An osmotic diuresis frequently occurs once fluid resuscitation has begun, and may delay achievement of a positive fluid balance. Once the intravascular volume has been restored, 0.45% saline at a rate of 150–200 cc/hr is appropriate maintenance therapy for the patient's normal cardiac and renal function.

The goal of insulin administration is reversal of ketogenesis and restoration of normal nutrient utilization. For these reasons, insulin is given as part of the initial treatment of DKA. The initial dose of insulin should be 10–15 units of regular insulin (or 0.15 units/kg) given as an intravenous bolus. Insulin is then usually given as a continuous infusion of 10 units/hr. Blood glucose levels should be utilized to guide initial adjustments in insulin dose.

levels are usually decreased, and serum chloride levels elevated, in patients with this disorder.

Management

Prompt identification of patients with hypercalcemia is essential, since hypercalcemia of malignancy is a life-threatening complication that can be controlled with medical intervention. Patients with hypercalcemia of malignancy who have a serum calcium level above 13 mg/dl or who are symptomatic require prompt medical attention, since the syndrome is often fatal if left untreated. One caveat, however, is the fact that hypercalcemia frequently presents as a late complication in the course of malignancy, and long-term management is difficult unless effective antineoplastic therapy remains an option. Therefore, the decision to treat the hypercalcemia should be based upon the patient's performance status and prognosis.

Acute management of hypercalcemia consists of measures that increase calcium excretion and decrease resorption of calcium from bone. The goal of treatment is alleviation of symptoms rather than rapid normalization of serum calcium level.

The first step is replacement of ECF volume. Initially, 0.9% saline should be infused at a rate of 300–500 cc/hr, with a reduction in rate after the ECF volume has been partially restored. A minimum of 3–4 L should be infused in the first 24 hours; a positive fluid balance of at least 2 L should be attained.

Fluid resuscitation is then followed by saline diuresis. A 0.9% saline infusion at a rate of 100–200 cc/hr should be given to promote excretion of calcium once ECF volume has been restored. Serum electrolytes, calcium, and magnesium should be monitored every 6–12 hours, with replacement as indicated by laboratory results. Cardiac status should be carefully monitored, and furosemide should only be administered in the event of cardiac failure. Thiazide diuretics should be avoided, since they impair calcium excretion.

An inhibitor of bone resorption should be given early in the treatment course. Mithramycin or pamidronate may be used; calcitonin is also an option. Glucocorticoids are most effective in inhibiting bone resorption due to breast carcinoma and multiple myeloma.

SELECTED READING

ACCP Consensus Conference: mechanical ventilation. *Chest* 1993; **104**: 1833.

American College of Chest Physicians/ Society of Critical Care Medicine Consensus Conference: definitions for sepsis and organ failure guidelines for the use of innovative therapies in sepsis. *Crit Care Med* 1992; **20**: 864.

Bernard GR, Artigas A, Grigham KL et al, The American–European Consensus Conference on ARDS: definitions, mechanisms, relevant outcomes, and clinical trial coordination. *Am J Respir Crit Care Med* 1994; **149**: 818.

Brochard L, Rauss A, Benito S et al, Comparison of three methods of gradual withdrawal from ventilatory support during weaning from mechanical ventilation. *Am J Respir Crit Care Med* 1994; **150**: 896.

Dupuis YG, *Ventilators: Theory and Clinical Applications*, 2nd edn. St Louis: Mosby-Year Book, 1992.

Fleckman AM, Diabetic ketoacidosis. *Endocrinol Metab Clin North Am* 1993; **22**: 181.

Gallup DG, Nolan TE, The gynecologist and multiple organ failure syndrome (MOFS). *Gynecol Oncol* 1993; **48**: 293.

Irwin RS, Cerra FB, Rippe JM (eds), *Irwin and Rippe's Intensive Care Medicine*, 4th edn. Philadelphia: Lippincott-Raven, 1999.

Ranson JH, Acute pancreatitis: pathogenesis, outcome and treatment. *Clin Gastroenterol* 1984; **13**: 843.

Silverman P, Distelhorst CW, Metabolic emergencies in clinical oncology. *Semin Oncol* 1989; **16**: 504.

Weinman EJ, Patak RV, Acute renal failure in cancer patients. *Oncology* 1992; **6**: 47.

Williams R, Gimson AES, Intensive liver care and management of acute hepatic failure. *Dig Dis Sci* 1991; **36**: 820.

"elective" cancer surgery for 3–4 weeks. Several cardiac-risk scoring systems have been developed, but one of the most widely used is the American Society of Anesthesiologists' scale of physical status (Table 6.3). This is a functional risk-assessment scale based solely on subjective assessment, yet gives a reproducible prediction of significant morbidity and mortality; for patients with an ASA class of V, mortality related to surgery may be as high as 50%. The importance of preoperative consultation with internists and cardiologists for patients in ASA Class III and higher cannot be overemphasized.

Hypertension affects over fifty million Americans, and therefore many women who are candidates for surgery will be taking antihypertensive medications at the time of their cancer diagnosis. Some of the more commonly pre-

Table 6.1 Risk factors for cardiovascular complications

Prior myocardial infarction
Angina
Congestive heart failure
Diabetes
Hypertension
Age >70 years
Arrhythmias
Valvular disease

Table 6.2 Noninvasive cardiac evaluation

Modality	Comments
Exercise ECG	Information about exercise tolerance, BP and arrhythmias
Exercise echocardiography	Observe contractility changes with exercise
Exercise thallium (^{201}Tl)	Used for uninterpretable ECG
Pharmacologic stress perfusion study Adenosine–thallium Adenosine ^{99m}Tc-sestamibi SPECT[a]	For 30–50% of patients who cannot achieve required exercise level

[a]Technetium-99m sestamibi single-photon emission computed tomography.

Table 6.3 American Society of Anesthesiologists' scale of physical status

Category	Functional status
I	No significant disease, good health
II	Mild one-system disease, no effect on function (e.g., obesity, smoking)
III	Multisystem disease that limits daily function
IV	Multisystem disease that incapacitates and threatens life
V	Death is imminent, surgery is last resort

Table 6.4 Commonly used antihypertensive agents

Agent	Mechanism	Dose	?Continue preop
Enalapril (Vasotec®)	ACE inhibitor	50 mg p.o. q.d.	Yes
Metoprolol (Lopressor®)	β-adrenergic antagonist	50 mg p.o. b.i.d.	Yes
Amlodipine (Norvasc®)	Calcium-channel blocker	5 mg p.o. q.d.	Yes
Prazosin (Minipress®)	α-adrenergic antagonist	1 mg p.o. b.i.d.–t.i.d.	Yes

scribed antihypertensives are listed with their mechanisms of action in Table 6.4. As a general rule, all antihypertensive medications should be continued until the day of surgery, except for monoamine oxidase (MAO) inhibitors, which should be stopped 2 weeks preoperatively. Continuing medication perioperatively is particularly important for patients using beta-blockers, to avoid rebound tachycardia and obtain the demonstrated survival benefit that perioperative use of these drugs has shown in patients at risk of coronary-artery disease.

Pulmonary

Although less common than cardiac disease, pulmonary disease, especially related to smoking, remains an important consideration in preoperative evaluation of candidates for gynecologic-cancer surgery. As with cardiac evaluation, a careful history and review of symptoms is the first step in screening for significant pulmonary problems. Table 6.5 lists commonly accepted risk factors for perioperative pulmonary complications ranging from atelectasis to acute respiratory-distress syndrome (ARDS). Of these risk factors, smoking is one that can be altered preoperatively to significantly reduce complication rates. Smoking cessation for at least 8 weeks preoperatively has been demonstrated to reduce the risk of pulmonary complications by as much as one-half. Stopping for less than 8 weeks, however, may paradoxically increase risk. Patients with chronic obstructive pulmonary disease or asthma should be considered for pulmonary function testing preoperatively to further characterize their risk. Commonly used indices of pulmonary function are detailed in Table 6.6. For patients at high risk based on history, physical-exam findings, or pulmonary-function testing, referral for expert consultation and treatment with a combination of bronchodilators, corticosteroids, antibiotics, and physical therapy is indicated to maximize pulmonary reserve prior to surgery. In both high- and normal-risk patients, lung-expansion techniques such as deep-breathing

Table 6.5 Risk factors for postoperative pulmonary complications

Smoking
Obesity
Chronic obstructive pulmonary disease
Asthma
ASA > II
Age > 70
Abdominal or thoracic surgery
Surgery duration > 3 hours

Table 6.6 Preoperative pulmonary-function tests

	Definition		High risk
FEV_1	Forced expiratory volume in 1 second	Ability to clear secretions	<50%
FVC	Forced vital capacity	Balance of muscle function and chest-wall forces	<50% predicted
RV/TLC	Residual volume/total lung capacity	↑ with air-trapping hyperinflation	>0.5
D_LO_2	Diffusing capacity for oxygen	↓ in restrictive or obstructive disease	<15 ml/min/mm

exercises or incentive spirometry markedly reduce pulmonary complications, and these measures should be standard preoperative patient teaching in all candidates for gynecologic-cancer surgery.

Diabetes

Adult-onset or type II diabetes is common in the age group of women affected by gynecologic malignancies. Diabetics have an estimated 50% greater surgical morbidity and mortality than nondiabetics, including increased risk for perioperative MI, infectious complications, impaired wound healing, and acute renal failure. Control of perioperative blood sugar may decrease these risks significantly. Table 6.7 lists common oral hypoglycemic agents, and Table 6.8 lists commonly used insulin preparations and their duration of action. Most oral hypoglycemic agents should not be given on the day of surgery, and long-

Table 6.7 Oral hypoglycemic agents commonly used

	Maximum dosage	Duration of action (hrs)
Glyburide (Micronase®)	10 mg p.o. b.i.d.	24–60
Glipizide (Glucotrol®)	20 mg p.o. b.i.d.	12–24
Chloropropamide (Diabinese®)	250 mg p.o. b.i.d.	60–90
Metformin (Glucophage®)	500 mg p.o. q.d.	12–24

Table 6.8 Types of insulin and duration of action

	Onset (hrs)	Peak (hrs)	Duration (hrs)
Rapid action:			
Regular	0.25–1	2–6	4–12
Semilente	0.5–1	3–10	8–18
Intermediate-action:			
NPH, Lente	1.5–4	6–16	14–28
Long-action:			
Ultralente	3–8	4–10	9–36
Protamine zinc	3–8	14–26	24–40

acting agents should be discontinued 2–3 days preoperatively. A patient using insulin should be given half of her usual a.m. dose on the morning of surgery, and whenever possible she should be scheduled as a first case. For the diabetic, even a type II diabetic, whose surgery is not scheduled as a first case, intravenous line placement and hydration with D5W with blood-glucose monitoring should be performed to avoid hypoglycemia. Postoperatively, type I and type II diabetics should have orders for glucose monitoring every 2–4 hours, and a sliding scale of insulin written to cover and maintain blood sugars in a normal range. As oral intake is resumed postoperatively, diabetic patients should resume their preoperative regimens of insulin or oral hypoglycemic agents to maintain euglycemia. Endocrine consultation to direct perioperative management of the diabetic patient is indicated for those with a history of poor control, ketoacidosis, or end-organ disease such as retinopathy or nephropathy.

Nutrition

Most women diagnosed with gynecologic cancer will not present with significant nutritional deficiencies as a result of their disease. An important exception is the patient with a malignancy that has impaired intestinal function for a prolonged period, such as an advanced ovarian cancer causing massive ascites and carcinomatosis. Most gynecologic-cancer patients will not be malnourished on presentation, but the increased morbidity associated with severe malnutrition makes assessment of nutritional status an essential part of the preoperative evaluation. History of weight loss, exam findings, and laboratory values listed in Table 6.9 can be used to assess the nutritional status of surgical candidates. Whether intervention for patients identified as malnourished preoperatively can reduce morbidity remains controversial; to date, no randomized, prospective, clinical trial has demonstrated a benefit for cancer patients treated with perioperative total parenteral nutrition (TPN). The decision to use perioperative TPN should be based both on the patient's nutritional status at time of surgery and on the surgical procedure's likely effect on gastrointestinal function. If surgery is likely to result in a prolonged period of inadequate caloric intake (greater than 7–10 days; 5–7 days in a malnourished patient), TPN should be considered. In order to be of benefit, TPN must be given for at least 7–10 days; for a severely malnourished patient with a bowel obstruction who is not likely to resume oral intake for at least this period of time, starting TPN in the preoperative period is indicated. For patients in whom enteral intake is restored in less than 7 days, the risks of TPN (increased infection, metabolic abnormalities) probably outweigh the potential benefit.

Thromboembolic prophylaxis

Prevention of thromboembolic complications – deep-vein thrombosis (DVT) and pulmonary embolism (PE) – is a critical part of the preoperative care of the patient with gynecologic cancer. Malignancy produces a hypercoagulable state, possibly due to production of as-yet-unidentified factors that disrupt the normal clotting and fibrinolytic cascades. Thus, women with gynecologic can-

Table 6.9 Assessment of preoperative nutritional status	
Evaluation	Possible malnutrition
History of weight fluctuation	5% weight loss in 1 month 10% loss in 6 months Current weight < 85% of ideal body weight
Physical exam	Muscle wasting Peripheral edema
Laboratory values	Serum albumin < 3.0 gm/dl Anergy to skin testing (*Candida*) Transferrin < 200 mg/dl Total lymphocyte count < 1,200 cells/μl

Table 6.10 Methods for thromboembolic prophylaxis[a]	
Mechanical	Pharmacologic
Pneumatic compression boots ×5 days	Heparin 5,000 units s.q. q 8–12 hrs starting 2 hrs preop ×7 days
IVC filter placement	LMWH (e.g., dalteparin), 5,000 IU s.q. q day, starting 2 hrs preop

[a]LMWH, low-molecular-weight heparin; IVC inferior vena cava.

cer undergoing surgery are at an increased risk of both DVT and PE periopera-tively, and should be considered at high risk for both of these complications. All candidates for gynecologic-cancer surgery should have perioperative thromboembolic prophylaxis; Table 6.10 lists both mechanical and pharmaco-logic methods commonly employed. Both pneumatic compression boots and low-molecular-weight heparin (LMWH) have been studied extensively, and clearly reduce the incidence of DVT and PE when used in cancer patients peri-operatively. Pneumatic compression boots are the method favored on most gynecologic oncology services because of lower cost and fewer side effects compared with unfractionated heparin, which is associated with thrombocy-topenia and increased retroperitoneal lymphatic drainage. For all methods of thromboembolic prophylaxis, treatment should continue for at least 5–7 days postoperatively to be effective. A subgroup of gynecologic-cancer patients, namely, those with recent or current thromboembolism on anticoagulant ther-apy, are candidates for preoperative inferior vena cava (IVC) filter placement to prevent pulmonary emboli.

Antibiotic prophylaxis and bowel preparation

Gynecologic-cancer patients undergoing surgery are at risk for perioperative infections, including pneumonia, urinary tract infections, and wound infec-tions. Although the benefit of universal antibiotic prophylaxis for "benign" procedures such as abdominal hysterectomy is controversial, the increased risk of infectious complications in the cancer patient justifies that standard preop-erative orders include administration of antibiotic prophylaxis in the majority of patients. Table 6.11 lists antibiotic regimens commonly used for prophylaxis on the gynecologic oncology service. Antibiotics should be administered no longer than 2 hours prior to incision to be maximally effective, and cephalosporins can be safely administered to patients with other than a type I (anaphylactic) penicillin allergy. When the duration of surgery exceeds the dosing interval of the agent used, or when excessive blood loss occurs, repeat doses of antibiotics should be given intraoperatively.

Table 6.11 Regimens for antibiotic prophylaxis

Procedure	Regimen
Bacterial endocarditis	Ampicillin 2 g i.v. + gentamicin 1.5 mg/kg i.v. before incision and repeat in 8 hr Penicillin allergy: vancomycin 1 g i.v. 1 hr before surgery + gentamicin
Laparoscopy, vaginal or abdominal hysterectomy	Cefazolin 1 g i.v. before incision Penicillin allergy: doxycycline 100 mg i.v. 1 hr before surgery
Bowel surgery, ovarian debulking, pelvic exenteration	Cefotetan 2 g i.v. before incision Penicillin allergy: clindamycin 600 mg i.v. + gentamicin 1.5 mg/kg i.v. before incision

Table 6.12 Preoperative bowel preparation

Procedure	Regimen
Laparoscopy	Preoperative day 1: clear liquid diet, 1.5 oz Fleet's Phospha Soda® mixed with 4 oz water NPO after midnight
Laparotomy	Preoperative day 1: clear liquid diet 1.5 oz Fleet's Phospha Soda® at 10 a.m. and 6 p.m. NPO after midnight Day of surgery: Fleet's enema on arrival to hospital
Radical hysterectomy, ovarian debulking, bowel surgery, pelvic exenteration	Preoperative day 1: same as for laparotomy *or* Golytely® 4 liters p.o. or per NG tube in 4 hrs *and* Neomycin 1 g p.o. at 2 p.m. and 11 p.m. metronidazole 1 g p.o. at 2 p.m. and 11 p.m.

Infectious morbidity associated with gynecologic-cancer surgery is also reduced by the use of preoperative bowel preparation. The most commonly used bowel regimens for different types of procedures are listed in Table 6.12. For procedures associated with a significant risk of large-bowel injury, a combination of mechanical cleansing and oral antibiotics is used. With studies showing equivalency of oral sodium phosphate regimen (Fleet's Phospha Soda®) to polyethylene glycol (Golytely®), the former is favored, since it requires less volume and thus has fewer side effects of nausea and bloating. For patients with suspected small-bowel obstruction, cathartic preparations should be avoided, and bowel cleansing should be limited to enemas to empty, but not overdistend, the distal colon. In cases of emergency bowel surgery in the unprepared patient, systemic antibiotics administered 2 hours before surgery and continued postoperatively for 24–48 hours can be combined with intraoperative lavage of the colonic segments with dilute povidone-iodine solution to decrease the burden of fecal material and debris.

Who should be admitted preoperatively?

Over the last few years, the rule that patients with gynecologic cancer are admitted to the hospital the night before surgery has become the exception. However, in some situations, preoperative hospitalization is still indicated. Patients with congestive heart failure, pulmonary hypertension, or severe valvular disease may require admission for invasive cardiac monitoring and adjustment of medications. Patients requiring anticoagulation are admitted 3–5 days before surgery for conversion from oral warfarin to an intravenous heparin infusion, which can be stopped 6 hours preoperatively, or they may have placement of an IVC filter. Patients with chronic obstructive pulmonary disease or asthma may need hospitalization preoperatively for steroid, bronchodilator, and antibiotic therapy.

PERIOPERATIVE COMPLICATIONS

General postoperative care

The first step in postoperative care is writing orders that clearly and completely communicate the treatment plan to the nursing and ancillary staff who will care for the patient. To ensure that nothing is omitted, housestaff should use a repetitive system for order writing such as the "A-D-C-V-A-N-D-I-M-S-L" mnemonic in Table 6.13. After briefly describing the nature of the procedure

Table 6.13 Postoperative orders	
Admit to	Drains
Diagnosis	Intravenous fluids
Condition	Medications (cardiac, thyroid, diabetes)
Vital signs	Sleep and sedation (analgesia)
Activity	Laboratory tests
Allergies	
Nutrition	

and the condition of the patient, the orders should specify the frequency and parameters for vital signs, the activity level, and diet. Typical observations that justify "call MD for..." include hypotension, tachycardia, tachypnea, decreased urine output, and fever. To decrease the incidence of pulmonary complications, early ambulation is indicated for all patients, with the exception of those having a radical vulvectomy or pelvic exenteration. Gynecologic-cancer patients were historically kept NPO (nothing by mouth) and often maintained with nasogastric (NG) suction after surgery until definitive signs of intestinal function such as flatus or bowel movement appeared. Several recent trials have demonstrated that those patients given a diet "as tolerated" and managed without NG tubes have more rapid return of bowel function and shorter length of hospital stay compared with patients managed in the "traditional" manner.

Similarly, the routine use of postoperative closed suction drains in cases of retroperitoneal lymph-node dissection, once the standard of care, has been largely abandoned in light of data from recent randomized trials. Intravenous-fluid orders must be written with careful attention to the patient's current volume status and expected fluid shifts in the immediate postoperative period. Continuing cardiac medications, particularly beta-blockers, in the perioperative period is important for preventing perioperative ischemia and arrhythmias. Providing adequate analgesia reduces the incidence of pulmonary complications, and the use of patient-controlled analgesic pumps and epidural analgesia are excellent approaches for patients undergoing extensive pelvic surgery.

Intraoperative and postoperative hemorrhage

Because many of the surgical procedures in gynecologic oncology involve dissection of major blood vessels and resection of hypervascular tumors, familiarity with the steps necessary to prevent and treat intraoperative hemorrhage are essential in the care of the gynecologic-cancer patient. Preoperative screening for coagulopathy, and discontinuing medications and supplements associated with increased bleeding risk (aspirin, NSAIDs, gingko biloba, St John's Wort) are simple measures to prevent intraoperative hemorrhage. Familiarity with blood-component therapy (Table 6.14) is essential in the management of operative hemorrhage, and although general guidelines for transfusion exist (hemoglobin < 8 g/dl), the threshold for transfusion must be individualized. In elderly patients or those with significant cardiac disease, keeping the hemoglobin above 10 g/dl is necessary to maximize oxygen-carrying capacity. For otherwise-healthy patients, the risks of transfusion, including infection with hepatitis B (1 in 80,000 units), hepatitis C (1 in 3,000 units), and HIV (1 in 500,000 units), must be weighed against the benefits. Just as definitions of the volume of blood loss constituting hemorrhage varies, so does the incidence of hemorrhage reported in series of radical pelvic surgery. When excessive bleeding is encountered intraoperatively, a series of steps should be followed to

Table 6.14 Blood component therapy

Component	Dosage/volume	Indications
Packed red blood cells	1 unit = 250–300 cc should ↑ Hb by 1 g/dl, ↑ Hct by 3%	Hemoglobin < 8 g/dl Loss of >30% total blood volume (TBV = 75 cc/kg body wt)
Platelets	1 pack = 8–10 units 1 unit should ↑ count by 10,000	Platelets < 50,000 in patients with normal counts preop and ongoing hemorrhage, <20,000 in patients with low platelets preop
Fresh-frozen plasma	1 unit = 225 ml contains 200 units of factors VIII and V and other factors	Correct bleeding from multiple factor deficiencies (liver disease, massive blood loss)
Cryoprecipitate	15 ml contains 80 units factor VIII, 150 mg fibrinogen	von Willebrand's disease, massive transfusion

Table 6.15 Controlling intraoperative hemorrhage

Direct pressure
Repair or ligation of blood vessel
Topical hemostatic agents
Packing
Embolization

restore hemostasis (Table 6.15). Direct pressure applied to the source of bleeding is the simplest and often most effective measure that can be taken. Repair of a damaged vessel, use of hemostatic agents, packing with planned return to the OR, and even angiographic arterial embolization are all measures that may be required in cases of massive intraoperative bleeding.

Postoperative hemorrhage is encountered less often; however, the effects can be devastating if not recognized and treated early. Signs of postoperative hemorrhage in the gynecologic-cancer patient may include tachycardia, oliguria, hypotension, rapidly increasing abdominal girth, sudden bleeding from drains placed in the pelvis or retroperitoneum, and flank discoloration (in the case of retroperitoneal hemorrhage). Diagnosis is confirmed with serial hematocrits.

The choice of treatment for postoperative hemorrhage is based on the patient's hemodynamic state, including the presence of coagulopathy and the transfusion requirement. For brisk vaginal bleeding, a pelvic examination at the bedside or under anesthesia should be performed to exclude a vaginal cuff "pumper" that can be stopped with simple application of a clamp or suture without re-exploration. When the patient requires re-exploration for postoperative hemorrhage, the guidelines for controlling intraoperative hemorrhage described above should be followed.

Oliguria

Being called to evaluate decreased urine output in the immediate postoperative period is a frequent request of housestaff on the gynecologic oncology service. To appropriately evaluate and treat postoperative oliguria, both the intravascular volume and total body fluid status of the patient must be determined, and central venous pressure measurements may be required. Although oliguria may reflect hemorrhage or renal failure, a more common cause of oliguria in patients undergoing ovarian-cancer debulking surgery is "third-spacing," or sequestration of excess total body fluid in the extravascular compartment. For such patients, the usual response to oliguria of ordering a crystalloid fluid bolus will likely be ineffective. Administration of 250 cc of 5% albumin followed by 10 mg of furosemide may decrease the extravascular volume, at least temporarily. For otherwise healthy patients, "third-spacing" usually resolves within 48–72 hours.

Cardiac complications: arrhythmias and myocardial infarction

Gynecologic cancer often strikes elderly women who have higher rates of obesity, diabetes, and hypertension. This increased baseline risk, combined with the hemodynamic stresses caused by radical pelvic surgery, makes evaluation and triage of cardiac complications an integral part of perioperative care. Since the majority of perioperative cardiac ischemic events are asymptomatic, routine postoperative ECG studies should be ordered for high-risk patients, including those aged over 70 years and those with a history of myocardial infarction, angina, or coronary artery revascularization surgery. Unexplained hypotension, dyspnea, chest pain, or arrhythmias may signal ongoing ischemia, and should trigger appropriate evaluation and consultation as outlined in Table 6.16. Atrial fibrillation is the most commonly occurring arrhythmia in the perioperative period, and although common causes include electrolyte abnormalities and valvular disease, pulmonary embolus must be considered as a possible etiology.

Table 6.16 Diagnosis of postoperative myocardial infarction

Symptoms/signs	Evaluation	Suspect MI
Hypotension	Physical exam	Serial enzymes
Dyspnea	Chest radiograph	Cardiology/ICU
Chest pain	12-lead ECG: compare with preop	consult
Arrhythmias	Arterial blood gas,	
	electrolytes, hematocrit	

Thromboembolic events: deep-vein thrombosis and pulmonary embolus

Despite using thromboembolic prophylaxis in every patient, deep vein thrombosis (DVT) and pulmonary embolus remain significant causes of perioperative morbidity and mortality on the gynecologic oncology service. The symptoms and signs of DVT are nonspecific, and include fever, pain, and edema of the extremities. Recognizing signs of DVT against the background of the edema and pain associated with pelvic surgery may be difficult, and there should be a low threshold for diagnostic imaging to exclude DVT. Duplex Doppler ultrasound to visualize thrombus and measure blood flow through vessels has replaced venography as the "gold standard" for diagnosis of proximal lower-extremity DVT. The treatment of DVT has been revolutionized by the introduction of low-molecular-weight heparin (LMWH) regimens such as that outlined in Table 6.17. Although clinical trials are ongoing, studies have demonstrated improved survival in cancer patients treated with LMWH, providing an additional reason to choose this regimen over the traditional unfractionated heparin for treatment of DVT. For the cancer patient, anticoagulation should be continued for as long as she has detectable thrombosis or measurable tumor burden.

Recognition and treatment of pulmonary embolus is made difficult by the similarity of signs and symptoms to those of more common pulmonary complications such as atelectasis or pneumonia (Table 6.18). Isolated tachycardia or tachypnea may signal pulmonary embolus, and arterial blood-gas measurements should be performed even for these subtle signs. Ventilation–perfusion (V/Q) scanning is the most common method of diagnosis, but use of spiral CT scanning is increasing and may be more sensitive than V/Q scanning, particularly when underlying lung pathology such as pleural effusion or atelectasis hampers interpretation of the V/Q scan. Because of the morbidity associated with pulmonary embolus, if diagnostic studies cannot be performed immediately, anticoagulation is instituted until the studies are complete. Treatment of pulmonary embolus is identical to the unfractionated heparin infusion for DVT outlined in Table 6.17, but higher doses of heparin are often required to attain the desired aPTT value. Although no trials have established their use in cancer

Table 6.19 Diagnosis of postoperative fever	
Timing after surgery	Differential diagnosis
0–48 hours	Atelectasis, aspiration pneumonia, thrombophlebitis
2–7 days	Urinary-tract infection, wound infection, nosocomial pneumonia
7–21 days	Abscess, ureteral injury, bowel anastomotic leak, vaginal-cuff cellulitis

Table 6.20 Antibiotic choices for common postoperative infections		
Infection	Common organisms	Antibiotic
Wound cellulitis	Staphylococci, streptococci	Cefazolin or vancomycin
Urinary-tract infection	Gram-negative rods, enterococci	Cefazolin, trimethoprim–sulfamethoxazole, ciprofloxacin
Pneumonia	Gram-negative rods	Ticarcillin/clavulanate, ciprofloxacin
Intra-abdominal: abscess or peritonitis	Enteric gram-negative rods, anaerobes	Cefotetan, imipenem, ampicillin + gentamicin, metronidazole

bowel function is related to the type and extent of surgery, but is also influenced by patient factors such as diabetes, prior surgery, and analgesic requirements. Determining when intestinal symptoms become a complication and distinguishing between postoperative ileus and obstruction is one of the challenges of perioperative care. The major differences between postoperative ileus and obstruction relate to timing and persistence of symptoms despite gastric decompression (Table 6.21). In both situations, x-ray findings may lag clinical findings by 1 or 2 days, so greater weight should be given to results of frequent serial abdominal examinations. A CT scan in patients who do not improve with conservative measures can determine the approximate site of obstruction, if present, or exclude an abscess or ureteral injury as a cause of ileus. Although having no advantage over a nasogastric tube in relieving obstruction, a

Table 6.21 Postoperative ileus versus postoperative obstruction

	Ileus	Obstruction
Timing	48–72 hours	5–7 days
Symptoms	Constant pain from distention	Episodic, cramping pain
Physical exam	Abdominal distention, absent or hypoactive bowel sounds	Abdominal distention, hyperactive bowel sounds, rushes and high-pitched
X-ray findings	Distended small- and large-bowel loops, air in colon	Distended small-bowel loops with air–fluid levels, no air in colon
Treatment	Gastric decompression NG tube, correct electrolyte abnormalities, enemas, suppositories	Gastric decompression NG tube, correct electrolyte abnormalities, surgical exploration

7
Nutrition and TPN

Mark A Schattner, Moshe Shike

Cachexia and weight loss are common manifestations of cancer and exert major impacts on quality of life and survival. Malnutrition is a complex, multifactorial phenomenon that leads to progressive weight loss and deficiency of specific nutrients. Both the cancer and its various therapeutic modalities contribute to cachexia. Advances in understanding nutritional requirements and intermediary metabolism, and major technologic progress in the ability to provide nutritional support, have made it possible to feed almost any patient with cancer. Nevertheless, the indications for and appropriate use of the various modalities of nutritional support are still evolving, and many questions remain unanswered.

Malnutrition in most patients with cancer is usually a manifestation of general calorie–protein deficits that result in progressive weight loss and weakness. It is important to recognize, however, that in some patients specific nutrient deficiencies, such as magnesium deficiency or vitamin B_{12} deficiency, can be present even in the absence of weight loss and can contribute significantly to morbidity and even mortality.

Gynecologic malignancies and their multimodal therapies may be associated with severe malnutrition. Although some nutritional problems occur in patients with cervical and endometrial cancer, they are most commonly seen in those with ovarian cancer, particularly in cases of advanced-stage disease, in which intra-abdominal metastases severely impair gastrointestinal function. Because of the high incidence of malnutrition and its impact on the patient with cancer, nutritional assessment and appropriate therapy should be integral parts of the overall treatment plan.

NUTRITIONAL ASSESSMENT

Nutritional assessment in cancer patients is an ongoing process. It should be part of the patient's initial evaluation and updated periodically thereafter. It is especially important to determine the patient's nutritional state prior to therapeutic interventions as well as during and after an acute illness, with the goal

135

The etiologic factors of malnutrition in the cancer patient, whether caused by the tumor or antitumor therapies, can be classified into three major categories: decreased food intake, malabsorption, and metabolic derangements that result in inefficient, wasteful metabolism.

Impaired food intake and absorption

Both tumor and cancer treatment modalities can lead to decreased food intake through direct effects on the gastrointestinal tract or systemic effects leading to anorexia. Obstruction of the gastrointestinal tract can be caused by any gynecologic malignancy through external compression, or, more rarely, by direct invasion. Although, at times, localized obstructions can be relieved surgically, the obstruction due to peritoneal carcinomatosis often seen in advanced ovarian cancer is particularly difficult to manage surgically. Often, draining gastrostomy with parenteral nutrition (when appropriate) is the only option for providing nutrition and symptomatic relief.

Therapies used for gynecologic malignancies often result in complications that impair nutrient intake and absorption. Surgical interventions can lead to fistulae, short-bowel syndrome, infections, and ileus, all of which impair oral intake significantly. In a review of 12 years of colonic surgery in gynecologic oncology patients, the rate for major systemic complications (myocardial infarction, pulmonary embolism, renal failure, sepsis) was 13.7%, and the rate of major bowel complications (abscess, fistulae, hemorrhage, obstruction) was 12.1%. Adjuvant irradiation and chemotherapy have been shown to increase the incidence of major complications after pelvic exenteration.

Radiation therapy can lead to various derangements in the structure and function of the gastrointestinal tract. Damage to the gastrointestinal tract following radiation to the abdomen and pelvis most commonly affects the small bowel, followed by the transverse colon, sigmoid, and rectum. Predisposing risk factors include previous abdominal surgery, pelvic inflammatory disease, thin body habitus, hypertension, and diabetes mellitus. In general, a dose of 50 Gy is the threshold for significant injury. In the acute phase of radiation enteritis, virtually all patients experience anorexia, nausea, and vomiting, which are thought to be mediated by effects of serotonin on the gut and the central nervous system. This is followed 2–3 weeks later by diarrhea caused by direct injury to the intestinal mucosa, resulting in mild to moderate malabsorption. Most patients will have complete resolution of these acute symptoms. However, a significant minority of patients who received radiation therapy will experience chronic dysfunction of the gastrointestinal tract. There is often a latent period of 1–2 years, and possibly as long as 20 years, before the symptoms of chronic radiation enteropathy surface. In a review of 102 patients with radiation enteritis after treatment for cervical or endometrial cancer, the median time to development of severe symptoms, such as obstruction or perforation, was 18 months.

Chronic radiation enteropathy is characterized pathologically by transmural injury leading to submucosal fibrosis, edema, lymphatic ectasia, and oblitera-tive endarteritis, which can induce colicky abdominal pain, diarrhea, steator-rhea, ulceration, perforation, stricture, and fistula formation. In 47 patients with gynecologic malignancies who had gastrointestinal complaints lasting more than 4 months after radiation therapy, Kwitko et al found 19 partial small-bowel obstructions, 11 cases of malabsorption, and 5 fistulae. The mor-tality rate from radiation damage to the small bowel in this report was 32%. Improved fractionation of radiation therapy and protective shielding of the intestine where possible have reduced these complication rates.

Chemotherapy is often associated with decreased food intake. Odynophagia, oral ulcers, and diarrhea are commonly seen during therapy with cytotoxic agents that affect the replicating cells of the intestinal mucosa, such as 5-flourouracil, methotrexate, and bleomycin. The vinca alkaloids can cause ileus and constipation mediated by toxic effects on gastrointestinal neural pathways, while cisplatin and the nitrosoureas are highly emetic. Significant nausea, vomiting, stomatitis, and diarrhea occur in 15% of patients receiving intra-venous paclitaxel and 55% in those receiving the drug orally.

The psychological impact of a malignancy and its associated therapies can also lead to decreased nutrient intake. Depression is a frequent cause of anorexia in this population, and learned food aversions are a common conse-quence of irradiation or chemotherapy. These learned behaviors are character-ized by a psychological association between the consumption of a particular food and a temporally related unpleasant reaction to the therapy such as nau-sea and vomiting. Such reactions result in future avoidance of that particular food item.

Metabolic derangements

Even with normal nutrient intake, patients with cancer are at risk for malnutri-tion due to inefficient nutrient utilization and wasteful metabolic pathways. Compared with simple starvation, cancer cachexia is associated with altered metabolism of carbohydrates, fat, protein, vitamins, and minerals. Therefore, in order to optimize nutritional support in the cancer patient, it is imperative to consider metabolic derangements along with problems of ingestion, diges-tion, and absorption.

Increase in basal energy expenditure (BEE) has been reported in many but not all studies of patients with malignancy. Elevated basal energy expenditure may drop after tumor resection. There are limited data on the metabolic rate in patients with gynecologic cancers. Dickerson et al used indirect calorimetry to determine the resting energy expenditure in 31 patients with ovarian cancer and 30 patients with cervical cancer. Fifty-five percent of those with ovarian cancer were found to be hypermetabolic (BEE > 110% predicted by the Harris–Benedict equation), while only 13% of patients with cervical cancer were hypermetabolic. These differences could not be explained by differences in the extent of disease, nutritional status, body temperature, or nutrient intake.

The role of TPN in the perioperative period has been extensively studied. In an early study by Mueller et al, 10 days of preoperative TPN was associated with nutritional improvement and significant reduction in major postoperative complications and mortality. These impressive results have not been confirmed in subsequent studies. At Memorial Sloan-Kettering Cancer Center, a prospective study of 117 patients undergoing curative resection for pancreatic cancer randomized to receive TPN or intravenous fluids in the postoperative period showed no benefit from routine use of postoperative TPN. The group receiving TPN had a significant increase in postoperative infectious complications. The largest prospective randomized trial investigating the role of TPN in the perioperative setting was the Veterans Administration Cooperative Study. In this study, 395 patients were randomized to receive either TPN or oral feeding plus intravenous fluids for 7–15 days preoperatively and 3 days postoperatively. TPN did not improve morbidity or 90-day mortality. However, subgroup analysis showed that patients considered to be severely malnourished had fewer infectious complications if they received TPN. The authors concluded that the routine administration of preoperative TPN should be limited to patients who are severely malnourished unless there are other specific indications.

These data and others provide the basis for the consensus statement from the National Institutes of Health, the American Society for Parenteral and Enteral Nutrition, and the American Society for Clinical Nutrition regarding the use of perioperative TPN, which states the following: (1) 7–10 days of preoperative TPN in a malnourished patient with gastrointestinal cancer results in a 10% reduction in postoperative complications; (2) routine use of postoperative TPN in malnourished surgical patients who did not receive preoperative TPN results in a 10% *increase* in complications; (3) if, by postoperative day 5–10, a patient is unable to tolerate oral or enteral feedings, TPN is indicated to prevent the adverse effects of starvation (Table 7.1).

Composition of TPN solutions

Once the decision to proceed with parenteral nutritional support has been made, access to a large-bore central vein should be obtained. This access allows the use of calorically dense, hypertonic solutions, which are often necessary in severely ill patients who may have restrictions on the amount of intravenous fluids they can receive. When possible, this line should be used exclusively for TPN infusion and should be treated with strict aseptic technique. The composition of the TPN solution should be individualized based on the patient's condition and requirements, preferably by a dedicated nutritional support team. The solution must provide the protein and caloric needs, fluid, minerals, trace elements, and vitamins. Although indirect calorimetry and nitrogen balance can be used to determine energy and protein requirements, they are too costly and cumbersome for routine use. There are numerous formulas, charts, and tables that can provide estimates of protein and calorie requirements. Estimates of nutritional requirements are based on weight and

Table 7.1 Indications for TPN in patients with gynecologic cancers	
Perioperative	• 7–10 days preoperatively in a malnourished patient (who cannot be fed enterally) • Postoperative complications that prevent oral or enteral intake for more than 7–10 days • Enterocutaneous fistula • *No* indication for routine use
During radiation or chemotherapy	• Maximization of performance status prior to therapy in a malnourished patient who cannot be fed enterally • Severe persistent (more than 7–10 days) mucositis, diarrhea, ileus, or emesis • *No* indication for routine use
General	• After 7–10 days of inability to tolerate oral or enteral feeding due to any cause
Home TPN	• Severe chronic radiation enteropathy • Short-bowel syndrome • Persistent enterocutaneous fistula • Selected patients with obstruction due to peritoneal carcinomatosis (selection based on performance status and potential for further chemotherapy)

adjusted for the degree of physiologic stress encountered by the patient. Generally, patients require 30 kcal/kg nonprotein calories, 1 g/kg amino acids, and about 2,000 ml of fluid. As illness severity increases and organ function changes, adjustments may be required. Thus, patients with kidney or liver failure require decreased amounts of amino acids, while those with heart failure require restriction of sodium and fluids. Nonprotein calories can be provided as dextrose or lipids, and the relative amounts of these should also be individualized. Lipids provide 9 kcal/g, compared with 3.4 for dextrose. (In dextrose solutions, the glucose is present as glucose monohydrate; hence, a gram contains less than 4 kcal.) Lipid calories are particularly useful in patients who have high caloric requirements but cannot tolerate a large fluid load. In addition, lipids are useful in patients with severe pulmonary or hepatic dysfunction, since glucose metabolism produces more carbon dioxide, which can add to the burden of the ailing lung and can lead to fatty infiltration of the liver. Up to 60% of caloric requirements can be provided as lipids, but serum triglyceride levels must be monitored closely. Appropriate electrolyte content of TPN solutions is of critical importance. The amounts must be tailored to the patient's requirements and organ function. Care must be taken to prevent potentially fatal hypokalemia or hypophosphatemia (particularly in the patient with severe weight loss), which can be precipitated by insulin-induced transport of the minerals to the intracellular space when inadequate amounts are given. Other electrolyte disorders such as cisplatin-induced hypomagnesemia and SIADH (syndrome of inappropriate secretion of antidiuretic hormone) are common in the patient with gynecologic malignancy, and must be addressed when ordering TPN. The TPN solution must also contain vitamins, minerals, and trace elements. Typically, these are available as standard commercial combination products. Certain patients, however, require specific modifications. For example, a patient with persistent diarrhea requires zinc supplementation in excess of the amounts present in standard trace-element solutions.

Complications

TPN-induced complications can be classified as catheter-related, metabolic, or infectious. Catheter complications most often occur during placement of a central venous catheter, and include pneumothorax, hemothorax, arterial injury, and hematoma. Metabolic derangements are frequently encountered during support with TPN, and the prescribing physician must be well versed in the pathophysiology of these disorders. Hyperglycemia is the most common abnormality, and if not corrected can lead to an osmotic diuresis, dehydration, acidosis, and hyperosmolar coma. Patients receiving parenteral nutrition should have continuous monitoring for glycosuria, and if the dipstick is positive, the blood sugar concentration should be determined and sliding-scale insulin coverage should be provided. Other metabolic complications that are encountered include hypomagnesemia in a patient after platinum-based chemotherapy, metabolic acidosis due to severe diarrhea, and hyponatremia secondary to SIADH.

One metabolic complication that deserves special mention is the "refeeding syndrome." In chronically ill patients with severe malnutrition, there is often a depletion of total-body phosphorus and potassium. The phosphorus deficits may be masked by increased renal phosphorus absorption designed to maintain normal serum levels. When TPN is initiated, the infusion of a large glucose load, with the subsequent surge in insulin, leads to an increased cellular uptake of phosphorus and potassium that may induce severe life-threatening hypokalemia and hypophosphatemia. These disorders cause widespread tissue and organ dysfunction, including muscle weakness, rhabdomyolysis, heart failure, cardiac arrhythmias, and respiratory failure, and, in extreme cases, may result in death. Therefore, in patients with evidence of severe undernutrition, TPN should be initiated with small amounts of dextrose calories, supplemental phosphorus and potassium, and careful monitoring of serum phosphorus and electrolytes.

TPN has been associated with cholestatic liver disease as well as with fatty infiltration of the liver and glycogen deposition. These abnormalities have been attributed to infusion of excessive glucose calories, imbalance of amino acids, and, in rare cases, fatty acid deficiency. Elevation of serum aminotransferases may occur, but it is generally mild. Severe liver dysfunction in adult TPN recipients is rare and requires a search for causes other than TPN.

Infections are particularly serious complications in patients with malignancy who are receiving TPN. In an evaluation of seven studies comparing TPN plus chemotherapy with chemotherapy alone, Koretz found four studies that showed an increase in infectious complications in patients receiving TPN. A meta-analysis by the American College of Nutrition showed a fourfold increase in infections when patients receiving chemotherapy were given TPN. In a prospective, randomized study of TPN following pancreatic resection, recipients of TPN had significantly more infectious complications. Data from a Veterans Administration randomized cooperative study showed that patients with mild to moderate malnutrition given perioperative TPN had increased rates of infections, while those with severe malnutrition developed significantly fewer infections when supported with TPN. Infectious complications are related to both central venous catheters and a variety of sites (wound infection, abscess, and pneumonia).

Home TPN

Long-term TPN in the home can be a life-saving treatment in an appropriately selected group of patients. It is clear that cancer patients who have had severe gastrointestinal injury, such as massive intestinal resection or severe radiation enteritis, and in whom the cancer has been cured or is well controlled, benefit from long-term TPN at home. Survival rates and TPN-related complications in such patients are comparable to those seen in patients with benign diseases (Crohn's disease, intestinal necrosis) who require home TPN. Among patients with widely metastatic disease and poor prognosis, home TPN offers very limited benefit. Only 15% of such patients survive longer than 1 year on home TPN. Techniques for placing feeding tubes make it possible to hydrate and feed patients enterally, even in the presence of upper gastrointestinal obstruction, and thus obviate the need for home TPN in such patients. In terminally ill patients, TPN should be avoided. The concern that such patients should not be "starved to death" is not a justification for TPN. An uncontrolled study of terminally ill cancer patients hospitalized at a long-term care facility suggests that these patients did not experience hunger or thirst, and that in those who experienced such symptoms, small amounts of food alleviated the symptoms. In such patients, the utilization of TPN, either in the home or at healthcare facilities, cannot be justified.

It is often difficult to determine which patients with inoperable bowel obstruction due to metastatic ovarian cancer will benefit from home TPN. In a review of 9,897 days of home TPN administered to 75 patients with various cancers and intestinal obstruction, it was shown that a Karnofsky performance status greater than 50 at the initiation of TPN could predict which patients would have improved quality of life while on home TPN. The authors concluded that home TPN should be avoided if the performance status is below this level (50). In addition, patients with a life expectancy of less than 2–3 months will not benefit from home TPN. In a study from Yale–New Haven Hospital of 17 patients with inoperable bowel obstruction due to malignancy, patients with ovarian cancer had the shortest survival (39 days) compared with patients with colon cancer (90 days) and appendiceal cancer (184 days). Therefore, only a highly selected minority of patients with inoperable bowel obstruction can potentially benefit from home TPN. Currently, the best selection criteria for such patients are a fair or better performance status and the potential for further antitumor therapy.

Enteral nutrition

Enteral feeding delivers a liquid-nutrient formula into the gastrointestinal tract through tubes placed into the stomach or small intestine. As in oral feeding, an adequately functioning small intestinal mucosa is required for absorption of nutrients. Enteral feeding can overcome many difficulties encountered in patients with a wide variety of gastrointestinal-tract dysfunction. A proximal gastrointestinal obstruction can be bypassed; tubes can be placed distal to obstructions as far as the jejunum, thereby circumventing obstructing lesions of the oral cavity, esophagus, stomach, duodenum, or proximal jejunum. The liquid-nutrient formula can be delivered as a slow, continuous infusion, thus maximizing absorption by a limited intestinal surface that can be overwhelmed by the higher volume delivered during oral or bolus feeding. Such an approach may be useful in patients with radiation enteritis, short-bowel syndrome (with adequate remaining short bowel, usually 3–4 feet), or partial obstruction of the bowel.

Route of administration and nutrient formula

Short-term (<2 weeks) access to the gastrointestinal tract can be obtained through nasogastric or nasoenteric tubes. Patients requiring longer nutritional support should have a gastrostomy or jejunostomy tube placed endoscopically, radiologically, or surgically. In comparison with nasal tubes, gastrostomy or jejunostomy tubes are wider (15–24 French) and therefore less likely to be obstructed by medications or nutrient solutions. In addition, they are fixed in the stomach or the upper intestine and do not migrate into the esophagus. Thus, the risk of aspiration is considerably decreased. These tubes are more comfortable and aesthetically more pleasing. Their benefits were demonstrated in a randomized study of patients who had had an acute dysphagic stroke; this trial showed that patients fed with a gastrostomy tube had greater optimal provision of nutrients, achieved a better nutritional state, and had lower mortality than those fed with nasogastric tubes. Patients with gastrostomy tubes have been shown in prospective studies to receive over 90% of prescribed feedings, compared with only 55% in patients fed through nasal tubes. These differences are largely attributed to nasogastric tube dislodgment.

The endoscopically placed percutaneous gastrostomy tube (PEG) has become the procedure of choice for placement of enteral feeding tubes because of its ease and safety, and the fact that it can be performed on an outpatient basis. Percutaneous jejunostomy (PEJ) tubes can also be placed endoscopically; these allow for continued enteral feeding in patients with gastric resection, gastric outlet obstruction, or gastroparesis. Major complications (bleeding, peritonitis, abdominal-wall abscess, colonic perforation, and aspiration) from PEG and PEJ placement are rare, occurring in 0–2.5% of patients, while minor complications (wound infection, tube migrations, or leak) are seen in 5–15%. This compares favorably with the 2.5–16% complication rate and the 1–6% mortality rate with laparotomy, required for surgical placement of feeding tubes.

More than 100 different enteral feeding formulas are currently commercially available. They are designed to provide either complete nutrition, single nutrients, or fluids and electrolytes only. Formulas differ in protein concentration, calories, osmolarity, and percentage of nonprotein calories delivered as carbohydrates or fats. Enteral feeding formulas that provide 1,500–2,000 kcal/day normally contain all of the necessary nutrients, including proteins, vitamins, minerals, and trace elements. In addition, there are disease-specific formulations for patients with diabetes or hepatic, renal, or pulmonary dysfunction. The choice of formula should be individualized, and often helps to minimize problems such as diarrhea, bloating, and hyperglycemia.

Enteral solutions may be administered either by bolus feedings or by continuous infusion. Bolus feeding is possible when the tip of the feeding tube is in an intact stomach. Up to 500 ml of a feeding formula can be infused over a 10- to 15-minute period by syringe or gravity into the stomach. The pyloric sphincter regulates flow into the duodenum. All bolus feedings should be done with the patient sitting upright in order to minimize the risk of aspiration. When the tip of the feeding tube is distal to the pylorus, continuous feeding must be employed to avoid abdominal distention and diarrhea. Rates as high as 150 ml/hr are generally well tolerated.

Efficacy

Data from randomized trials examining the efficacy of enteral nutrition given as an adjuvant therapy in patients receiving chemotherapy for a variety of cancers have failed to demonstrate a clear benefit in terms of survival or response to treatment. The validity of the conclusions of these studies, however, is limited by their small size and poor design. Similar difficulties plague the studies examining the role of standard enteral nutrition in the perioperative period. Complication rates, mortality, and length of hospital stay are not affected by early postoperative enteral feedings. Therefore, routine use of enteral nutrition support in patients receiving chemotherapy or undergoing operations for cancer cannot be justified. Accepted indications for enteral nutrition in cancer patients include: (1) obstruction of the upper digestive tract in those who are not candidates for an operation, (2) the presence of chronic malnutrition due to inadequate oral intake, and (3) perioperative support of the malnourished patient.

Complications

Enteral nutrition is generally safe if careful attention is paid to the following: (1) choice of an appropriate formula; (2) infusion into an appropriate portion of the gastrointestinal tract; (3) use of the correct infusion method; (4) ongoing clinical and metabolic monitoring of the patient. The most serious complication of enteral feeding is aspiration, which occurs in 1–32% of patients. The risk is minimized by keeping patients upright during bolus feedings and using jejunal feedings if there is predisposition for aspiration, gastroparesis, or an impaired gag reflex. Diarrhea is reported in 5–30% of patients receiving enteral nutrition. While the diarrhea may be related to underlying disorders of the gastrointestinal tract such as radiation enteritis or short-bowel syndrome, a commonly overlooked cause is medication. Patients on enteral feeding often receive magnesium-containing antacids or antibiotics, both of which may induce diarrhea. Metabolic complications include dehydration, azotemia, hyperglycemia, and hyperkalemia. These are usually due to the patient's underlying disease, and can be avoided with the proper choice of formula and careful monitoring.

Home enteral nutrition

Home enteral nutrition (HEN) is increasingly being used to provide nutrients and fluids outside the hospital. Cancer is the most common indication for its use, and accounts for 42% of all patients receiving HEN. It is a safe therapy in patients with cancer, with only a 0.4% annual rate of complications requiring hospitalization. The overall 1-year survival rate for cancer patients on HEN is 30%; however, in patients with cancer of the head and neck who have been successfully treated, HEN has provided good nutrition for periods exceeding 7 years. Regular medical follow-up is essential to ensure appropriate functioning of the feeding tube and optimization of the nutrition regimen. This form of therapy is useful in patients with gynecologic malignancies who have upper gastrointestinal tract obstructions that cannot be treated surgically.

Oral dietary therapy

Patients who are able to eat but have impairment of the gastrointestinal tract or have special metabolic requirements may benefit from a specialized oral dietary therapy. Often, this may obviate the need for more costly and complex interventions such as parenteral nutrition. In oral dietary therapy, the regular diet is modified based on the pathophysiologic changes induced by the underlying disorder, with the goal of providing the most optimal nutrition possible. When the main problem is inadequate food consumption, various commercial oral supplements can be used, but usually for only short periods because of taste fatigue. Some preparations provide complete nutrition while others are intended to supplement deficits of specific nutrients. Problems common in patients with gynecologic malignancies such as partial small-bowel obstruction, chronic radiation enteritis, and short-bowel syndrome may all be amenable to dietary therapies. In partial small-bowel obstruction or motility dysfunction, a diet comprising frequent, small, calorically dense meals with minimal amounts of fiber is indicated. Patients with radiation enteritis should receive a low-fat, low-fiber, and lactose-free diet. Dietary management of patients with short-bowel syndrome includes frequent small meals, limitation of fiber, lactose, and simple sugars, taking liquids separately from meals, and supplementation of calcium and zinc orally, and magnesium and vitamin B_{12} parenterally.

The successful implementation of a prescribed diet depends to a large extent on a dietician converting the prescribed diet into a meal plan and working with the patient to implement it.

Pharmacologic agents

Agents that will reverse the wasting seen in patients with advanced-stage cancers have long been sought to complement or avoid the need for the provision of nutrients via the enteral or parenteral route. Hormones, appetite stimulants, and, most recently, cytokine antagonists have been examined. Studies of growth hormone, insulin-like growth factor I (IGF-I) alone, and IGF-I with insulin in cancer-bearing rodent models showed significant attenuation of tumor-induced weight loss. In human clinical trials, these agents provided a modest gain in weight, but no improvement in quality of life and no other benefits.

Appetite stimulants

Anabolic steroids have no proven efficacy in treating cancer cachexia. In a murine model, administration of norandrolone propionate resulted in weight gain, but this was largely due to fluid retention. In human trials, steroids produced transient improvement of nutritional parameters and appetite, but continued use is associated with negative nitrogen balance, net calcium loss, glucose intolerance, and immunosuppression.

Megestrol acetate is a progestational agent that has been shown to improve appetite and ameliorate weight loss in numerous but not all studies of patients with cancer and cachexia. Doses in these studies ranged from 160 to 1,200 mg/day, and maximal weight gain was generally seen within 8 weeks. However, the change in weight was largely due to increased adipose tissue and edema. Nevertheless, improvement in quality of life has consistently been demonstrated in several large prospective studies in patients with cancer cachexia who were treated with megestrol acetate. It is generally well tolerated but can exacerbate underlying diabetes mellitus and can lead to adrenal suppression in rare cases. Dronabinol, a marijuana derivative, has shown some promise in small studies, improving appetite and causing weight gain; however, large randomized trials are lacking. Food and Drug Administration (FDA) approval is currently limited to treatment of nausea and vomiting during chemotherapy and for cachexia in HIV-positive patients.

SELECTED READING

Abu-Rustum NR, Barakat RR, Venkatraman E, Spriggs D, Chemotherapy and total parenteral nutrition for advanced ovarian cancer with bowel obstruction. *Gynecol Oncol* 1997; **64**: 493.

American College of Physicians Position Paper, Parenteral nutrition in patients receiving cancer chemotherapy. *Ann Intern Med* 1989; **110**: 734.

August DA, Thorn D, Fisher RL, Welchek CM, Home parenteral nutrition for patients with inoperable malignant bowel obstruction. *JPEN* 1991; **15**: 323.

Baker JP, Detsky AS, Wesson DE et al, Nutritional assessment: a comparison of clinical judgment and objective measurements. *N Engl J Med* 1982; **306**: 969.

Burnett AF, Potkul RK, Barter JF et al, Colonic surgery in gynecologic oncology. Risk factor analysis. *J Repro Med* 1993; **38**: 137.

Danielson A, Nhylin H, Persson H et al, Chronic diarrhoea after radiotherapy for gynaecological cancer: occurrence and aetiology. *Gut* 1991; **32**: 1180.

Dickerson RN, White KG, Curicllo PG, King SA, Resting energy expenditure of patients with gynecologic malignancies. *J Am Coll Nutr* 1995; **15**: 448.

Donato D, Angelides A, Irani H et al, Infectious complications after gastrointestinal surgery in patients with ovarian carcinoma and malignant ascites. *Gynecol Oncol* 1992; **44**: 40.

Howard L, Ament M, Fleming R et al, Current use and clinical outcome of home parenteral and enteral nutrition therapies in the United States. *Gas-*

troenterology 1995; **109**: 355.

Klein S, Kinney J, Jeejeebhoy MB et al, Nutrition support in clinical practice: review of published data and recommendations for future research directions. *Am J Clin Nutr* 1997; **66**: 683.

Klein S, Koretz RL, Nutrition support in patients with cancer: What do the data really show? *Nutr Clin Pract* 1994; **9**: 91.

Kwitko Ao, Pieterse AS, Hecker R et al, Chronic radiation injury to the intestine: a clinico-pathological study. *Aust NZ J Med* 1982; **12**: 272.

Orr JW Jr, Wilson K, Bodiford C et al, Nutritional status of patients with untreated cervical cancer. I. Biochemical and immunologic assessment. *Am J Obstet Gynecol* 1985; **151**: 625.

Ottery FD, Walsh D, Strawford A, Pharmacologic management of anorexia/cachexia. *Semin Oncol* 1998; **25**(2 Suppl 6): 35.

Philip J, Depczynski B, The role of total parenteral nutrition for patients with irreversible bowel obstruction secondary to gynecological malignancy. *J Pain Sympt Manag* 1997; **13**: 104.

Shils ME, Olsen JA, Shike M, Ross AC (eds), *Modern Nutrition in Health and Disease*, 9th edn. Philadelphia: Williams & Wilkins, 1999.

Terada KY, Christen C, Roberts JA, Parenteral nutrition in gynecology. *J Repro Med* 1988; **33**: 957.

Veterans Affairs Total Parenteral Nutrition Cooperative Study Group, Perioperative total parenteral nutrition in surgical patients. *N Engl J Med* 1991; **325**: 525.

Weisner RL, Krumdieck CL, Death resulting from overzelous total parenteral nutrition: the refeeding syndrome revisited. *Am J Clin Nutr* 1981; **34**: 393.

Zoetmulder FA, Helmerhorst TJ, Van Coevorden F et al, Management of bowel obstruction in patients with advanced ovarian cancer. *Eur J Cancer* 1994; **30A**: 1625.

8

Procedures in gynecologic oncology

Judith K Wolf

CENTRAL-VENOUS CATHETER INSERTION

Indications

Primary indications for central-venous access include (1) access for fluid therapy, (2) access for drug therapy, (3) parenteral nutrition, and (4) central-venous pressure (CVP) monitoring. The most common uses in gynecologic oncology are for patients needing chemotherapy, patients with ascites after surgery who are experiencing fluid shifts (usually ovarian cancer patients), and patients receiving intravenous hyperalimentation. Secondary indications for central-venous catheter (CVC) access include (1) the need to aspirate air in case of embolism during neurosurgical procedures in the sitting position, (2) placement of pacemakers, and (3) hemodialysis access.

Contraindications to CVC are only relative, and include (1) bleeding diatheses and (2) contraindications to specific sites, such as vessel thrombosis, local infection or inflammation, or distortion by trauma or previous surgery.

Clinical utility

The clinical utility of CVC insertion includes venous access and the ability to measure CVP. A properly placed catheter can be used to measure right atrial pressure, which, in the absence of tricuspid-valve disease, will reflect the right end-diastolic pressure. It cannot be used to assess left ventricular function in critically ill patients, since there is often ventricular disparity and independence of right and left atrial pressures in these patients. The CVP is only a single parameter, however, in contradistinction to the more complete information concerning pressures, flow, and venous gas measurements available with pulmonary artery catheters.

Sites of catheterization

There are several choices for placement of the CVC. The patient's anatomy and the operator's experience are the major factors influencing site selection. Each site has advantages and disadvantages. The subclavian vein is probably the most common site. Its advantages include:

- a high rate of successful cannulation;
- the greatest ease of access in profound volume depletion;
- relative ease of securing catheter and dressings.

Its disadvantages include:

- a higher risk of pneumothorax;
- inability to compress the vessel if bleeding occurs.

Another common site is the internal jugular vein. Its advantages include:

- a high rate of successful cannulation;
- a lower rate of pneumothorax;
- the ability to compress the insertion site if bleeding occurs;
- the fact that the right jugular provides a straight path to the superior vena cava, facilitating placement of catheters and pacemakers.

Its disadvantages include:

- greater difficulty in cannulation in profound volume depletion;
- greater difficulty in fixation and dressing of catheters.

The external jugular vein has the advantage of:

- a lower incidence of complications.

However:

- there is a higher incidence of failure of cannulation;
- it is more difficult to fix and dress;
- it is not suitable for prolonged access.

The femoral vein is rarely used, because it has a theoretical increased risk of infection and thrombosis. The antecubital fossa has the advantages of:

- a lower incidence of pneumothorax;
- easy dressing fixation and care.

However:

- it is difficult to place;
- it has an increased incidence of thrombophlebitis.

Technique of CVC insertion

General principles
As with all procedures, the patient is first counseled, and written consent is obtained. General principles of CVC insertion include first determining the

depth of catheter placement. To do this, measure the depth from the planned point of insertion to the following surface markers on the chest wall:

(1) the sternoclavicular joint correlating to the subclavian vein;
(2) the midmanubrial area correlating to the brachiocephalic vein;
(3) the manubriosternal junction correlating to the superior vena cava;
(4) five centimeters below the manubriosternal junction correlating to the right atrium (note that the tip of the catheter is correctly placed in the subclavian vein, not the right atrium – placement in the atrium increases the risk of arrhythmias and myocardial perforation).

After determining the depth of catheter placement, place the patient in a supine, Trendelenberg position of at least 15° to reduce the chance of air embolism. The Trendelenberg position does not distend the subclavian vein in the euvolemic patient. Next, turn the patient's head away from the side of the venipuncture just enough to provide sufficient access to the puncture site. Rotation of the head beyond 45° should be avoided, because it can increase the incidence of catheter malposition. It is not helpful to place a towel between the shoulders to extend the head and make the clavicles more prominent, because this decreases the space between the clavicle and first rib, making the subclavian vein less accessible.

Once the patient has been positioned, clean and drape the area using sterile technique. If the patient is awake, infiltrate the skin with 1% lidocaine. Mount the needle on a syringe containing 0.5–1.0 ml of saline or lidocaine. After the skin has been punctured with the bevel of the needle upward, flush the needle to remove any possible skin plug. As the needle slowly advances, maintain negative pressure on the syringe. When the vein is entered, advance the needle a few millimeters farther to obtain free flow of blood. Rapid backward movement of the plunger and the appearance of bright red blood indicate that the artery has been entered. If this occurs, completely remove the needle and apply pressure for at least 10 minutes.

If the vein is not entered despite inserting the needle to the appropriate depth, maintain negative pressure on the syringe and slowly withdraw the needle. If no blood appears, completely remove the needle and reinsert it, directing it at a slightly different angle.

Once the vein has been canalized, remove the syringe from the needle, occluding the needle with a finger to prevent air embolism. If the patient is breathing spontaneously, do this during expiration; if patient is being mechanically ventilated, do it during inhalation. Next, insert the guide wire through the needle to a predetermined point and remove the needle. The guide wire is in too far if the patient complains of her heart beating fast or feeling funny; in this case, just pull it back a little.

After the needle has been removed, use the dilator to enlarge the skin and subcutaneous tunnel for the catheter. Then remove the dilator and pass the premeasured catheter over the guide wire into the vein. Remove the guide wire, affix the catheter to the skin with suture, and place a sterile dressing.

triangle. Use three fingers to trace the course of the artery; the vein should be just lateral to this position. You can also find the vein by using a small-gauge locator needle. Direct the needle caudally at an angle of 45° to the frontal plane. It should be just lateral and parallel to the artery's pulse. If the pulse is not palpable, direct the needle parallel to the medial border of the clavicular head of the SCM muscle. The vessel is normally entered at a depth of about 2 cm. If you go past 4 cm, slowly withdraw the needle and watch for blood return. If the vein is still not entered, the needle can be redirected a few degrees medially, but not across the sagittal plane (and the carotid artery).

All of these approaches require chest x-ray prior to use of the catheter to check position and to rule out pneumothorax.

MANAGEMENT OF PLEURAL EFFUSIONS

Pleural effusion

The pleural space is normally only a potential space lying between the visceral pleura investing the lung and the parietal pleura of the chest wall. The introduction of fluid or air breaks this dynamic coupling and converts the potential space into a real space. Normal respiratory mechanics are impaired in proportion to the size of the space created and the pressure within it. A pleural effusion is an accumulation of fluid in the pleural space. Alterations in systemic hydrostatic or colloid osmotic pressure that disturb the balance of forces across normal pleural surfaces produce an effusion that consists of protein-poor ultrafiltrate of plasma and is classified as a transudate. Changes in capillary permeability caused by inflammation or infiltration of the pleura produce a protein-rich effusion that is classified as an exudate. Common sources for transudates and exudates are listed in Table 8.1. Characteristics of the fluid obtained by diagnostic thoracentesis can be helpful in distinguishing between transudative and exudative effusions. These characteristics are described in Table 8.2. There can, however, be considerable overlap in the findings that separate transudates and exudates, and any chronic effusion tends to develop "exudative" characteristics. The clinical picture of the patient gives the most clues to the etiology of the effusion. The most common cause of transudative effusions is congestive heart failure, and the most common cause of exudative effusions is malignancy. A concave meniscus in the costophrenic angle on an upright chest x-ray suggests the presence of at least 250 ml of pleural fluid. A lateral decubitus view can detect a smaller volume and confirm that fluid is free in the pleural space if it is shown to layer out along a dependent surface. A subpulmonic effusion (one completely contained between the base of the lung and the diaphragm) can be difficult to distinguish from an elevated hemidiaphragm or a subpulmonic process. On the left side, the position of the stomach bubble can provide a useful clue. Adhesions can compartmentalize an effusion into loculations that assume a wide variety of radiographic configurations,

Table 8.1 Common sources of pleural effusions

Transudates	Exudates
Congestive heart failure	Malignancy (primary or metastatic)
Nephritic syndrome	Infection
Cirrhosis	Infarction
Hypoproteinemia	Sympathetic (pancreatitis, subphrenic abscess)
Myxedema	Traumatic
Peritoneal dialysis	Collagen vascular diseases (e.g., rheumatoid arthritis)

Table 8.2 Characteristics of transudates and exudates[a]

	Transudate	Exudate
Color	Clear, serous	Cloudy, tan
WBC count	$<1,000/mm^3$	$>10,000/mm^3$
RBC count	$<10,000/mm^3$	$>10,000/mm^3$ (blood-tinged) $>100,000/mm^3$ (gross blood)
Glucose	Normal serum level	Sometimes low
Protein	<3.0 g/dl	>3.0 g/dl
Pleural:serum protein ratio	<0.5	>0.5
Specific gravity	<1.016	>1.016
LDH pleural:serum ratio	<0.6	>0.6
pH	Same as arterial	<7.2 (usually with empyema)
Culture	Negative	Sometimes positive
Cytology	Negative	Sometimes positive

[a]WBC, white blood cells; RBC, red blood cells; LDH, lactate dehydrogenase.

frequently requiring multiple views or computed tomography scanning for definition. Thoracentesis is the mainstay of diagnosis.

Pleural effusions can produce dyspnea but can also be surprisingly asymptomatic at rest. Therapeutic drainage is rarely indicated for transudative effusions, since the fluid will rapidly reaccumulate until the underlying condition is improved. Most exudative effusions warrant a more aggressive approach.

Malignant pleural effusion

More than half of all patients with malignancy will have a pleural effusion at some time in their course. Up to 20% of gynecologic cancer patients will have an effusion. This occurs most commonly in ovarian cancer patients, but also this is a general rule, patients often do experience some irritation and coughing beyond 1,200–1,500 ml of fluid removal, and the process should stop at that point. Once the fluid has been removed, the catheter is removed and pressure is placed over the insertion site for several minutes. A chest x-ray is then performed to check for pneumothorax and to see how much fluid remains.

Pleurodesis

For patients who will require repeated thoracentesis for relief of pleural effusion, standard therapy is tube thoracostomy and pleurodesis. Another option is placement of a Denver catheter. A Denver catheter is a small catheter that is left in place and can be drained as needed with a suction drain. Patients or caregivers can learn to do this at home.

Pleurodesis creates an inflammatory fusion between visceral and parietal pleura that eliminates the potential pleural space. An essential first step is complete evacuation of the fluid and reexpansion of the lung, accomplished by inserting a chest tube connected to a water seal drainage system. If loculations or inaccurate tube placement prevent complete fluid removal and lung expansion, pleural coalescence will not occur uniformly, and pleurodesis is much less likely to succeed. This is probably more important than the choice of chemical agent used in the next step. The basic principle of this approach is that the chest tube drains the pleural space and the sclerosing agent creates a pleuritis that joins the visceral and parietal pleura and prevents fluid reaccumulation. Agents that are effective sclerosing agents share the property of causing a chemical pleuritis. Although many antitumor agents have been used successfully as sclerosing agents, it appears that the mechanism of control of effusion is related to their ability to induce a pleuritis rather than to their antitumor activity.

Table 8.3 lists some of the more commonly used sclerosing agents. Tetracycline controls the effusion in 33–84% of patients treated. The standard dose used is 1 g intrapleurally. Tetracycline distributes well throughout the pleural space, even without rotating the patient. It is not beneficial to do repeat instillations. The chief side effects are fever (33%) and pain (41%). The use of intrapleural lidocaine may substantially reduce local pain following instillation of tetracycline. Tetracycline is a low-cost, effective therapy that is well tolerated. Unfortunately, the parenteral formulation is no longer available in the USA. Doxycycline, prepared as 500 mg in 30 ml of saline, which has been reported to be successful in up to 80% of patients, or minocycline (300 mg in 50 ml normal saline) can be used.

Bleomycin has also been used as a sclerosing agent. The standard dose is 60 units intrapleurally; higher doses may be associated with increased toxicity, especially in the elderly. Effectiveness ranges from 60–80% at 1 month. Side effects include fever and pain, similar to tetracycline. The major drawback is cost.

Quinacrine is a highly effective sclerosing agent (64–100%). It is one of a

Table 8.3 Sclerosing agents for the pleura
Tetracycline Doxycycline Bleomycin Quinacrine *Corynebacterium parvum* Thoracoscopy Biologic (interferon-β and interleukin-2)

number of compounds that have historically shown effectiveness, but which are no longer widely in use. Most trials with quinacrine used multiple instillations. The reported toxicities include fever (95%) and pain (40%).

Corynebacterium parvum extract administered weekly in a dose of 4 mg has controlled 90–100% of maximal possible effect at 4 weeks. Randomized trials have shown that *C. parvum* has activity that is at least as good as, if not superior to, tetracycline and bleomycin. Fever and pain were significantly more common with *C. parvum*, however, and the agent is not widely available in the USA.

Talc produces an intense, reactive pleuritis that is highly effective in producing a chemical pleurodesis. This is the most commonly used method in the UK. When instilled directly onto the pleural surface via poudrage, talc is effective in close to 100% of cases. In the past, this approach was used with a rigid thoracoscope under local or general anesthesia. Video-assisted thoracoscopic surgery has made this approach much easier to perform. There are several advantages to thoracoscopic talc poudrage. Thoracoscopy allows visualization of pleural surfaces. Small adhesions can be broken with instruments, allowing apposition of the pleural surfaces. Patients who have an extensive pleural rind that will never reexpand can be identified and spared a prolonged attempt at sclerosis. Talc poudrage can be performed with thoracoscopy under local anesthesia, but generally one-lung anesthesia is preferred. Major difficulties in using talc include the need to sterilize it in a moisture-free environment and occasional reports of acute respiratory-distress syndrome following talc administration.

More recently, biologic agents have been used for pleurodesis with some success. Studies have found efficacy with both interferon-β and interleukin-2.

PARACENTESIS

Indications

Indications for paracentesis are either diagnostic or therapeutic. In gynecologic oncology, either case may occur. Many new ovarian patients present with symptomatic ascites, and the diagnosis of cancer is confirmed by paracentesis. Many ovarian-cancer patients as well as the occasional endometrial-cancer patient have symptomatic ascites later on in their course that requires therapeutic drainage.

Technique

The patient is first counseled, and written consent is obtained. The patient is placed in a supine position. Selection of the site for aspiration must take into consideration the anatomy of the abdominal wall and the course of the inferior epigastric vessels. The area for catheter insertion, generally lateral to the rectus abdominis muscles, is selected. The area is marked, prepared, draped, and anesthetized. First, a small, thin-walled needle is inserted into the abdominal cavity, with constant negative pressure applied to an attached syringe until fluid is aspirated. The larger trocar is then inserted. To help evacuate the abdominal fluid, a device with a vaccuum bottle and stopcock, similar to that used in the thoracentesis procedure, may be used (Figure 8.3). After the proce-

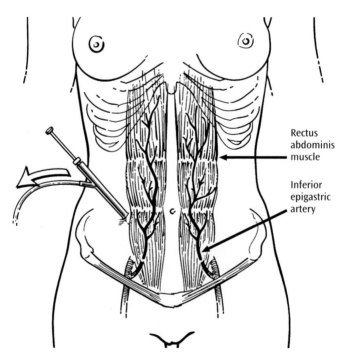

Rectus abdominis muscle

Inferior epigastric artery

Figure 8.3
Paracentesis.

dure, the patient's vital signs should be taken, and the patient should be observed for orthostatic symptoms. The procedure note is written, and the amount and color of fluid removed are documented. When doing paracentesis for diagnosis, fluid should be sent for Gram's stain, culture, and pathologic evaluation.

Complications

Paracentesis is simple, with relatively few complications, and these are preventable by avoiding the epigastric vessels. Rectus abdominis sheath hematoma is probably the most common complication. Especially with ascites, the risk of intestinal injury is slight, and studies have shown that penetration of the bowel with an 18-gauge needle is harmless, since the bowel seals off quickly without leakage. In patients with known or suspected malignant ascites, a common result of paracentesis is seeding of the tract with malignant cells, resulting in tumor growth in the insertion site. Because these patients already have metastatic disease, however, this occurrence usually has little impact on outcome.

CYSTOSCOPY

Indications

Routine preoperative cystoscopy is not necessary for most gynecologic oncology patients; however, if bladder invasion is suspected, it can be useful. Cervical cancer may involve the bladder by direct extension, and, therefore, cystoscopy can be used in the staging evaluation for patients with large cervical tumors or those for whom bladder involvement is suspected. Another common use of cystoscopy in gynecologic oncology is in cases of patients with previous pelvic irradiation and hematuria secondary to hemmorhagic cystitis.

Technique

The patient is first counseled, and written consent is obtained. The patient is placed in the lithotomy position, prepped, and draped in a sterile manner. A cotton-tipped applicator with 1% topical lidocaine gel can be placed in the urethra for 3 minutes prior to the procedure for anesthesia. Once this has been removed, the cystoscope introducer with lubrication can easily be passed through the urethral orifice. The introducer is removed from the sheath, and the scope is passed into the bladder. A scope with a 30° angle is commonly used. The bladder is filled with sterile saline (usually 200–250 ml), then visualized. The entire bladder wall can be visualized, and lesions of the bladder as small as 1–2 mm can be seen. One can also visualize the configuration and location of the ureteral orifices at the trigone. It is important to look for efflux

9
Supportive care: pain and symptom management

Andrea B Hamilton, Richard Payne,
Penny Damaskos, Juan Santiago-Palma

PAIN AND SYMPTOM MANAGEMENT

Pain prevalence

Pain is a highly prevalent symptom in patients with cancer. Studies from the Eastern Cooperative Oncology Group (ECOG) have reported that 67% of 1,308 ambulatory cancer patients experience pain, with 19% of those patients reporting severe pain, and 36% reporting pain significant enough to impair function. Pain complicating gynecologic cancers is similarly prevalent, ranging from 85% for cervical cancers in one review, to 80% of all gynecologic cancers surveyed in a hospice population. A survey of inpatients and outpatients with ovarian cancer at Memorial Sloan-Kettering Cancer Center reported pain preceding the onset or recurrence of cancer in 62% ($n = 151$) of patients. The same study also reported that 42% of the patients reported persistent or frequent pain during the proceeding 2 weeks. Pain as a presenting symptom occurs in approximately 4% of patients with endometrial cancer.

Despite our current level of sophistication in treating cancer pain, it is estimated that cancer pain is undertreated. For example, 29% of patients with cancer suffer from moderate to severe pain despite analgesic therapy. Forty-two percent of ambulatory cancer patients received insufficient analgesics for the level of their reported pain, by World Health Organization (WHO) standards.

There are many barriers leading to inadequate management of cancer pain. Among those most readily identified are poor pain-assessment skills on the part of healthcare providers, patient reluctance to report pain to physicians, physician reluctance to prescribe medications (related to concerns about side effects associated with the use of potent analgesics), and inadequate dosing of analgesics in an attempt to avoid addiction.

Pain assessment

The appropriate management of pain requires proper assessment. The key principles to pain assessment are listed in Table 9.1. Knowledge of the biology

Table 9.1 Clinical points in assessment of cancer pain

I.   Take a complete history:

   A. Fully evaluate the pain complaint:
       (1) Use simple self-report scales (0–10 scales or visual analogue scales)
       (2) Evaluate factors that make pain better or worse
            (a) Ask about incident- or movement-related pain
            (b) Ask about other breakthrough episodes of pain

   B. Evaluate the cancer history:
       (1) Was pain an initial symptom of cancer?

   C. Evaluate psychosocial aspects of the pain and the meaning of the pain for
       the patient:
       (1) How distressed is the patient?
       (2) Is there a history of chronic pain from a nonmalignant origin? How has
            the patient coped with chronic pain in the past?
       (3) Is there a history of depression or other affective illness or of substance
            abuse?
       (4) Evaluate patient and family attitudes toward the use of controlled
            substances (especially opioids).

II. Perform a careful physical and neurological examination:

   A. Evaluate pain sites and other common referral sites
   B. Evaluate for primary or secondary sources of musculoskeletal pain
   C. Perform focused neurological examination to assess motor, sensory, and
       autonomic findings associated with pain of neuropathic origin

III. Review radiographic and laboratory studies to stage disease and confirm
     cause and nature of pain

IV. Re-evaluate pain and responses to treatment at frequent intervals and
     reassess the extent of disease for all new or worsening reports of pain

V.   Assess the impact of pain on psychological well-being and physical function

---

of gynecologic tumors and the natural history of specific cancer types, including familiarity with the common pain syndromes seen in endometrial and ovarian cancer, is important in establishing the medical assessment of patients (Table 9.2). Another key to assessment is to identify the patterns of pain throughout the day. As many as 66% of cancer patients report a mixture of constant pain and superimposed episodes of breakthrough pain, representing exacerbations on a background of continuous pain. This typical pattern requires the use of continuous or around-the-clock analgesics as well as supplemental or so-called rescue analgesics.

Assessment is fundamental to treatment; the major therapeutic goal is to relieve or minimize pain in a manner that allows the patient to be as active and pain-free as possible.

Table 9.2 Common intractable pain syndromes in the cancer patient

Pain syndrome	Clinical characteristics
I. Musculoskeletal pain • Bone-pain syndromes	Metastatic bone pain is the most common pain syndrome associated with direct tumor involvement.
(1) Vertebral-body metastasis	Focal pain in neck or back. Risk of spinal-cord compression.
(2) Pelvis and long-bone metastasis	Risk of pathologic fracture with weight bearing; early orthopedic consultation usually required.
(3) Skull-base metastasis	Head pain usually severe with associated cranial nerve defects.
II. Neuropathic pain • Plexopathies	Pain usually severe and associated with spread of tumor from lymph nodes and organs to peripheral nerve structures.
(1) Brachial plexopathy	Most common with breast and lung cancer; pain in shoulder, radiating into arm and hand, with associated numbness and weakness. Bilateral pain indicates risk for spinal-cord compression. Can be a complication of radiation therapy to the region.
(2) Lumbosacral plexopathy	Most common with renal, uterine, and ovarian and colon cancers; pain in back radiating into leg. Bilateral pain indicates risk for spinal-cord compression. Can also be a complication of radiation therapy to the pelvis.
• Spinal-cord compression	Neurological emergency. Pain proceeds neurological dysfunction by days or weeks. Most common with prostate, breast, and lung cancers that metastasize to spinal vertebral bodies.
• Meningeal carcinomatosis	Pain can be focal or radicular in nature. Most common with lymphomas, leukemias, breast, and sarcomas.
• Postsurgical pain syndromes	Chronic chest-wall pain in region of surgical scar; associated sensory loss, with or without hyperpathia.
(1) Post-thoracotomy	Recurrent tumor must be excluded.
(2) Postmastectomy	May occur in up to 20% of women; more common with axillary dissection. Injury to intercostal–brachioradial nerve implicated. Can be distinguished from brachial plexopathy.

Table 9.2 Continued

Pain syndrome	Clinical characteristics
(3) Postradical neck surgery	Etiology is unclear. Often associated with recurrent tumor. Chronic infection may also be a source of pain in some patients.
(4) Postamputation stump and phantom pain	Stump pain common. Phantom phenomenon almost universal, although pain is not universal (but also not uncommon).
III. Abdominal and pelvic visceral pain	Pain usually associated with tumor infiltration or radiation therapy to abdominal and pelvic organs. Very common with local spread of gynecological cancers. Pancreatic and upper-gastrointestinal sources of pain produce periumbilical crampy pain often referred to back. Pain is often associated by small- and/or large-bowel obstruction with nausea and vomiting.
	Perineal and perirectal pain produced by infiltration of tumor or radiation-induced fibrosis of presacral spaces involving the sacral plexus. Sitting exacerbates perineal pain in most patients.

Pain mechanisms

Somatic pain

Patients with cancer experience pain as a result of tumor infiltration of organs and viscera and as a result of toxic effects of antineoplastic therapies. Somatic pain results from tissue injury in cutaneous, bony, and other musculoskeletal structures. Metastatic bone disease is the most common pain syndrome in patients with cancer, and even occurs, in rare cases, as the initial presentation of endometrial carcinoma.

Activation of specific pain fibers, called *nociceptors,* in somatic tissues is the mechanism by which the nervous system encodes pain. Tissue injury related to tumor infiltration, surgical trauma, chemotherapy-related toxicity, etc, causes the release of inflammatory and other chemical mediators that play an important role in the activation and sensitization of these nociceptors. Prostaglandin E is a particularly important chemical mediator of pain generally, and this is especially so in the case of bone metastasis; it is known to mediate osteolytic and osteoclastic metastatic bone changes, as well as to sensitize nociceptors and produce hyperalgesia.

Visceral pain

Pain receptors also exist in visceral tissues, and these receptors are generally stimulated by the same chemical mediators that activate somatic nociceptors. Stretching and distention of tissues also activate visceral nociceptors. Visceral pain is particularly common in gynecologic cancers. Visceral pain is poorly localized and is often referred to remote cutaneous sites (unlike somatic pain). This is the reason why many patients with pelvic tumor report back and even shoulder pain from peritoneal and retroperitoneal lesions.

Referred pain results from convergence of visceral and somatic afferent information onto common neuronal pools in the dorsal horn of the spinal cord. Recent studies suggest that experimentally induced visceral pain in animal models may be particularly responsive to a specific class of opioid analgesics (agonist–antagonist drugs such as butorphanol, buprenorphine, and nalbuphine), which are agonists at κ- and antagonists at μ-opioid receptors. To date, however, there are no data establishing the unique efficacy of agonist–antagonist opioids in clinical visceral pain.

Pain emanating from pelvic visceral structures also differs from somatic pain in another important way. Recent neuroanatomic studies have observed that neural impulses from pelvic visceral nociceptors reach the brain through a newly discovered pathway in the dorsal columns of the spinal cord, as opposed to the classic spinothalamic tract in the anterolateral column of the spinal cord utilized by somatic nociceptive afferents. This supports selective ablation of the dorsal columns via a midline or punctate myelotomy as a means of producing analgesia in patients experiencing intractable pelvic pain.

Neuropathic pain

Neuropathic pain represents another major pain pathophysiology. This type of pain occurs not as a direct result of nociceptor activation, but rather as a result of injury to the peripheral or central nervous system. Neuropathic pain is often qualitatively different from somatic or visceral (so-called *nociceptive*) pain for this reason. The hallmark of neuropathic pain is paroxysms of burning or electric-shock sensations, which may result, at least in part, from spontaneous discharges in the peripheral and central nervous systems.

Conventional analgesic therapies may not be as efficacious in neuropathic pain as they are in nociceptive pain. For example, some experts have argued that opioids are ineffective in the treatment of neuropathic pain. Although this view has been recently challenged – and indeed, there are controlled clinical trials demonstrating the effectiveness of opioids in the treatment of neuropathic pain – it is nonetheless observed that larger doses of opioids may be required in the management of neuropathic pain than are required in the management of nociceptive pain. These clinical observations are consistent with recent experimental observations that report a fourfold decrease in the potency of morphine when primary afferent fibers are severed. In addition to the use of nonsteroidal anti-inflammatory analgesic drugs (NSAIDs) and opioid analgesics, neuropathic pain is often managed with adjuvant analgesic drugs, particularly those in the antidepressant and anticonvulsant classes (Table 9.3).

Table 9.3 Adjuvant analgesic drugs used to treat cancer-related pain

Drug class and category	Usual dose	Indications
(1) General purpose, nonspecific		
• Tricyclic antidepressants	Amitriptyline 10–25 mg p.o. q.h.s. up to 150 mg/day Nortriptyline 25 mg p.o. q.h.s. up to 100–150 mg/day	Neuropathic and musculoskeletal pain
• Corticosteroids	Dexamethasone 4–16 mg/day p.o. in 2–4 divided doses Prednisone 60–80 mg/day p.o. in 2–4 divided doses	Essential for spinal-cord compression and brain herniation; also useful in malignant bone and nerve pain
• Phenothiazine	Methotrimeprazine 10–15 mg i.m. q 6 hrs	Useful for opioid sparing in very tolerant patients and in opioid-induced ileus
(2) Neuropathic pain		
• Anticonvulsants	Carbamazepine 200–800 mg/day p.o. in divided doses Valproic acid 15–60 mg/kg per day p.o. in divided doses Gabepentin 900–1,200 mg p.o. t.i.d. Clonazapam 0.5–1.0 mg p.o. t.i.d.	Useful for dysesthetic and paroxysmal lancinating pain. Gabapentin may require doses 2,700–3,600 mg/day
• Antiarrhythmics and local anesthetics	Lidocaine 5 mg/kg i.v. as continuous infusion over 30 minutes Mixelitine 450–600 mg/day p.o. in divided doses	Usually reserved for neuropathic pain refractory to anticonvulsants and opioids
• Topical creams, ointments, patches	Lidocaine patches 700 mg per patch Capsaicin 0.075% cream applied to site of pain at least 4 times a day Eutectic mixture of local anesthetics (EMLA) cream applied to site 60–90 min before procedure	Capsaicin most often used for postherpetic neuralgia. EMLA used often in children

3. Bone pain		
• Radiopharmaceuticals	Strontium-89 4 μCi per dose i.v. Samarium-153 1.0 μCi/kg	Dose may be repeated if positive response and adequate marrow reserve. Not useful as acute pain treatment
• Bisphosphonates	Pamidronate 90 mg i.v. over 2 hrs, monthly	Inhibits bone resorption and reduces bone pain
4. Visceral pain		
• Octreotide	Octreotide 100–600 μg/day s.q. bolus or infusion	Useful for secretory diarrhea and malignant bowel obstruction
5. Psychostimulants		
• Over-the-counter preparations	Caffeine 100–200 mg/day p.o.	One cup of coffee or 12 oz caffeinated beverage containing 65 mg caffeine
• Controlled substances	Methylphenidate 5–20 mg/day p.o. Dextroamphetamine sulfate 5–15 mg/day p.o. Pemoline	Act additively with opioids for analgesia and improve alertness

Persistent activation of pain fibers or pain caused by neural injury can be associated with sensitization of central neurons. This sensitization may be associated with the clinical phenomenon of pain evoked by normally non-noxious stimuli (allodynia), or an increased sensitivity to a painful stimulus (hyperalgesia). It is now known that activity of N-methyl-D-aspartate (NMDA) receptors in the spinal cord and brain is particularly important for these phenomena. Antagonism of the NMDA receptor can produce analgesia in nociceptive and neuropathic pain. It has been shown that drugs such as dextromethorphan, ketamine, and the *d* optical isomer of methadone noncompetitively antagonize the NMDA receptor, and may be associated with analgesia, particularly in the case of clinical neuropathic pain. The results, however, are inconsistent.

Complex pain

Some patients with somatic, visceral, or neuropathic pains will develop a particularly challenging pain syndrome with cutaneous hypersensitivity, peripheral edema, vascular abnormalities, and severe pain that is intractable to the usual analgesic therapies. This syndrome was called *reflex sympathetic dystrophy, or major or minor causalgia* (when accompanied by nerve injury), but it is now called *complex regional pain syndrome* because of the inconsistent involvement of the sympathetic nervous system in the basic pathophysiology of this disorder. Some patients with complex regional pain syndrome respond to regional sympathetic nerve blocks or the administration of adrenergic antagonists such as intravenous phentolamine, indicating some role of the sympathetic nervous system in this disorder; however, many other patients do not.

Management of chronic pelvic pain and associated symptoms

Local spread of ovarian and endometrial tumors frequently causes pain resulting from compression of nerves, infiltration of adjacent pain-sensitive tissues, and bowel obstruction (Figure 9.1). Furthermore, the occurrence of vesical–cutaneous fistulae in patients with progressive or even quiescent gynecologic cancers can be a source of significant morbidity as a result of pain, incontinence, nausea, vomiting, and infection.

Lumbosacral plexopathy

The lumbosacral plexus runs within the substance of the psoas muscle and is commonly invaded by gynecologic cancers.

Assessment and diagnosis

Lumbosacral plexopathy (LSP) presents frequently with pain (91%), which can be local (pain in the sacrum, sacroiliac joint, lower back, or groin) or radicular and/or referred (pain in the lateral, posterior, or anterior leg). Oncologists who

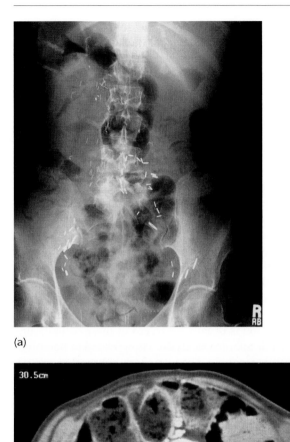

(a)

(b)

Figure 9.1

(a) Plain abdominal x-ray and (b) computed tomography scan of a 63-year-old woman with advanced ovarian cancer and partial small-bowel obstruction. She presented with nausea, vomiting, and abdominal pain. Her symptoms responded to conservative treatment with antiemetics and a morphine intravenous infusion by means of self-controlled analgesia.

are not familiar with this entity may miss this diagnosis, since pain and sensory symptoms frequently predominate early in the course, sometimes before radiographic evidence of tumor recurrence. Incontinence is unusual, but autonomic symptoms due to involvement of the paravertebral sympathetics are common. Tumors that compress the proximal lumbosacral plexus in the paraspinal region may also grow through the neural foramina to compress the cauda equina and conus medullaris. This will produce bilateral findings.

Treatment

Treatment of pain in LSP is best accomplished by instituting radiation therapy and other antitumor treatments appropriate for the tumor type. Radiation-therapy portals must encompass any coexistent epidural tumor in order to prevent paralysis or other neurological complications. Lumbosacral plexopathy often occurs in advanced cancer, however, when no further antineoplastic therapy is possible. In addition, even if one can reverse tumor growth, if irreversible neural injury has occurred, significant pain may persist. Spinal opiate infusions may be appropriate for bilateral pain below the level of the umbilicus if the adverse effects of systemic opioids limit their usefulness. In addition, unilateral incident pain complicating LSP may be treated with percutaneous cordotomy. Because bowel and bladder function is usually preserved in these patients, and because of the risks of irreversible sphincteric dysfunction related to neurolytic anesthetic approaches (e.g., subarachnoid phenol), these approaches are not usually acceptable to the patient.

As noted above, however, the recent discovery of a dorsal-column pathway specific for pelvic visceral afferents has led to the limited use of punctate myelotomy for treatment of intractable pelvic pain. Although this procedure requires myelotomy under general anesthesia, motor and sphincteric dysfunction should not occur.

Symptoms other than pain in pelvic tumors

Bowel obstruction

Pelvic tumors causing bowel obstruction produce nausea, vomiting, and colicky pain. Nearly 100% of patients with malignant bowel obstruction complain of vomiting, which may be severe in more than 80%. Decompression of the bowel obstruction is, of course, the most effective way to manage symptoms. Phenothiazines and other centrally acting antiemetics can control nausea, but they usually do not eliminate vomiting. Colicky abdominal pain is reported in 76% of patients with malignant bowel obstruction. Anticholinergic drugs (e.g., atropine and hyoscine), antiserotonergic drugs (e.g., octreotide), and antiperistaltic drugs (e.g., senna and metoclopramide) have all been used with variable effectiveness. Much recent interest has focused on octreotide, which can be administered subcutaneously, once or twice a day, as an effective means of medical management of malignant bowel obstruction. The mechanism of action is presumed to be related to reduction in secretions.

Ascites

Symptomatic malignant ascites occurring in advanced ovarian cancer may be treated with diuretics, such as furosemide or spironolactone, and with paracentesis. At the time of paracentesis, the installation of sclerosing agents such as bleomycin or thiotepa may prevent reaccumulation of fluid. Ascites may respond to treatment of the cancer with antineoplastic drugs.

Fistulae

Fistulae are a significant cause of morbidity for patients with advanced gynecologic tumors. The associated infection should be treated; it is often necessary to provide anaerobic coverage with metronidazole. The use of bulking agents for the stool may be helpful but could worsen constipation in patients on opioids. Other local measures such as catheterization of the bladder, vaginal packing, and the use of colostomy bags to collect fluids and absorb offensive odors should be used when possible. Surgery to close fistulae or to perform diverting colostomies or ileostomies should be considered whenever possible but are usually not feasible in patients with very advanced cancer who are near the end of life.

Table 9.3 lists the adjuvant drugs commonly used for treating pain and other symptoms in gynecologic malignancies.

Pharmacological management of pain

Pharmacotherapy is the cornerstone of cancer-pain treatment, and can provide satisfactory pain relief for most patients. Therapy must be individualized to maximize pain relief and minimize adverse effects. The WHO has developed a *three-step analgesic ladder* for the treatment of cancer pain. This approach matches the patient's reported pain intensity with the potency of analgesic to be prescribed:

- **Step 1:** Begin with a nonopioid drug for mild pain.
- **Step 2:** For moderate pain that is not controlled by a nonopioid alone, a weak opioid is administered in addition to the nonopioid drug. (Opioids that are classified as weak include codeine and hydrocodone, especially when they are formulated in fixed combinations with acetaminophen or aspirin.)
- **Step 3:** For severe pain that is not relieved by weak opioids, a strong opioid is used, either alone or in combination with a nonopioid drug.

At all levels of the ladder, certain adjuvant analgesics may be used for specific indications. Patients presenting with severe pain should be started at the third step of the ladder, rather than being "walked" up the ladder from the first step. In fact, using an assessment tool called the *pain management index* (which relates the potency of the analgesic regimen prescribed to the patient's reported pain intensity) as a measure, 46% of ambulatory cancer patients are undertreated for pain. Although imperfect, this approach provides a useful framework for the management of cancer pain and has proven to be effective in most cases.

The validation studies noted above have been criticized, however, because they generally have not included blind control trials to test the effectiveness of the WHO ladder concept. Moreover most have used relatively small numbers of patients, and the drop-out rate from the study analysis is sizeable. Nonetheless, these data are consistent with clinical experience, which has shown empirically that pain can be treated effectively in the vast majority of patients.

Nonopioid analgesics

Acetaminophen and NSAIDs are considered to be in this class. There is a ceiling on the analgesic efficacy of these drugs; thus, when used as single agents, they are useful for mild to moderate pain only. They can, however, be used in any stage of the WHO analgesic ladder and are often formulated or otherwise combined with opioid and adjuvant analgesics to treat moderate and severe pain. Table 9.4 lists the commonly used NSAIDs for cancer-related pain.

Table 9.4　Partial list of nonopioid drugs used for cancer pain

Drug type	Brand names	Typical starting dose
Acetaminophen	Tylenol and others	650 mg q 4 hrs p.o.
Aspirin	Multiple	650 mg q 4 hrs p.o.
Ibuprofen	Motrin and others	200–800 mg q 6 hrs p.o.
Choline–magnesium trisalicylate	Trilisate	1,000–1,500 mg t.i.d. p.o.
Diclofenac sodium	Voltaren	50–75 mg q 8–12 hrs p.o.
Diflunisal	Dolobid	500 mg q 12 hrs p.o.
Etodolac	Lodine	200–400 mg q 8–12 hrs p.o.
Flurbiprofen	Ansaid	200–300 mg q 4–8 hrs p.o.
Naproxen	Naprosyn	250–750 mg q 12 hrs p.o.
Naproxen sodium	Anaprox	275 mg q 2 hrs p.o.
Oxprozin	Daypro	600–1,200 mg once daily p.o.
Sulindac	Clinoril	150–200 mg q 12 hrs p.o.
Piroxicam	Feldene	10–20 mg once daily p.o.
Nabumetone	Relafen	1,000–2,000 mg once daily p.o.
Ketoprofen	Orudis	50 mg q 6 hrs p.o.
Ketorolac	Toradal	10 mg q 4–6 hrs p.o. (not to exceed 10 days)
Ketorolac		60 mg (initial), then 30 mg q 6 hrs i.v. or i.m. (not to exceed 5 days)
Celecoxib[a]	Celebrex	100 mg b.i.d. p.o. or 200 mg b.i.d.
Rofecoxib[a] (pain)	Vioxx	12.5 mg (arthritis); 25 mg once daily p.o.

[a]Selective for cyclo-oxygenase-2 isoenzyme.

Nonselective cyclo-oxygenase inhibitors

Inhibition of the enzyme cyclo-oxygenase (COX), which is required for the synthesis of prostaglandins, is an important mechanism of analgesia for NSAIDs. For cancer patients in general, the nonselective COX-inhibitor NSAIDs have many limitations, including the risk of gastrointestinal ulceration, perforation, and bleeding. Although the risk of these toxicities are not well known for cancer patients, it is reported that among arthritis patients taking NSAIDs chronically, the risk for gastrointestinal perforation or bleeding is 1% per year. Furthermore, gastrointestinal ulcerations or hemorrhage can occur without warning symptoms.

Selective cyclo-oxygenase inhibitors

The COX enzyme exists in two forms: COX-1, which is constitutively expressed in most cells, and COX-2, which is an inducible form. Selective inhibitors of COX-2, rofecoxib and celecoxib, are now available. These drugs offer the advantage of providing analgesia without causing the gastrointestinal ulceration and prolongation of bleeding due to platelet dysfunction that are caused by COX-1 inhibition. Celecoxib and rofecoxib represent a major advance because of the improved safety they afford during acute and chronic use. As COX-2 is constitutively expressed in the renal vasculature, however, COX-2-selective drugs do not protect against renal dysfunction. Although both of the COX-2-selective drugs are indicated for chronic use with osteoarthritis and rheumatoid arthritis, only rofecoxib has been approved by the Food and Drug Administration for the short-term (up to 5 days) management of pain. The drugs are available in oral formulation only, but "second-generation" parenteral drugs are in development.

Opioid analgesics

The opioid analgesics represent the mainstay of therapy for cancer pain (Table 9.5). These drugs produce analgesia by binding to specific opioid receptors in the brain and spinal cord. The opioid drugs may be classified as pure agonists or agonist–antagonists on the basis of their interactions with the opioid receptors.

The agonist–antagonist drugs include butorphanol, nalbuphine, pentazocine, and dezocine; they produce analgesia by activating κ receptors but act as antagonists (i.e., they have a naloxone-like effect) on μ receptors, precipitating withdrawal in physically dependent patients. In addition, agonist–antagonist opioids commonly produce psychotomimetic effects at increasing doses; for these reasons, drugs in the agonist–antagonist class of opioids are of limited usefulness in the treatment of patients with cancer. They are, however, used in postoperative pain management, and it has been found that agonist–antagonist drugs might produce more robust analgesia in women than in men.

Principles of opioid analgesia

Certain principles should be followed when using opioid analgesics in the treatment of cancer pain:

Table 9.5 Guidelines for the use of opioids in chronic-pain management

(1) Select opioid on the basis of the patient's reported pain intensity and with consideration of availability, convenience of use, and ease of compliance.

   (a) Use long-acting preparation unless contraindicated.
   (b) Prescribe short-acting analgesic for rescue medications to treat breakthrough pain.
   (c) Avoid agonist–antagonist opioids and meperidine for chronic administration.

(2) Administer opioids around-the-clock after initial dose titration.

(3) Individualize dose by titrating to pain relief or dose-limiting side effect.

(4) Treat side effects prophylactically and aggressively.

(5) Do not confuse the concepts of tolerance, physical dependence, and addiction (psychological dependence).

   (a) Withdraw chronic opioids slowly to avoid precipitation of abstinence syndrome.
   (b) Administer naloxone in a dilute solution when required to reverse respiratory depression.

(6) Use equianalgesic dose calculations when switching between drugs and routes of administration (see below and Table 9.6).

   (a) Start with 50% of the calculated equianalgesic dose to account for incomplete cross-tolerance.

Drug	Dose (i.v.)	Dose (p.o.)
Morphine	10 mg	30 mg
Hydromorphone	1.5 mg	7.5 mg
Oxycodone	–	30 mg
Methadone	10 mg	20 mg
Fentanyl	0.1 mg	25 μg/hr

- When pain is continuous, as is often the case, medications should be administered on an around-the-clock basis.
- The schedule of medication administration should be based upon a sound knowledge of the pharmacokinetics of the drug being used, including its usual duration of action.
- Administering medications on an as-needed basis often results in the patient experiencing multiple episodes of pain during the day, and so is generally undesirable.

- In spite of around-the-clock dosing, many patients will continue to experience *breakthrough pain* (transitory increases in pain above the baseline level). For such pain, an as-needed *rescue dose* of a short-acting opioid should be available. A rescue dose equal to 10–20% of the total scheduled daily dose is usually satisfactory for treating breakthrough pain.
- Unlike NSAIDs, there is no ceiling effect with the pure opioid agonist drugs. The dose of the drug used should be titrated upwards until satisfactory analgesia is achieved or until intolerable side effects occur.
- There is no maximum dose; the right dose for an individual patient is the dose that controls the pain without unacceptable side effects. There is substantial variation between individuals in the dose that is necessary to provide adequate analgesia, even among patients with similar pain syndromes.

Routes of administration

Oral

Oral controlled-release preparations currently exist for morphine, hydromorphone, and oxycodone, while a controlled-release transdermal delivery system is available for fentanyl. These formulations facilitate compliance and should be utilized whenever possible.

Oral administration is the preferred route because of its convenience and cost-effectiveness.

Rectal

Rectal suppositories are available for several opioids. Although this is an effective means of drug delivery, many patients prefer not to use these preparations.

Transdermal and transmucosal

Fentanyl is available as a transdermal patch, which delivers the drug at a fixed rate for 72 hours and may be effective for patients who are unable to take oral medications. As noted below, transmucosal fentanyl is used for patients requiring a drug with a rapid onset but a short duration of action for the treatment of acute procedure-related pain. In cancer patients, it is also used for the treatment of breakthrough pain.

Parenteral

For selected patients who are unable to take oral opioids, such as those with intractable nausea and vomiting or nonfunctional gastrointestinal tracts, opioids may be administered by continuous infusion, either subcutaneously or intravenously. The subcutaneous route has been recommended because it provides equally effective analgesia at lower cost, especially in patients treated at home. Portable programmable infusion pumps provide the opportunity for patient-controlled analgesia and allow for successful outpatient pain management.

Intraspinal
Epidural and intrathecal opioid administration is generally preserved for patients who have dose-limiting side effects to systemic opioids or who require the addition of a nonopioid drug such as a local anesthetic or α-adrenergic analgesic (e.g., clonidine) to manage pain below the level of the midthorax. The addition of local anesthetic drugs such as bupivacaine or tetracaine to an opioid may be particularly helpful in managing pain that is intractable to the use of systemic opioids alone.

Opioid selection

Weak opioids
Many opioid analgesics are available (Table 9.6). The WHO ladder advocates the use of a so-called *weak opioid* for moderate pain that is not controlled by a nonopioid agent. In reality, the distinction between *weak* and *strong opioids* is an artificial one, since these drugs lack a ceiling effect and equianalgesic doses are known for all of the opioids.

A number of opioid–nonopioid combination products exist, however, whose maximum daily dose is limited by the potential toxicity of the nonopioid. These products are appropriate for the second step of the WHO ladder. However, it is often more practical to use an opioid and a nonopioid separately rather than as a combination product in order to allow freer titration of the opioid so as to achieve pain relief while avoiding the risk of acetaminophen or aspirin toxicity.

Strong opioids
Morphine is the most widely used agent for moderate to severe pain because of its availability, its well-defined pharmacology, and its relatively low cost. The choice of drug must be tailored to the individual patient's needs, however, and for those patients who are unable to tolerate morphine, many useful alternatives exist (see Table 9.3). It is often useful to "rotate" patients from morphine to another opioid to minimize toxicity and to gain added pain relief. For example, rotation of morphine to hydromorphone, or hydromorphone to methadone or morphine, reduces cognitive failure. Fentanyl is particularly interesting in this regard. It is available as a transdermal patch that delivers the drug at a fixed rate for 72 hours and may be effective for patients who are unable to take oral medications. Recent evidence also suggests that fentanyl and morphine may act on different subtypes of μ-opioid receptor, pointing to a reason to rotate to fentanyl when patients are intolerant of side effects with morphine and other classical μ-agonists.

Fentanyl is the only opioid available as a transmucosal formulation for anesthetic premedication in children and for the treatment of procedure-related pain in children and adults in monitored settings before general or regional anesthesia and painful procedures. A second formulation of transmucosal fentanyl, Actiq®, is available for the treatment of breakthrough pain in opioid-tolerant individuals.

Table 9.6 Opioid analgesics used for acute and chronic pain

Opioid	Usual starting dose	Comment
WHO Step 2 opioid		
Codeine (with APAP or ASA) Tylenol # 2 (15 mg codeine) Tylenol # 3 (30 mg codeine) Tylenol # 4 (60 mg codeine)	60 mg q 3–4 hrs p.o.	(1) Fixed combination with ASA and APAP scheduled as DEA III; single entity as DEA II schedule. (2) Usually 250 mg APAP or ASA per tablet. Take care not to exceed toxic doses of APAP and ASA. (3) Sustained-release codeine formulations in clinical development.
Hydrocodone (with APAP or ASA) Lorcet; Lortab; Vicodan; others	10 mg q 3–4 hrs p.o.	(1) Same as for codeine; Vicodin-ES has 750 mg ASA per tablet.
Oxycodone (with APAP or ASA) Percocet; Percodan; Tylox; others	10 mg q 3–4 hrs p.o.	
Tramadol Ultram	50 mg q.i.d. p.o.	(1) Recently approved in the USA. (2) Although a μ-opioid agonist, it is not scheduled as an opioid because of alleged low abuse potential. Also blocks catecholamine reuptake. Nausea common side effect. (3) Seizures may occur in doses over 400 mg/day.
WHO Step 2/3 opioids		
Morphine Immediate-release (MSIR) Sustained-release (MS Contin, Oramorph, Kadian)	30 mg q 3–4 hrs p.o. 10 mg q 3–4 hrs i.v. 30 mg q 12 hrs p.o.	(1) Standard to which all other opioids are compared. (2) Morphine is also available as suppository. (3) MSIR is preferred rescue analgesic for controlled-release preparations. (4) Some clinicians do not view MS Contin and Oramorph as therapeutically interchangable; MS Contin is available in 15, 30, 60, 100 and 200 mg tablets; Oramorph available in 15, 30, 60 and 100 mg tablets only.

Continued

Table 9.6 Continued

Opioid	Usual starting dose	Comment
		(5) Kadian has 24-hr duration of action; available in 20, 50, and 100 mg capsules.
		(6) Kadian may retain its controlled-release properties if the capsule is broken and sprinkled on apple sauce.
Oxycodone OxyContin (sustained release) Roxicodone (immediate release)	20 mg q 12 hrs p.o.	(1) Twice as potent as morphine; available in 10, 20, 40 mg tablets. (2) Immediate-release oxycodone also considered step 2 or 3 opioid and recommended as rescue medicine for OxyContin.
Hydromorphone Dilaudid; others	4–6 mg q 3–4 hrs p.o.	(1) Sustained-release formulation recently approved in USA (Pallidone). (2) Comes in 2, 4, and 8 mg tablets. (3) Available as a suppository 4 mg.
Fentanyl Duragesic (transdermal) Sublimaze, other Oralet Actiq	50 µg/hr q 72 hrs 50 µ/hr by continuous infusion 100–400 µg/unit 200 µg/unit	(1) The only opioid available for transdermal administration; many patients require oral rescue doses; comes in 25, 50, 75, and 100 µg/hr patches. (2) Oral potency ratio relative to morphine close to 100:1. (3) Fentanyl Oralet approved for treatment of acute pain complicating procedures and for conscious sedation in monitored settings. Actiq approved for treatment of breakthrough pain in opioid-tolerant patients; available in 200, 400, 600, 800, 1,000, 1,200, and 1,600 µg unit doses. (4) The dose of Actiq required for treatment of breakthrough pain must be determined by titration, and is not predictable based on the patient's baseline opioid requirements.
Methadone Dolophine; others	20 mg q 6–8 hrs p.o. 10 mg q 6–8 hrs i.v.	Excellent analgesic but very stigmatized because of use to treat heroin addiction.
Levorphanol Levo-Dromoran	2–4 mg q 6–8 hrs p.o.	Relatively long-acting; may have higher incidence of psychotomimetic effects than other opioids.

Other opioids[a]

Meperidine (Demerol)	75–100 mg i.v. q 3–4 hrs	(1) Oral potency is low (e.g., 75 mg i.m. = 300 mg p.o.). (2) Central-nervous-system stimulation occurs as a function of metabolite, normeperidine. Not recommended for chronic use. (3) Do not use naloxone to reverse normeperidine toxicity (see text).
Propoxyphene (Darvon, others)	65 mg p.o. q 4–6 hrs	(1) Useful for mild pain only. Also can be formulated with APAP as Darvocet-N-100 (propoxyphene 100 mg–APAP 650 mg). (2) One study observed found propoxyphene to be no different from placebo[b] (3) Norpropoxyphene metabolite may be associated with toxicity.

Agonist–antagonist opioids

Butorphanol (Stadol)	2 mg i.m. q 4–6 hrs 1–2 mg each nostril q 2–3 hrs	Opioids in agonist–antagonist class may precipitate opioid abstinence syndrome in physically-dependent patients. This class of opioids does not depress respiratory drive when given acutely. As a class, psychotomimetic effects are more commonly seen then with pure opioid agonists. Drugs in this class reported to be more effective in women than men in a dental pain study.[c]
Nalbuphine (Nubain)	10 mg i.m. q 4–6 hrs	
Buprenorphine (Buprenex)	0.4 mg i.m. q 4–6 hrs 0.8 mg sublingual q 4–6 hrs	
Dezocine	2.5–5.0 mg i.m. or i.v. q 2–4 hrs	
Pentazocine (Talwin NX)	50 mg pentazocine–0.5 mg naloxone q 4–6 hrs	Butorphanol NS indicated for treatment of migraine headache. Buprenorphine is the only commercially available sublingual opioid preparation, but is not available in the USA.

APAP, acetaminophen; ASA, aspirin.

[a] These opioids may be used for acute pain but are not generally recommended for chronic administration or to manage severe pain because of toxicity (e.g., multifocal myoclonus with meperidine) or lack of efficacy (partial agonist–antagonist class).

[b] Mortel CG et al, *N Engl J Med* 1972; **286**: 813.

[c] Gear RW et al, *Nature Med* 1996; **2**: 1248.

Treatment of opioid-related side effects

Frequently reported opioid-related side effects include sedation, confusion and hallucinations, myoclonus, respiratory depression, nausea and vomiting, constipation, dry mouth, urinary hesitancy, and pruritus. Although any of the opioids may produce any of these adverse effects, individuals vary in their responses to the different drugs. A patient who experiences intolerable dose-limiting side effects with one opioid may tolerate an equianalgesic dose of another opioid without significant adverse effects.

Sedation

Sedation is frequent at the start of treatment or after a dose increase, but it often resolves within a few days. Persistent sedation may be treated with low doses of pemoline, methylphenidate, or dextroamphetamine.

Confusion and hallucinations

Confusion and hallucinations are much less common, but may sometimes occur and necessitate a switch to an alternative opioid analgesic. It is important to remember, however, that delirium has many other potential causes in the cancer patient, including metabolic derangements, infection, and neoplastic involvement of the central nervous system. An opioid-treated cancer patient with a change in mental status may therefore require a careful evaluation before the delirium can be confidently attributed to the opioid.

Myoclonus

Myoclonus is another potential central-nervous-system effect of opioid analgesics, and, if frequent or bothersome, may require treatment with clonazepam.

Respiratory depression

Respiratory depression is a widely feared complication of the opioids, but it is uncommon, particularly in the opioid-tolerant patient. Pain acts as a physiologic antagonist to the depressant effects of opioids. Respiratory depression caused by opioids is always associated with sedation, so measures, such as physical stimulation, that arouse the patient may prevent the need for pharmacological reversal with an opioid antagonist. Also, most sick patients are on multiple psychoactive medications or have many reasons for sedation or altered respiratory drive, so that reflex administration of naloxone is often a mistake. When naloxone is administered to patients who have taken opioids chronically, a dilute solution (0.4 mg naloxone mixed in 10 cc of normal saline) should be given by slow intravenous administration and titrated against the respiratory rate and pupillary diameter to minimize precipitation of an overt abstinence syndrome and the return of pain.

Nausea and vomiting

Nausea and vomiting are frequent, but, again, often resolve within a few days of continued treatment. The regular use of an antiemetic drug may be required in some cases to control this side effect.

Constipation

Constipation is an almost universal accompaniment of chronic treatment with opioids, and should be anticipated and treated prophylactically. Patients should receive regular laxatives and instructions to maintain adequate intake of fiber and fluids. A typical bowel program would involve daily use of a senna-based laxative supplemented as needed by lactulose or milk of magnesia.

Other side effects

Other frequently reported adverse effects include dry mouth, urinary hesitancy, and pruritus. Again, any of the opioids may produce any of these adverse effects, and individuals vary in their responses to the different drugs; a patient who experiences intolerable dose-limiting side effects with one opioid may therefore tolerate an equianalgesic dose of another opioid without significant adverse effects.

Tolerance, physical dependence, and addiction

Tolerance

Tolerance refers to the need to increase the dose of the drug in order to maintain the same analgesic effect. In the clinical setting, tolerance to the analgesic effects of the opioids is rarely a major problem for patients with stable pain syndromes. In the cancer patient, the need for increasing doses of opioid to maintain analgesia often implies worsening pain caused by progressive disease, and it should not simply be attributed to tolerance. N-methyl-D-aspartate antagonists prevent and reverse tolerance related to change in opioid-receptor responsiveness.

Physical dependence

Physical dependence refers to the development of a withdrawal syndrome with abrupt discontinuation of therapy or substantial dose reduction; this phenomenon potentially occurs whenever repeated doses of opioids are administered for more than a few days.

Addiction

Tolerance and physical dependence do not imply drug addiction. Addiction is a psychological and behavioral syndrome characterized by compulsive drug use and continued drug use despite harm to the user. In the treatment of cancer pain with chronic opioid therapy, addiction develops extremely rarely, although physical dependence is almost universal. Unwarranted fears of addiction, both on the part of the physician and the patient, are one of the main barriers to adequate pain treatment in the cancer patient.

Adjuvant drugs for management of pain and other symptoms

Adjuvant drugs are compounds that were introduced for treatment of specific conditions but have been shown to be empirically effective for the management of pain and other symptoms such as nausea, bowel obstruction, and sedation (see Table 9.3). These drugs may also be used as coanalgesics when administered in combination with traditional opioid and nonopioid drugs.

THE MANAGEMENT OF PSYCHIATRIC SYMPTOMS AND PSYCHOLOGICAL ISSUES

The diagnosis of gynecologic cancer represents a significant threat to life that is accompanied by feelings of helplessness, uncertainty, and fear. Most women respond to the initial diagnosis with acute anxiety. In the majority of cases, however, women are able to adapt to the stress of cancer without experiencing persistent psychiatric symptoms. About 30% of women with gynecologic cancer will experience levels of emotional distress that warrant psychiatric intervention. Women who struggle to adapt often benefit from referrals to a variety of supportive interventions, including, but not limited to, support groups, individual psychotherapy, and psychotropic medications to manage anxiety and depressive symptoms. There are rare instances of psychiatric emergencies and severe psychiatric illness that warrant intensive intervention. Additionally, gynecologic cancer patients often complain of sexual dysfunction, menopausal symptoms, emotional distress related to infertility, body-image concerns, and relationship discord. It is important for medical staff to be able to identify and manage psychological distress so that the patient receives expedient care.

Normal psychological reactions to the diagnosis of cancer

Most women respond to the initial diagnosis of gynecologic cancer with a brief period of acute psychological distress. Women will express distress differently, depending upon individual personality and coping style. Symptoms of distress that frequently occur in the setting of cancer diagnosis include:

- insomnia
- loss of appetite
- panic attacks
- crying spells
- emotional numbness
- helplessness
- indecision
- intense fear
- social withdrawal
- dissociation and derealization

Table 9.7 Characteristics that distinguish between adapters and nonadapters to the stress of cancer	
Characteristics of adapters	Characteristics of nonadapters
• Engaged with social support • Optimistic • Confident • Seek information	• Socially withdrawn • Pessimistic • Helpless and hopeless • Avoidant

After a period of days to weeks, however, these acute symptoms resolve for most people, and the process of adaptation begins. Brief treatment of acute anxiety and insomnia with a benzodiazepine (e.g., lorazepam, 0.5–1 mg p.o. at bedtime) or a mild sedative (e.g., zolpidem tartrate, 5–10 mg p.o. at bedtime) often helps patients to cope with the stress of initial diagnosis if symptoms are severe. If adaptation is successfully achieved, motivation to achieve a cure replaces the acute shock.

Adaptation to the stress of cancer

There are differences between those patients who adapt successfully to the stress of cancer and those who have a more difficult time doing so. These differences are outlined in Table 9.7. It is important to help women who show signs of poor adaptation to organize a support network that will assist them with practical and emotional support during treatment.

Management of psychological distress

Owing to the stressful nature of a cancer diagnosis, cancer patients remain vulnerable to psychological distress throughout their cancer experience and beyond. There are no stress-free aspects of the cancer experience. Several phases of gynecologic cancer treatment, however, are particularly challenging. These include the initial diagnosis, the recurrence of disease, the loss of a normal physical function (e.g., the placement of a colostomy or the loss of fertility), and the termination of cancer therapy.

Signs and symptoms
Patients will not always communicate their distress in ways that are clear to the treatment team. There are usually signs, however, that signal psychological stress. These include:

• noncompliance with treatment
• apathy or disinterest
• depressed mood

- expressions of hopelessness (e.g., "I'll never get better," "I don't know if I can go on with this any longer.")
- excessive guilt
- ruminative thoughts of death and dying
- irritability
- indecision
- expressions of loneliness or isolation

These symptoms can be mild to severe and transient or persistent. It is important to understand that these are warning signs of psychological distress in the patient and to respond to them by offering increased support.

Interventions for mild distress

When psychological distress is mild (one or two transient symptoms in reaction to a specific event), additional time in which to discuss her concerns may be all that the patient needs to decrease her anxiety. Medical staff should let the patient know that they are aware of her distress and help to identify its source. This usually requires only a few minutes of inquiry. Open-ended questions, rather than direct ones, yield a greater amount of information and, contrary to what is generally believed, do not take up more time. Questions such as "I notice that you are having trouble making a decision about what to do, how can I help?" or "I am concerned because you have missed several appointments for treatment. What's making it hard to get here?" are very helpful.

If the patient needs additional support, members of the medical team should refer patients to clergy, psychoeducational programs, patient-to-patient volunteers, social workers, and support groups. Patients should also be informed about additional psychosocial services that are available, and they should be encouraged to utilize more intensive forms of support if necessary.

Interventions for moderate to severe distress

When distress is moderate or severe (several symptoms that persist for more than 1 week), more intensive intervention is required. In addition to the steps discussed above, patients should be reassured that treatment designed to ease their emotional suffering is available. Referrals to social workers, psychiatric nurse clinicians, psychologists, and psychiatrists should be strongly encouraged.

Psychotherapy provided by a trained professional in an individual or group setting effectively decreases the emotional distress experienced by most gynecologic cancer patients. Psychotropic medications relieve symptoms of depression and anxiety with minimal side effects. Serotonin-specific reuptake inhibitors and benzodiazepines are most commonly prescribed drugs to relieve anxiety and depressed mood (Table 9.8). As with physical pain, patients should not suffer because of emotional distress without intervention.

Table 9.8 Commonly prescribed medications used to control anxiety and depressed mood			
Antianxiety medication	Starting daily dose (mg, p.o.)	Antidepressant medication	Starting daily dose (mg, p.o.)
Alprazolam	0.5–1	Fluoxetine	10
Clonazepam	0.25–0.5	Sertraline	25
Diazepam	5–10	Paroxetine	10
Lorazepam	0.5–1	Citalopram	10
Temazepam	15–30		

Management of psychiatric emergencies

There are several psychiatric conditions that require the urgent attention of medical staff and mental-health specialists. Most common are delirium, agitation, and suicidal ideation. These conditions require the following immediate crisis intervention:

- Secure the environment (remove sharp implements, medications, and other harmful items from patient's surroundings).
- Initiate one-to-one observation.
- Administer medications (e.g., haloperidol, lorazepam) to treat agitation.
- As a last resort, restrain the patient to ensure her safety and that of staff.
- Request an emergency psychiatric consultation.

Delirium
Delirium is a disturbance in the level of consciousness accompanied by cognitive impairment. Symptoms develop rapidly, usually over the course of hours or days, and wax and wane in intensity. Delirium is the consequence of physiological changes associated with a medical condition, substance intoxication or withdrawal, medications, toxin exposure, or a combination of the above.

During an episode of delirium, a patient may be hypoactive or hyperactive or may alternate between the two. The patient may experience disorientation, visual or auditory hallucinations (or both), delusions, inability to attend, and memory loss, and may exhibit unusual or bizarre behavior. Hypoactive delirium often goes untreated, because symptoms are mistaken for emotional withdrawal, depression, or fatigue. Delirium and other forms of mental disorientation are sometimes accompanied by agitation.

Agitation
Agitation is excessive, nonpurposeful motor movement accompanied by severe distress. It is often present during abrupt changes in mental status, and requires immediate attention to ensure patient and staff safety. Delirium and

agitation are most effectively treated with neuroleptic medication. Neuroleptic medication should also be used in the case of hypoactive delirium, despite the common belief that these medications will contribute to the patient's sedation. If agitation is severe, and if the neuroleptic alone is inadequate in sedating the patient, a benzodiazapine may be added.

Suicidal ideation

Suicidal ideation most frequently presents during severe depression, when a patient feels desperate, worthless, and hopeless about the future. An expression of a desire to take one's own life may be subtle, emphatic, or dramatic. All suicidal patients need immediate crisis intervention and an evaluation by a trained mental-health professional. The mental-health professional will perform a thorough review of the patient's thoughts about suicide and determine the degree to which the patient is at risk of harming herself. They will make further recommendations to staff regarding how to ensure the continuation of the patient's safety.

Risk factors for attempted suicide

Encouraging the patient to talk about her suicidal ideation is crucial. Contrary to myth, asking about suicide will not increase the likelihood of an attempt. In fact, patients who openly discuss their suicidal ideation with others are less likely to commit suicide. The following characteristics increase the patient's risk of making a suicide attempt:

- social withdrawal
- anhedonia
- hopelessness
- worthlessness
- agitation
- mental confusion
- age over 40 years
- being unmarried
- living alone
- unemployment
- bereavement
- family stressors
- terminal illness
- drug or alcohol abuse
- attempting to conceal suicide attempts
- taking action to secure means of attempting suicide
- pain
- family history of suicide

Table 9.9 is a reference for interventions appropriate for psychiatric emergencies and other levels of psychological distress.

Table 9.9 Interventions for the treatment of psychological distress		
Level of distress	Staff interventions	Referrals
Mild distress	Inquire about source of distress Provide information Clarify misconceptions	Clergy Psychoeducational programs Patient-to-patient volunteers Support groups

Moderate to severe distress	Inform patient of available
	   treatments
	Encourage follow-up with
	   mental-health professional
		Social-work evaluation
		Psychiatric evaluation
		Psychiatric-nurse
		   intervention

Psychiatric emergency	Secure the environment
	Place patient on one-to-one
	   observation
	Sedate and restrain the patient
	   if appropriate
		Emergency psychiatric
		   evaluation

Psychiatric disorders

The majority of women with gynecologic cancer do not experience psychiatric disorders, and such disorders in this population should be considered to be outside the range of "normal" and expected reactions to cancer. Approximately 30% of gynecologic cancer patients do, however, experience a pattern of symptoms that would meet criteria for a psychiatric disorder. Therefore, screening for psychiatric disorders among gynecologic cancer patients is recommended, since it facilitates early intervention and thereby decreases the individual's suffering. Women with symptoms that warrant a psychiatric diagnosis are experiencing significant degrees of suffering, and they should be followed closely by a mental-health professional during their treatment.

Risk factors

Risk factors related to age, stage of disease, treatment intensity, treatment side effects, and psychosocial stressors may place patients at risk for developing a psychiatric disorder during their cancer experience. Such risk factors include the following circumstances:

- premorbid history of psychiatric illness
- family history of psychiatric illness
- advanced stages of cancer
- multiple life stressors other than cancer
- radical surgical procedures
- treatment-induced menopause
- treatments with side effects that affect mood and behavior

Table 9.10 Prevalence of psychiatric diagnoses in the gynecologic oncology population	
Diagnosis	Prevalence (%)
Adjustment disorder	43
Major depression	15
Delirium	11
Mood disorder due to general medical condition	9
Dementia	9
Substance abuse	7
Bipolar disorder	2
Somatoform disorder	2
Schizophrenia	2

Prevalence

The most prevalent psychiatric disorder diagnosed in the gynecologic cancer population is an *adjustment disorder with depressed and/or anxious mood*, followed by *major depression* and *delirium* (Table 9.10). *Mood disorders* are by far the most frequently diagnosed psychiatric disorders in the gynecologic cancer setting. The most effective intervention for these psychiatric conditions is a combination of psychotherapy and psychotropic medication. Treatment for anxiety and depressed mood related to a medical condition may require medical intervention in combination with psychiatric treatment. For example, depressed mood following surgically induced menopause may respond best to a combination of hormone replacement and antidepressant therapy in situations where it is not medically contraindicated.

Managing sexual dysfunction

Sexual dysfunction occurs in up to one-third of women with gynecologic cancer. Even when women are focused on curing their disease during treatment, they continue to view sexual function as a significant issue. Hypoactive sexual desire, decreased arousal, and dyspareunia are most frequently reported. The consequences of gynecologic cancer treatment also contribute to menopausal symptoms, infertility, and problems related to body image, all of which impact on sexual functioning and relationships.

Doctor–patient communication

Issues related to sexual dysfunction cause distress and warrant attention, but many physicians and patients are embarrassed to ask questions about sexual health. Physicians ease patients' distress about these issues when they ask direct questions about sexual functioning and menopausal symptoms and make referrals to specialists in sex therapy and couples or family counseling in response to complaints by patients of problems with sexual functioning.

Hypoactive sexual desire and decreased arousal

Treatment often involves a combination of couples psychotherapy, hormonal therapy, and vaginal-dilator use. Estrogen and testosterone replacement, when not medically contraindicated, and alternative preparations of hormone therapies (e.g., testosterone cream, Estring®) are recommended to enhance sexual desire and arousal and to decrease menopausal symptoms. Psychotherapy helps the patient to cope with the underlying body-image concerns, self-esteem issues, and relationship problems that contribute to sexual dysfunction.

Dyspareunia

Dyspareunia can be prevented by *consistent* use of a vaginal dilator. It is important for medical staff to:

- Have dilators of different sizes available.
- Recommend the use of water-based vaginal lubricants with the dilator.
- Give verbal and written instructions on how to use the dilator effectively – insert it for 10 minutes, and use it daily for 10 days and then three times per week for 1 year.
- Encourage consistent use by asking about frequency of use and pain.
- Recommend stopping use if it is painful, and suggest a smaller size of dilator.
- Instruct patients to avoid painful intercourse.
- Do not instruct patients to have intercourse in lieu of vaginal-dilator use. It may be painful and it places an unrealistic expectation on the patient and her partner that leads to sexual avoidance.

PROVIDING SUPPORT AND MANAGING PRACTICAL NEEDS

Communicating medical information to the patient

The severe psychological distress that occurs at the time of diagnosis interferes with the patient's ability to process information. Therefore, it is important to take steps to assist the patient in communicating about important aspects of her treatment plan. If the patient does not object, important diagnostic and treatment information should be provided in the presence of a family member or close friend because they will retain information that the patient is unable to process. Present treatment information in a manner that is clear and concise. Allow the patient an opportunity to ask questions and express concerns. Important quality-of-life issues such as fertility, sexual functioning, hormonal treatments, and surgical reconstruction often come up at home, when the patient is more relaxed and discussing her situation with friends and family. For this reason, encourage patients to call with questions that emerge after the consultation. When imparting information about a cancer diagnosis, further treatment, or change in treatment plan, keep in mind that most of what you say may not be retained. The following suggestions facilitate patient–physician communication:

- Give the patient written educational material that she can take home and read.
- Let the patient take home informed-consent documents to read under less stressful circumstances.
- Suggest that a family member or companion accompany the patient when discussions about medical treatment are to take place.
- Expect to repeat information, and be available to answer questions.
- Refer to support staff who are available to spend time with the patient at critical times in her medical treatment and diagnosis.
- Refer to staff who will orient the patient and her family to the hospital or ambulatory-care facility.

Most patients achieve acceptance of the diagnosis and treatment over a period of days; cognitive functioning returns to baseline, and the patient becomes increasingly able to participate in her care.

Practical needs

Transportation
Most patients need assistance traveling to and from the hospital. Inadequate or unaffordable transportation prevents access to medical care. Transportation benefits vary depending on the patient's situation. Medicaid benefits include transportation expenses as part of the insurance coverage for medical treatments. The physician or nurse practitioner needs to provide authorization. The patient can travel by public transportation, car service, ambulance, or ambulette. Most private insurers and Medicare benefits do not cover the cost of transportation. Patients with this type of insurance need additional assistance to cover transportation costs. Social workers can help patients apply for philanthropic funds through agencies such as the American Cancer Society. The hospital may also have funds specifically dedicated to this service, but patients need assistance in the application process. Helping a patient negotiate access to medical treatment increases the likelihood that she will follow through with treatment, and reduces anxiety in a very concrete and direct manner.

Housing
Cancer treatments are increasingly administered in the ambulatory-care setting. Therefore, if patients must travel a distance to receive treatments, they may need lodging for a night or longer. This can be very expensive and, in a large city, difficult to accomplish within a reasonable budget. The social worker can assist with housing for both the patient and her primary caretakers, and provide them with a list of safe, low-cost hotels in the area. For those patients in need of financial assistance, an assessment is made, and if a finan-

cial need is determined, the hospital can provide housing by means of a voucher system and arrangements with local hotels.

Home care

Home care or visiting-nurse services are often provided to patients after surgery and/or adjuvant treatments. The level of home care services that is provided depends on the patient's needs. Home care may consist of a registered nurse, a home health aid, and a physical therapist. In some cases, a nurse specializing in the administration of i.v. antibiotics or wound care is required. A patient can also request that a social worker make a home assessment of psychosocial supports or of a stressful home environment that could impact on her overall care. The assessment for home care occurs either in the hospital or in an ambulatory setting, and is conducted by the primary doctor and nurse. The case manager evaluates the patient's medical needs and confirms the insurance coverage for the recommended services. Some patients may insist on home care even if it is not medically indicated. This request often reflects the patient's fears about coping with cancer at home. The social worker can work with the medical team and the patient to facilitate coping and to determine the patient's actual needs during this adjustment process.

Financial burden

Patients are often overwhelmed by the enormity of their medical bills and need help in navigating the complexities of the hospital billing system. With the help of a hospital patient representative, the social worker can guide the patient through this financial morass. An assessment of financial resources is of primary importance. If the treatment takes place in a private hospital, patients will need health insurance or the means to pay for services independently. The social worker can help the patient apply for insurance through private agencies or through government-subsidized programs such as Medicaid or Medicare. If she is denied coverage, she may be eligible to apply to a financial-assistance program through the hospital that defrays the cost of the hospital bills only.

Many patients apply for disability benefits as either short- or long-term financial assistance. Disability can be first obtained through a patient's employer and, once that has been completed, through government-sponsored programs. For both applications, an assessment from the doctor is required. Ongoing disability is difficult for most patients, because it represents a loss of autonomy. Social workers provide emotional support and practical assistance to help patients cope during this stressful transition period.

Social support

Support groups
Support groups provide education and social support in an environment in which participants can learn from, teach, and listen to each other. Support groups provide a valuable opportunity to dispel myths and clarify misconceptions about

cancer care. Support groups are led by healthcare professionals and, in some cases, a collaboration of staff and cancer survivors. Support groups are appropriate for a variety of populations, including patients in treatment, patients post-treatment, care givers, and hospital staff.

Peer support
Survivors are a unique, invaluable source of education and social support. They help patients to cope with initial diagnosis by providing a source of hope. Whenever possible, patients should be matched to peers who have gone through similar medical experiences. There are many national organizations that provide individual and group peer support. Social workers provide patients with the names and contact information of these organizations.

Hospice care
End-of-life care is central to the patient's quality of life and emotional well-being. For most patients, this phase of their disease necessitates hospice care and augmentation of supportive services. Patients and their families can benefit from grief counseling to help them to cope with the tremendous losses at this time.

Communicating with the patient and her primary care givers about hospice care is usually difficult and complex. It is recommended that the healthcare team have a meeting to discuss further course of treatment and hospice care with the patient and her family. It is a misconception that hospice care comprises a nurse who tends to the patient for 24 hours per day. This is not the case, and often both staff and patients undergo a process of education when discussing this aspect of care.

With the help of a hospice agency, the family may be able to provide hospice care at home. The agency provides some visiting-nurse and home health-aide assistance, but the majority of the care for the patient is left up to the family. The hospice provides supportive services (e.g. religious, psychological) for the family and the patient, to help them to cope with the end-of-life process.

The hospice staff are also trained in pain management, which is a primary concern and issue with cancer patients at this stage. Physicians should have a discussion with the patient about the *Do Not Resuscitate (DNR) order* before hospice care. A DNR order is not a requirement to initiate hospice care, but it is advisable, since the philosophy of hospice is not to prolong life, but rather to help the patient maintain a good quality of life that is as pain-free and as peaceful as possible.

If the patient cannot go home safely, there are also inpatient hospice units in skilled nursing facilities. Most insurance policies pay for hospice care, both inpatient and outpatient. The transition to hospice care can be difficult and stressful for the patient and medical staff alike, and both can feel like failures. The social worker can help facilitate communication between them to ensure the most comfortable and suitable end-of-life care for the patient.

SELECTED READING

Cleeland CS, Gonin R, Hatfield AK et al, Pain and its treatment in outpatients with metastatic cancer. *N Engl J Med* 1994; **330**: 592.

Holland JC, *Psycho-oncology*. New York: Oxford University Press, 1998.

Jacox A, Carr DB, Payne R et al, *Clinical Practice Guidelines* (No. 9). *Management of Cancer Pain*. Rockville, MD: Agency for Healthcare Policy and Research, 1994.

Portenoy RK, Kornblith AB, Wong G et al, Pain in ovarian cancer patients. Prevalence, characteristics, and associated symptoms. *Cancer* 1994; **74**: 907.

Sterns N, *Oncology Social Work: A Clinician's Guide*. Atlanta, GA: American Cancer Society, 1993.

10
Preinvasive disease of the lower female genital tract

Diane C Bodurka, Michael W Bevers

The squamous intraepithelial neoplasias of the vulva, vagina, and cervix represent a spectrum of preinvasive disorders of the squamous epithelium that may regress, persist, or progress to invasive cancer. These squamous neoplastic disorders are characterized by disordered maturation and nuclear abnormalities such as loss of polarity, pleomorphism, coarsening of nuclear chromatin, irregularities of the nuclear membrane, and mitotic figures at various levels in the epithelium above the basement membrane. The degree of epithelial abnormality present, as measured from the basement membrane to the surface, serves as a histopathologic grading system for the severity of the lesion (Table 10.1). Lesions are classified as follows:

- lesions of the vulva are referred to as *vulvar intraepithelial neoplasia (VIN)*;
- lesions of the vagina are referred to as *vaginal intraepithelial neoplasia (VAIN)*;
- lesions of the cervix are referred to as *cervical intraepithelial neoplasia (CIN)*.

Table 10.1 Histopathologic classification of intraepithelial neoplasia

Classification	Location of atypia
VIN 1	Lower 1/3
VIN 2	Lower 2/3
VIN 3–carcinoma in situ	Upper 1/3–entire epithelium
VAIN 1	Lower 1/3
VAIN 2	Lower 2/3
VAIN 3–carcinoma in situ	Upper 1/3–entire epithelium
CIN 1	Lower 1/3
CIN 2	Lower 2/3
CIN 3–carcinoma in situ	Upper 1/3–entire epithelium

VULVAR INTRAEPITHELIAL NEOPLASIA (VIN)

Incidence

The incidence of VIN has increased over the last decade. The mean age at diagnosis is 43 years, and appears to be falling. The most significant increase has been seen in women in the third decade of life.

Risk factors

No definitive etiologic agent has been identified. Epidemiologic data suggest that human papillomavirus (HPV) infection, smoking, history of other genital-tract dysplasia or malignancy, and immune suppression are risk factors for VIN.

Clinical features

Clinically, patients can be divided into two groups. While patients in one group are usually premenopausal women with HPV-positive multifocal disease, the second group consists of postmenopausal patients with HPV-negative unifocal disease. The most common presenting complaint found in 60% of patients with VIN is pruritus. The remainder of patients are asymptomatic and VIN is diagnosed at the time of routine gynecologic exam.

The lesions of VIN are typically found on the non-hair-bearing surface of the vulva, and may also be present on the perineum and perianal areas. Lesions are often visible to the naked eye, and may appear pigmented, erythematous, beige, black, brown, or white. They are sharply demarcated from the surrounding epithelium, raised, and, after the application of acetic acid, turn white ("acetowhite lesions"). Lesions of particular concern for VIN include those with excessive hyperkeratosis, elevated lesions, lesions demonstrating a blood vessel pattern of angiogenesis (punctation, mosaicism, or other atypical vessels), and lesions with an ulcerated surface.

Diagnosis

The goal of evaluation and diagnosis is to rule out a malignant process. Evaluation of suspicious areas includes application of 3–5% acetic acid for 5 minutes to the vulva, perineum, and perianal areas. Colposcopy is accomplished with a hand lens or colposcope, and representative punch biopsies are obtained from suspicious areas. In addition, the remainder of the lower genital tract should be carefully evaluated, including the vagina and cervix (if present).

Treatment

Patients 45 years and older should undergo excision of VIN, since the incidence of microinvasive cancer increases at this age. Once invasive disease has

Table 10.2 Common modalities used to treat VIN		
Treatment	Clinical data	Failure rate (%)
Laser	No suspicion of invasion; VIN 1, VIN 2, and selected patients with VIN 3; up to 22% of patients with VIN 3 will have underlying carcinoma	10–20
Wide local excision with clear margins	Suspicion of invasion or VIN 3	15–25

been ruled out, the goal of treatment of VIN is preventing progression to invasive cancer. The two most widely used treatment modalities for biopsy-proven VIN are laser ablation and wide local excision (Table 10.2).

Follow-up

Recurrence of VIN is common, especially in the subgroup of patients who smoke. Long-term observation with colposcopy is required. A general follow-up schema following treatment is to repeat the exam at 3- to 4-month intervals during the first year, then every 6 months during years 2 and 3, and annually thereafter.

VAGINAL INTRAEPITHELIAL NEOPLASIA (VAIN)

Incidence

The exact incidence of VAIN is unknown, but the number of cases appears to be increasing. The mean age at diagnosis is 50 years, and, as is the case with VIN, the mean age is decreasing.

Risk factors

The most consistent risk factor for VAIN is a prior history of cervical intraepithelial neoplasia. Other risk factors include HPV infection, prior irradiation for pelvic malignancy, smoking, and immune suppression.

Clinical features

Patients with VAIN are primarily asymptomatic. Mucosal abnormalities are detected in the majority of cases following a screening Pap smear. Occasionally, women may complain of postcoital bleeding or an abnormal vaginal

Table 10.3 Common modalities used to treat VAIN		
Treatment modality	Clinical data	Failure rate (%)
Laser	No suspicion of invasion	22
5-FU 5% cream daily for 7 days and repeat at 3-week intervals for 3 cycles	No suspicion of invasion	15
Partial vaginectomy with clear margins	Suspicion of invasion	10

discharge. VAIN tends to be multifocal in nature. It is commonly located in the posterior upper one-third of the vagina. Lesions may appear as acetowhite lesions with punctation, or they may be leukoplakic, velvety, or ulcerated.

Diagnosis

The evaluation of patients with suspected VAIN includes colposcopy of the vagina, cervix (if present), and vulva. Colposcopy of the vagina may be performed with 3–5% acetic acid applied to the vagina for 5 minutes and/or with Lugol's solution. The speculum should be rotated and the entire vaginal surface evaluated. Representative biopsies of suspicious areas should be performed to establish the histologic diagnosis and to rule out an invasive neoplasm.

Treatment

The most common treatment modalities include 5-fluorouracil (5-FU) cream, laser ablation, and partial vaginectomy (Table 10.3).

Postmenopausal women may have abnormal Pap smears attributable to vaginal/cervical atrophy. A trial of topical estrogen cream and repeat Pap smear may be considered as front-line treatment if the exam supports atrophy and the results are not otherwise suspicious. Older patients and those with Pap smears suspicious for invasion should undergo partial vaginectomy.

CERVICAL INTRAEPITHELIAL NEOPLASIA (CIN)

Terminology and The Bethesda System

The Bethesda System (TBS) was conceived in 1988 by a National Institutes of Health consensus panel and revised in 1991. Prior cytologic classification systems devised by Papanicolaou and later by the World Health Organization (WHO) did not allow direct cytohistologic correlations to be made (Table

Table 10.4 The World Health Organization system and The Bethesda System (TBS) for cervical cytology

WHO system	TBS
Normal	Within normal limits
Atypical	Benign cellular changes or atypical squamous cells of undetermined significance (ASCUS) or atypical glandular cells of undetermined significance (AGUS)
Dysplasia Mild dysplasia Moderate dysplasia Severe dysplasia	Squamous epithelial abnormality Low-grade squamous intraepithelial lesion (LGSIL) High-grade squamous intraepithelial lesion (HGSIL) High-grade squamous intraepithelial lesion (HGSIL)
Carcinoma in situ	High-grade squamous intraepithelial lesion (HGSIL)
Squamous-cell carcinoma	Squamous-cell carcinoma
Adenocarcinoma	Adenocarcinoma

Table 10.5 TBS and histopathologic correlation

TBS epithelial abnormality	Histopathologic correlation
Low-grade squamous intraepithelial lesion (LGSIL)	CIN 1
High-grade squamous intraepithelial lesion (HGSIL)	CIN 2
High-grade squamous intraepithelial lesion (HGSIL)	CIN 3
Squamous-cell carcinoma	Squamous-cell carcinoma
Adenocarcinoma	Adenocarcinoma

10.4). The terminology of TBS correlates closely with histopathologic terminology (Table 10.5). In addition, this reporting system states the adequacy of the specimen, general categorization, and a descriptive diagnosis. TBS also makes provisions for glandular-cell abnormalities.

Incidence

Approximately 50,000,000 Pap tests are performed annually, with 5–7% being reported as abnormal. It is estimated that ASCUS represents 2,000,000 smears, LGSIL 1,250,000 smears, and HGSIL 250,000 smears. Only the biopsy incidence of carcinoma in situ is known, and accounts for 70,000 cases.

Risk factors

Epidemiologic evidence has long suggested that cervical neoplasia behaves like a sexually transmitted disease. In support of this hypothesis, several measures of sexual behavior are consistently associated with increased risk of neoplasia. The most common associated risk factors include high-risk sexual behavior, HPV infection, smoking, nonbarrier contraception, immunosuppression, socioeconomic status, and reproductive history.

It appears that HPV infection coupled with another cofactor may account for cervical neoplasia. At present, there are more than 70 subtypes of HPV. These subtypes include the high-risk (HPV-16, -18, -45, and -56) and intermediate-risk (HPV-31, -33, -35, -51, -52, and -58) types. The most common subtypes associated with cervical dysplasia are HVP-16, -18, -31, -33, and -35.

Clinical features

The majority of patients with squamous intraepithelial lesions of the cervix are asymptomatic. Symptoms that may, however, be associated with these lesions include postcoital bleeding, vaginal spotting, and abnormal vaginal discharge. Areas of the cervix with abnormal DNA content appear white when viewed through the colposcope following application of acetic acid, and are referred to as acetowhite epithelium. Vessels beneath the surface of this acetowhite epithelium can be seen through the colposcope with a green filter. Vascular atypia in the form of angiogenesis is often present in the acetowhite epithelium. The vascular atypia takes many forms, including punctation and mosaicism.

Diagnosis

The Pap smear is the screening tool used to detect squamous intraepithelial lesions. An adequate smear is obtained by using a wooden or plastic spatula and an endocervical brush followed by immediate fixation of the cells on a single slide. The triage of patients is then based on the results of the cytologic abnormalities noted on the slide (Table 10.6). Once an abnormal lesion is detected, histological evidence must be obtained prior to treatment. The mainstays of diagnosis are colposcopy, biopsy, and endocervical curettage. The caveat in diagnosing squamous intraepithelial lesions, as with VIN and VAIN, is to rule out an invasive lesion. Several criteria can be used to help exclude an invasive neoplasm (Table 10.7).

As the predictive capability of the colposcope is disputed, its main purpose should be to focus the site of biopsy. Following application of 3–5% acetic acid for 5 minutes, the cervix is visualized through the colposcope. Acetowhite areas are biopsied, especially if they are associated with atypical vessels. The colposcopy is graded as satisfactory (entire transformation zone visualized and lesion seen in its entirety) or unsatisfactory (entire transformation zone not visualized or lesion not seen in its entirety). The colposcopically directed biopsies are followed with an endocervical curettage (ECC). It is estimated that up

Table 10.6 Triage options for patients with an abnormal Pap smear

Cervical cytology results	Triage options
ASCUS diagnosis not further qualified or qualified by favor neoplastic process	HPV testing, and if positive, proceed to colposcopic evaluation, indicated biopsies, and endocervical curettage or Repeat Pap every 4–6 months until three consecutive negative smears
ASCUS diagnosis associated with severe inflammation	Treatment of underlying infection and repeat Pap in 2–3 months
ASCUS diagnosis in a post-menopausal patient not on hormone replacement therapy	Estrogen therapy followed by a repeat Pap in 2–3 months
LGSIL	Colposcopic evaluation, indicated biopsies, and endocervical curettage or Repeat Pap every 4–6 months until three consecutive negative smears. If repeat smears demonstrate persistent abnormalities, colposcopic evaluation, indicated biopsies, and endocervical curettage are indicated
HGSIL	Colposcopic evaluation, indicated biopsies, and endocervical curettage

Table 10.7 Criteria for excluding an invasive neoplasm

(1) Transformation zone fully visible
(2) Lesion seen in its entirety
(3) Endocervical curettage negative for dysplasia
(4) No discrepancy between Pap smear and biopsy
(5) No suspicion of invasion on Pap, colposcopy, or biopsy

to 25% of lesions may be missed if the ECC is omitted; therefore, an ECC should always be performed as part of the diagnostic workup.

Treatment

The treatment of cervical dysplasia is based on the following: Pap smear, adequacy of colposcopy, colposcopically directed biopsies, and endocervical curettage results. Current treatment modalities include ablative and excisional procedures (Table 10.8).

The choice between ablative and excisional therapy (Tables 10.9 and 10.10) is based on whether all five criteria for ruling out an invasive lesion have been satisfied (Table 10.7).

Table 10.8 Ablative and excisional procedures for the treatment of cervical dysplasia

Ablative procedures	Failure rate (%)	Excisional procedures	Failure rate (%)
Cryotherapy	15–18	Loop electrosurgical excision procedure (LEEP)	15–18
Laser	15–18	Cold knife cone biopsy	2–5

Table 10.9 Treatment following satisfactory colposcopy, histologic confirmation of squamous intraepithelial lesion (SIL), and negative endocervical curettage

Biopsy diagnosis	Treatment
Low-grade SIL (CIN 1)	• 80% of these lesions may spontaneously regress; therefore, one option is serial exams at 4- to 6-month intervals for 2 years • 20% of these may progress, so ablation or excision is also appropriate therapy if lesions persist for 2 years
High-grade SIL (CIN 2, CIN 3, carcinoma in situ)	• Excision or ablation of the entire transformation zone and lesion

Table 10.10 Treatment following unsatisfactory colposcopy and/or positive endocervical curettage and/or microinvasion on biopsy

Biopsy diagnosis	Treatment
Unsatisfactory colposcopy	LEEP cone or cold knife cone and repeat endocervical curettage
Positive endocervical curettage	LEEP cone or cold knife cone and repeat endocervical curettage
Microinvasion on biopsy	Cold knife cone and endocervical curettage

Follow-up

The majority of recurrences occur during the first 2 years following therapy. The recommended follow-up interval is every 3–6 months for the first 2 years and, if evaluation is consistently negative, annually thereafter.

SELECTED READING

Aho M, Vesterinen E, Meyer B et al, Natural history of vaginal intraepithelial neoplasia. *Cancer* 1991; **68**: 195.

Audet-Lapointe P, Body G, Vauclair R et al, Vaginal intraepithelial neoplasia. *Gynecol Oncol* 1990; **36**: 232.

Basta A, Adamek K, Pitynski K, Intraepithelial neoplasia and early stage vulvar cancer. Epidemiological, clinical and virological observations. *Eur J Gynaecol Oncol* 1999; **20**: 111.

Benedet JL, Miller DM, Nickerson KG, Results of conservative management of cervical intraepithelial neoplasia. *Obstet Gynecol* 1992; **79**: 105.

Campagnutta E, Parin A, Piero GD et al, Treatment of vaginal intraepithelial neoplasia (VAIN) with the carbon dioxide laser. *Clin Exp Obstet Gynecol* 1999; **26**: 127.

Cheng D, Ng TY, Ngan HY, Wong LC, Wide local excision (WLE) for vaginal intraepithelial neoplasia (VAIN). *Acta Obstet Gynecol Scand* 1999; **78**: 648.

Huang LW, Hwang JL, A comparison between loop electrosurgical excision procedure and cold knife conization for treatment of cervical dysplasia: residual disease in a subsequent hysterectomy specimen. *Gynecol Oncol* 1999; **73**: 12.

Husseinzadeh N, Recinto C, Frequency of invasive cancer in surgically excised vulvar lesions with intraepithelial neoplasia (VIN 3). *Gynecol Oncol* 1999; **73**: 119.

Jones RW, Baranyai J, Stables S, Trends in squamous cell carcinoma of the vulva: the influence of vulvar intraepithelial neoplasia. *Obstet Gynecol* 1997; **90**: 448.

Jones RW, Rowan DM, Vulvar intraepithelial neoplasia III: a clinical study of the outcome in 113 cases with relation to the later development of invasive vulvar carcinoma. *Obstet Gynecol* 1994; **84**: 741.

Kurman RJ, Henson DE, Herbst AL et al, Interim guidelines for management of abnormal cervical cytology. The 1992 National Cancer Institute Workshop. *JAMA* 1994; **271**: 1866.

Mitchell MF, Tortolero-Luna G, Cooke E et al, A randomized clinical trial of cryotherapy, laser vaporization, and loop electrosurgical excision for treatment of squamous intraepithelial lesions of the cervix. *Obstet Gynecol* 1998; **92**: 737.

Modesitt SC, Waters AB, Walton L et al, Vulvar intraepithelial neoplasia III: occult cancer and the impact of margin status on recurrence. *Obstet Gynecol* 1998; **92**: 962.

Solomon D, Schiffman M, Tarone R, Comparison of three management strategies for patients with atypical squamous cells of undetermined significance: baseline results from a randomized trial. *J Natl Cancer Inst* 2001; **93**: 293.

Sugase M, Matsukura T, Distinct manifestations of human papillomaviruses in the vagina. *Int J Cancer* 1997; **72**: 412.

Sun Y, Hildesheim A, Brinton LA et al, Human papillomavirus-specific serologic response in vulvar neoplasia. *Gynecol Oncol* 1996; **63**: 200.

Trimble CL, Hildesheim A, Brinton LA et al, Heterogeneous etiology of squamous carcinoma of the vulva. *Obstet Gynecol* 1996; **87**: 59.

11
Vulvar cancer

Thomas W Burke

Primary malignant tumors of the vulva are uncommon neoplasms that account for only 3–4% of all gynecologic cancers. Prior to the development of surgical management strategies, vulvar cancers were rarely curable and produced significant morbidity through extensive local growth and regional lymphatic spread. A protracted clinical course characterized by pain, bleeding, and drainage was common. Historically, diagnostic and treatment delays were frequently encountered. The use of radical vulvectomy, and subsequent more conservative, surgical approaches, coupled with earlier diagnosis and multi-modal therapy, have greatly altered the outcome for women with vulvar cancer. Long-term survival rates of 80% or better can now be anticipated for those diagnosed with early disease.

EPIDEMIOLOGY

The incidence of vulvar cancer tends to have a bimodal distribution. The majority of tumors develop as solitary lesions in postmenopausal women, often in association with chronic vulvar dystrophy. More recent series have also identified a subset of tumors developing in younger women, usually in association with multifocal carcinoma in situ or manifestations of human papillomavirus (HPV) infection. The rarity of vulvar cancer makes detailed investigation of epidemiologic risk factors difficult. A number of potential associations have been suggested, however, and are summarized in Table 11.1. Current reviews suggest that history of preinvasive genital neoplasia, HPV infection, cigarette smoking, and, possibly, chronic dystrophy are the most significant factors.

HISTOLOGIC TYPES

Because the vulva is a cutaneous organ covered by skin, about 85% of vulvar malignancies are squamous-cell carcinomas. Melanoma is the second most

---

Table 11.1 Possible risk factors for vulvar cancer

Chronic medical illnesses
- Diabetes mellitus
- Hypertension
- Obesity
- Immunosuppression

Sexually transmitted disease/infections
- Granulomatous disease
- Syphilis
- Herpes simplex virus infection
- Human papillomavirus infection

Chronic inflammatory diseases
- Lichen sclerosus
- Hypertrophic dystrophy

Personal/lifestyle factors
- Cigarette smoking
- Multiple sexual partners
- Prior genital-tract neoplasia

---

common cancer, accounting for 5–10% of cases. The remaining tumors are a diverse set of rare lesions that include basal-cell carcinoma; adenocarcinomas arising from sweat glands, Bartholin's gland, or ectopic breast tissue; Paget's disease; and sarcomas arising from connective tissue. Metastases from adjacent organs – rectum, vagina, cervix, and bladder – will sometimes present as vulvar lesions. Most of the clinical and treatment information regarding vulvar cancer applies to squamous tumors.

PATTERNS OF SPREAD

Vulvar cancers spread by local extension and microembolization to regional lymph nodes. Hematogenous spread to distant sites is uncommon, except for melanoma. A well-defined in situ lesion has been described and is covered in Chapter 10. The earliest invasion of the subcutaneous tissue can be identified and measured microscopically. Measurement is made between the base of the nearest normal dermal papilla and the greatest depth of tumor infiltration. Cancers invading less than 1 mm are categorized as microcarcinomas. Grossly evident cancers spread by local tissue infiltration and extension to local structures. Smaller, early cancers typically invade the vulvar skin and supporting soft tissue. Larger lesions may extend to involve the vagina, urethra, anus, or pubic bones. Massive tumors infiltrate deeply to the upper urethra, bladder base, or rectum.

The lymphatic drainage of the vulva seems to follow a predictable, stepwise pattern (Figure 11.1). The cutaneous lymphatic channels course within the borders of the vulva to the ipsilateral superficial inguinal lymph nodes. No

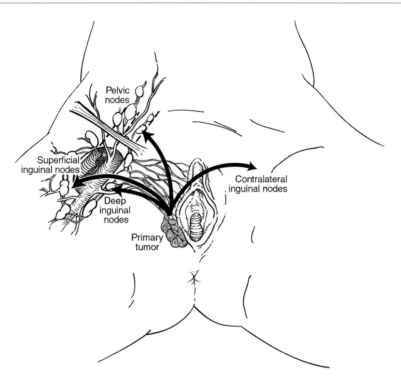

Figure 11.1
The major routes of lymphatic drainage progress from the primary tumor to the superficial inguinal lymph nodes, then to the deep inguinal nodes, and, finally, to the pelvic nodes. Variations in this pattern are occasionally identified, and may provide an explanation for unanticipated lymphatic treatment failure.

channels extend lateral to the labiocrural folds. Lymphatic fluid drains from the superficial inguinal to the deep inguinal nodes located beneath the cribriform fascia of the groin, and then on to the pelvic lymph nodes. For most women with vulvar cancer, these patterns of lymphatic drainage can be used as reliable predictors of nodal spread. These anatomic observations have allowed the development of less radical lymphatic dissection as a method for evaluating patients for lymph-node metastasis. Clinical experience, as well as current experimentation with intraoperative lymphatic mapping, suggests that a small percentage of women have anatomic variations of their lymphatic anatomy that deviate from the usual pattern, making prediction of lymphatic spread more difficult.

PRESENTATION OF DISEASE

Most women present with a pruritic vulvar lesion. Pain and bleeding may be present if surface ulceration has occurred. Diagnostic delays of 6–12 months are frequently seen, and usually represent a combination of the patient ignoring symptoms and the physician attempting topical therapy without establishing a definitive diagnosis. All clinically evident vulvar lesions should be biopsied. This procedure is easily accomplished in the clinic using infiltration of a local anesthetic and a Keyes punch-biopsy instrument. Colposcopic visualization of the vulva following a 5-minute application of dilute acetic acid (3–6%) may be helpful in selecting sites for cutaneous biopsy, particularly in women with extensive areas of preinvasive or inflammatory change.

Clinical examination and diagnostic biopsy will usually provide an accurate pretreatment evaluation of women with vulvar cancers. Additional studies may be helpful in special settings such as cases involving large primary tumor, obvious lymphatic spread, suspected involvement of adjacent organs, symptoms of distant metastases, or medical illnesses that might impact treatment decisions. The use of chest radiograph, computed tomography (CT), magnetic resonance imaging (MRI), barium enema, cystoscopy, proctoscopy, and other studies should be tailored to the specific clinical setting.

STAGING

The International Federation of Gynecology and Obstetrics (FIGO) employs a modified TNM and surgical staging scheme that was most recently modified in 1995 and which is outlined in Appendix 3 of this handbook. This staging system incorporates the major identified prognostic factors of increasing primary tumor volume, lymph-node metastasis, and distant spread. Assessment of lymphatic spread is based upon operative findings in the groin. This modification eliminates the major weakness of the previous staging scheme that employed clinical nodal assessment – a technique with a well-documented error rate of 20–30%. The FIGO staging system also includes a preinvasive category (Stage 0) for carcinoma in situ and a microinvasive category for lesions invading less than 1 mm (Stage IA). Depth of invasion is measured from the base of the nearest normal dermal papilla. Diagrammatic representations of the different stages of vulvar cancer are shown in Appendix 3.

THERAPY

It is convenient to separate treatment decisions into two categories – one aimed at eradicating the primary tumor on the vulva and the other directed at the assessment and treatment of the regional lymph nodes. Preinvasive lesions can be effectively treated with excisional biopsy, CO_2 laser ablation, or other local destruction techniques. Many preinvasive lesions are associated with HPV infection and have a propensity for recurrence. Close observation of treated patients is essential to detect new or recurrent lesions when they are small in size. This strategy minimizes the long-term impact of multiple

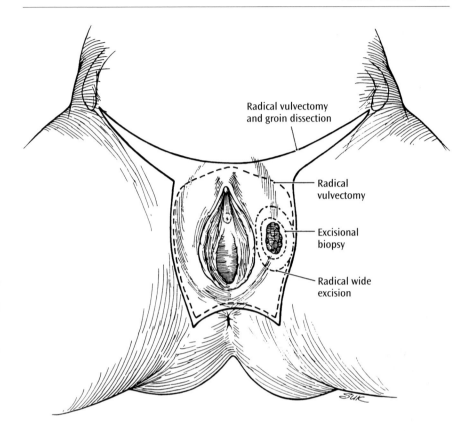

Radical vulvectomy
and groin dissection

Radical
vulvectomy

Excisional
biopsy

Radical wide
excision

Figure 11.2
Comparison of the typical excision lines for various excisional procedures. Note the
wide variation in the amount of uninvolved tissue retained as the radicality of the
resection increases.

episodes of treatment. Microinvasive cancers are almost always localized to the
vulva and can be adequately resected using a 1-cm margin of normal tissue. T1
and T2 tumors with obvious invasion can be excised via radical wide excision
with a 2-cm normal tissue margin or by radical vulvectomy. Typical incisions are
illustrated in Figure 11.2. The current trend is to use less-radical operations, particularly in women with T1 lesions. Larger tumors in the T3 and T4 categories
are difficult clinical problems. Resection often requires a combined abdominal
and perineal approach. Preservation of adjacent urinary or bowel structures may
not be feasible. A number of recent studies suggest that excellent tumor
responses can be obtained using external-beam irradiation or chemoradiation
followed by a more limited resection of residual tumor. This strategy has the
major advantage of organ preservation. Strategies for the treatment of women

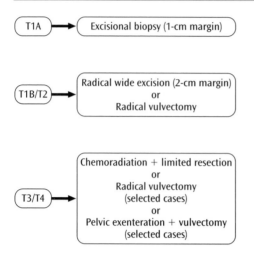

Figure 11.3

Algorithm for the treatment of primary tumors by stage.

with very large tumors are evolving and will likely change as more data become available. A summary of the treatment options for primary tumors is provided in Figure 11.3.

Groin dissection can be considered both diagnostic and therapeutic. The presence of lymph-node metastasis is the single most important prognostic factor in vulvar cancer. Detection of nodal spread at the time of initial diagnosis permits modification of the treatment plan and a better opportunity for cure. Unexpected late failure in the groin is virtually always fatal. The extent of groin dissection recommended is currently under debate. Some argue for a limited unilateral resection of the superficial inguinal nodes for lateralized tumors that preserves the ipsilateral deep-nodal group and all of the contralateral nodes. This approach is designed to minimize the morbidity associated with extensive disruption of the lymphatics from the lower extremities. Others consider superficial and deep dissection or bilateral dissection as necessary in order to reduce the incidence of unexpected groin failure. Many investigators use intraoperative lymphatic mapping and lymphoscintigraphy to better define lymphatic drainage in individual cases. These techniques may provide the data necessary to support more limited approaches to groin dissection but should be considered experimental at present.

Women with metastasis to inguinal nodes probably benefit from additional therapy. Postoperative irradiation is most commonly used to control tumor in the groin. Although some prefer to attempt more extensive nodal resection in node-positive cases, the combination of additional dissection and irradiation increases the potential for post-therapy lymphedema. Limited resection of obvious nodal disease supplemented by irradiation is less morbid. However, an optimal management plan for inguinal node metastases is not yet clearly defined. A synopsis of treatment options is provided in Figure 11.4.

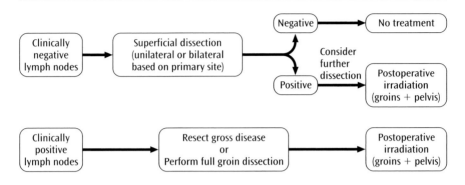

Figure 11.4
Algorithm outlining treatment options for the inguinal lymph nodes.

Treatment outcome is largely related to FIGO stage. Table 11.2 lists approximate survival percentages by stage.

It is useful to separate treatment morbidity into two separate categories for analysis purposes – one associated with the primary tumor site and the other associated with therapy of the regional nodes. Breakdown of the vulvar wound is the most common complication of surgical resection. Significant necrosis and wound separation is seen in about 50% of radical vulvectomy cases, in 15–20% of radical wide excisions, and in 5% of excisional biopsies. Desquamation of vulvar skin occurs to some degree in virtually all women who receive vulvar irradiation. This reaction may be more pronounced in those who receive concomitant chemotherapy. Despite its sometimes impressive visual appearance, desquamation regresses rapidly following completion of therapy and heals with an acceptable cosmetic result in most women.

Groin morbidity includes wound separation, lymphocyst formation, lymphangitis, and lymphedema. Complications related to groin therapy are poorly quantified and usually under-reported. The overall incidence rate for significant problems is about 25%. The likelihood of morbidity can be correlated with the extent of therapy: it is lowest in women who have unilateral superficial dissection and is greatest in those who have bilateral superficial and deep

Table 11.2 Survival by FIGO stage	
Stage	Approximate 5-year survival rate (%)
0	100
I	90
II	80
III	50
IV	15

authors describe primary vaginal lesions as those having no coexisting cervical or vulvar lesions either at the time of diagnosis of vaginal cancer or during the 10 years prior to diagnosis. Any malignant neoplasm that involves both the cervix and vagina and that is histologically compatible with origin in either organ is classified as a primary cervical cancer. Lesions vary in size from clinically occult to greater than 10 cm, and may be polypoid, indurated, ulcerated, or fungating upon gross examination. Squamous-cell carcinomas of the vagina resemble other squamous lesions histologically. While clinical stage is the most important prognostic indicator, histologic grade has not been linked to prognosis.

Verrucous carcinomas are extremely rare vaginal tumors and are classified as a variant of squamous-cell carcinoma. Grossly, the lesions are large, exophytic, and fungating. The diagnosis is based on the presence of bland cytologic features in broad bulbous masses of squamous cells at the stromal interface. These lesions have an indolent growth potential, with frequent local recurrence following incomplete excision. Lymph-node metastases rarely occur.

Melanomas

Malignant melanoma is the second most common vaginal cancer, accounting for 3–5% of all vaginal cancers. The mean age at diagnosis is 57 years, with a range from 22 to 83 years. Although these tumors may arise anywhere in the vagina, they occur most frequently in the lower third. Melanomas vary in color, shape, and size. They may be gray or black, fungating, nodular, or polypoid, and usually extend from 0.5 to 8 cm in diameter. Microscopically, the presence of junctional activity and of highly atypical melanocytes extending through the squamous epithelium is seen. When lesions are devoid of pigment, the immunoperoxidase staining pattern or ultrastructural findings may help establish the diagnosis. Positive staining with antibodies against S-100 protein is a sensitive but not specific indicator; HMB-45 is a less sensitive but more specific indicator of melanoma. Cells should not stain positive for desmin or keratin. Premelanosomes and melanosomes, along with abundant smooth and rough endoplasmic reticulum, can be seen ultrastructurally. The depth of tumor invasion is the best prognostic indicator. The method of Breslow is frequently used to assess tumor depth, while Chung's modification of Clark's levels has also been utilized.

Adenocarcinomas

Approximately 9% of primary vaginal neoplasms are adenocarcinomas. While the majority of these lesions occur in older women, vaginal clear-cell adenocarcinomas predominantly affect young women.

Vaginal clear-cell adenocarcinomas have been associated with maternal DES ingestion, and the average age at diagnosis is 19 years. The incidence of this lesion in women exposed to DES in utero ranges from 0.14 to 1.4 per 1000.

Approximately 65% of young women with vaginal clear-cell adenocarcinoma have been exposed to DES prenatally, while about 25% have not. To date, no correlation between the dose or duration of treatment and the incidence or pattern of cancer has been demonstrated.

The majority of DES-associated clear-cell adenocarcinomas occur in the upper third of the vagina and exocervix. Tumors vary in size from microscopic to large. While usually palpable, some small lesions may not be visible on colposcopic examination if covered by intact epithelium of normal appearance. Microscopically, these lesions are identical to clear-cell adenocarcinomas of the endometrium and ovary. Solid sheets of clear cells are usually seen; however, a pattern consisting of tubules and cysts lined by hobnail cells may also be observed. Atypical adenosis, typified by glands with hyperchromasia, nuclear pleomorphism, cellular stratification, and prominent nucleoli, is often seen at the periphery of these lesions.

Other rare histologies

Smooth-muscle tumors and primary sarcomas involving the vagina are extremely rare lesions. Embryonal rhabdomyosarcoma, or sarcoma botryoides, is the most common malignant tumor of the vagina in infants and children, with 90% of the lesions occurring in girls under 5 years of age. The average age at diagnosis is 2 years. The tumors are frequently located along the anterior wall of the vagina, and appear as small nodules or sessile, polypoid masses with an intact overlying mucosa. These lesions are gray or tan, edematous, and nodular. Large polypoid tumors may protrude through the introitus. Microscopically, this lesion is described as a polypoid growth pattern with a dense cambium layer of tumor cells that lies immediately adjacent to the surface epithelium. The term *cambium* is used to describe this dense layer of cells, since it has a growth pattern similar to that of the actively growing peripheral layer in tree trunks and branches. Small, round to spindle-shaped tumor cells are scattered in a dense collagenous or loose myxoid stroma within the cambium layer.

Other rare primary vaginal sarcomas include angiosarcoma, hemangiopericytoma, malignant fibrous histiocytoma, and sarcomas arising in endometriosis.

PATTERNS OF SPREAD

Vaginal cancer may spread locally, via lymphatics, or hematogenously. Owing to the absence of anatomic barriers, these lesions may extend directly to adjacent structures, including the bladder and rectum.

The pattern of lymphatic spread is usually dependent upon the location of the lesion in the vagina. If the lesion arises in the upper portion of the vagina, the pattern of lymph-node involvement is similar to that seen in cervical cancer, with metastasis first to the obturator, then iliac, then hypogastric nodes. If the lesion is located in the lower vagina, the pattern of spread is similar to that seen in vulvar cancer. Inguinal and femoral nodes are usually involved first, with subsequent involvement of deep pelvic nodes. Owing to the complexity of the lymphatic system of the vagina, exceptions to these patterns can exist, and any nodal group may be involved, regardless of the location of the primary lesion.

Hematogenous metastases may be present in the lungs or supraclavicular nodes. These are usually associated with advanced disease.

DISEASE PRESENTATION

Patients with primary vaginal cancer present with symptoms similar to those of cervical cancer. Vaginal discharge, frequently bloody, is the most commonly reported symptom. Patients may have postcoital spotting, or irregular or post-menopausal bleeding. Urinary symptoms may prompt evaluation in women with disease compressing or involving the bladder, while pelvic pain usually signifies advanced disease.

The diagnostic workup begins with a thorough history and physical examination. The pelvic examination includes visualization of the vagina, with careful rotation of the speculum as it is withdrawn in order to evaluate both the anterior and posterior vaginal walls, as well as bimanual and rectal examinations. While a Pap smear may detect squamous-cell lesions, the use of Lugol's solution and colposcopy is often required to detect submucosal clear-cell adenocarcinomas. A chest radiograph, cytoscopy, and proctoscopy should be performed on all patients with invasive vaginal cancer. Other imaging studies, including an intravenous pyelogram, barium enema, computed tomography (CT) scan, and magnetic resonance imaging (MRI), may be performed as clinically indicated.

STAGING

The staging of primary vaginal cancer is clinical rather than surgical and is based upon either the International Federation of Gynecology and Obstetrics (FIGO) or the American Joint Committee (AJC) staging system. Some authors advocate subdivision of FIGO Stage II lesions based on parametrial extension because of the more aggressive nature of tumors with parametrial extension; to date, this modification has not been formally adopted by FIGO (see Appendix 3 of this handbook).

THERAPY

The majority of cases of primary vaginal carcinoma are treated with radiation therapy. Specific treatment plans are based on the stage and extent of disease. Surgical resection remains an option for young women with Stage I clear-cell adenocarcinomas, nonepithelial lesions, and tumors that recur after irradiation. Chemotherapy is used only as salvage treatment. While chemoradiation is a potential treatment option for locally advanced disease, the data are too limited to address the efficacy of this intervention.

Stage 0

These lesions do not invade the basement membrane, and they are often multifocal. Surgical excision, laser ablation, and fluorouracil cream are all treatment options.

Stage I

These lesions are usually treated by radiation therapy, and treatment plans are tailored to the characteristics of the specific lesion. An intracavitary cylinder is generally used for 1–2 cm lesions, while an interstitial implant may be added for thick lesions localized to one vaginal wall. Whole-pelvic irradiation is usually followed by an interstitial implant in patients with larger, poorly differentiated or infiltrating lesions.

Surgery remains a viable treatment option for Stage I lesions involving the upper vaginal fornices. The procedure usually consists of a radical hysterectomy, pelvic lymphadenectomy, and partial vaginectomy.

Patients with Stage I clear-cell adenocarcinoma of the vagina may also be treated surgically. The procedure includes periaortic-node biopsies to assess possible extrapelvic lymphatic involvement, followed by vaginectomy with frozen-section biopsies to define the lower margins of surgical resection. This step is critical, since a common pathologic feature of clear-cell adenocarcinoma is microscopic subepithelial extension. Pelvic lymphadenectomy and radical hysterectomy are then performed, followed by vaginal reconstruction. Some authors advocate intracavitary irradiation rather than surgery for these lesions because of the similar control rates and the preservation of the vagina and ovaries that is possible with irradiation.

Stages II–IV

Radiation therapy is the standard treatment for patients with Stages II–IV vaginal cancer. External-beam radiation therapy is followed by intracavitary and/or interstitial therapy. Lesions of the distal one-third of the vagina are associated with a high frequency of inguinal nodal metastases. Gross adenopathy is usually resected, followed by irradiation.

Treatment of nonepithelial lesions

The optimal treatment of vaginal melanoma remains illusive. These lesions are highly aggressive, and survival after radical surgical resection remains dismal.

Table 12.1 Treatment of vaginal cancer by stage

Stage	Treatment
0	Surgical excision, laser ablation, and, in some cases, 5-fluorouracil
I	Lesions of the upper vaginal fornices: • Radical hysterectomy, pelvic lymphadenectomy, and upper vaginectomy; or • Radiation therapy consisting of intracavitary cylinder and/or interstitial implant with/without whole-pelvic radiation therapy
II, III, IV	• External-beam radiation therapy and intracavitary and/or interstitial therapy • Treatment of the groin if lower one-third of vagina involved with tumor
Recurrent	Treatment depends on extent of recurrence. Options include: • Wide local excision • Partial vaginectomy • Exenteration • Chemotherapy

Some authors perform wide local excision followed by irradiation. Recently, the addition of bioimmunotherapeutic agents to wide local excision and irradiation has been advocated.

Rhabdomyosarcoma of the vagina is treated with combination chemotherapy consisting of vincristine, dactinomycin, and cyclophosphamide (VAC), with or without radiation therapy. Radical surgery may be avoided in many patients owing to the efficacy of the above treatment regimen (Table 12.1).

PROGNOSIS

The prognosis is dependent upon the stage of the disease (Table 12.2).

Table 12.2 Five-year survival rate by stage

Stage	Survival rate (%)
I	80
II	45
III	35
IV	10

THERAPY FOR PERSISTENT OR RECURRENT DISEASE

The majority of recurrences appear within 2 years of primary therapy and are located in the pelvis. Locally recurrent or persistent vaginal cancer following irradiation can be treated with surgery; options range from wide local excision to exenteration. The numbers are too small to comment on specific cure rates. Although cisplatin chemotherapy may have a role to play in the treatment of recurrent disease, most patients who recur in a previously irradiated field do not respond to chemotherapy.

FUTURE THERAPY

Owing to the rarity of this disease, it is virtually impossible to conduct prospective, randomized studies. Future collaborative efforts should focus on the use of hypoxic sensitizers for radiation therapy, as well as the need for effective chemotherapeutic regimens.

SELECTED READING

Berek JS, Hacker NF, *Practical Gynecologic Oncology*, 2nd edn. Baltimore: Williams & Wilkins, 1994: 441.

Delclos L, Wharton JT, Rutledge FN, Tumors of the vagina and female urethra. In: *Textbook of Radiotherapy*, 3rd edn (Fletcher GH, ed). Philadelphia: Lea and Febiger, 1980: 812.

DiSaia PJ, Creasman WT, *Clinical Gynecologic Oncology*, 5th edn. St Louis: Mosby-Year Book, 1997: 233.

Herbst AL, Robboy SJ, Scully RE et al, Clear-cell adenocarcinoma of the vagina and cervix in girls: analysis of 170 registry cases. *Am J Obstet Gynecol* 1974; **119**: 713.

Kucera H, Vavra N, Radiation management of primary carcinoma of the vagina: clinical and histopathological variables associated with survival. *Gynecol Oncol* 1991; **40**: 12.

Morrow CR, Curtin JP, Townsend DE, *Synopsis of Gynecologic Oncology*, 4th edn. New York: Churchill Livingstone, 1993: 93.

Perez CA, Camel HM, Galakatos AE et al, Definitive irradiation in carcinoma of the vagina: long-term evaluation of results. *Int J Radiat Oncol Biol Phys* 1988; **15**: 1283.

Stock RG, Chen AS, Seski J, A 30-year experience in the management of primary carcinoma of the vagina: analysis of prognostic factors and treatment modalities. *Gynecol Oncol* 1995; **56**: 45.

Wilkinson EJ, Premalignant and malignant tumors of the vulva. In: *Blaustein's Pathology of the Female Genital Tract*, 4th edn (Kurman RJ, ed). New York: Springer-Verlag, 1994: 97.

13
Cervical cancer

Charles Levenback

The management of patients with cervical cancer is at the core of gynecologic oncology. Multidisciplinary planning is vital to optimize treatment selection. Superior surgical skills are required to perform radical hysterectomy and pelvic exenteration safely. Intimate knowledge of chemotherapy administration is mandatory in order to treat primary disease and recurrent disease. Finally, outstanding communication skills are recognized as essential in the care of dying patients, many of whom have young families and all of whom benefit from discussion of disease progression and end-of-life decision making.

EPIDEMIOLOGY

There were almost 12,900 new cases of cervical cancer and 4,400 deaths from the disease in the USA in 2001. The number of deaths in North America has been decreasing since the introduction of cytological screening in the 1940s. Unfortunately, this downward trend has flattened out in recent years, at least in part due to the persistence of unscreened populations. These include patients over 60 years of age and those in lower socioeconomic groups. Over 50% of patients with cervical cancer have not had a Pap smear within 5 years of diagnosis. Although cervical cancer is relatively uncommon in North America, it remains the most common malignancy among women in countries as diverse as Colombia and Vietnam.

One unusual aspect of cervical cancer is that it bears features of a sexually transmitted disease. Risk factors for the development of cervical cancer are listed in Table 13.1. Gonorrhea, genital herpes, and chlamydia have all been implicated in the past; however, the most recent molecular research indicates that incorporation of the E6 and E7 genes from human papillomavirus (HPV) into cells results in malignant transformation in over 90% of patients with cervical cancer. There are numerous HPV subtypes, with the high-risk subtypes 16, 18, 31, and 41 being those most commonly associated with malignancy.

It is estimated that over six million American women are infected with HPV, yet a relatively small proportion develop cancer. It is assumed that other

Table 13.1   Risk factors for the development of cervical cancer
• Infections with HPV • Multiple sexual partners • Early age of coitarche • Short interval between menarche and coitarche • Smoking • Sexual contact with men who have had partners with cervical cancer

factors, such as smoking, vitamin deficiency, and immunocompromise, play a role in the development of invasive disease.

In North America, cervical cancer is twice as common among black women as among white women. Black women with cervical cancer are three times as likely to die from their disease as white women. This "mortality gap" persists when mortality is controlled for demographic characteristics, prognostic factors, and type of treatment. These data suggest that improvements in screening alone may not close the mortality gap, and more data are needed to explain these survival differences among black and white women.

HISTOLOGIC SUBTYPES

The histologic subtypes of cervical cancer are listed in Table 13.2. In patients with invasive squamous carcinoma detected by cone biopsy, a depth of invasion from the nearest rete peg or full tumor thickness should be reported. The presence or absence of lymph vascular space (LVS) should be described, although there is no agreed-upon methodology to quantify the extent of LVS. The majority of squamous carcinomas are high-grade. Verrucous carcinoma is a form of low-grade carcinoma, which is of note because the tumor does not respond to radiation therapy.

There is a wide range in the biologic activity of adenocarcinomas of the cervix. Adenoma malignum is a very low-grade malignancy, and metastases are very rare. Poorly differentiated adenocarcinomas are highly malignant, and regional and distant metastases are much more common.

Recent changes in the nomenclature of neuroendocrine and small-cell tumors have led to some confusion among clinicians. There is a range of aggressiveness among neuroendocrine tumors, from carcinoid, which has a low risk of metastatic disease, to neuroendocrine tumors, which are highly malignant. Small-cell carcinomas are not the same as neuroendocrine tumors; however, both are very aggressive, with a high risk of metastasis and death from even the smallest tumor.

Table 13.2 World Health Organization classification of cervical cancer

Squamous-cell carcinoma
Keratinizing
Nonkeratinizing
Verrucous
Papillary transitional
Lymphoepithelioma-like

Adenocarcinoma (glandular)
Mucinous:
   Cervical-type
   Intestinal-type
   Signet-ring
Endometrioid
Clear-cell
Minimal deviation (adenoma malignum)
Well-differentiated villoglandular (papillary)
Serous
Mesonephric

Other epithelial
Adenosquamous
Glassy-cell
Adenoid cystic
Adenoid basal
Carcinoid tumor (adenocarcinoma with features of carcinoid)
Small-cell
Undifferentiated

Mixed histology is common in the cervix. Adenosquamous carcinomas are the most common mixture, and the adenocarcinoma is invariably high grade. In addition, high-grade adenocarcinomas can have a neuroendocrine component.

PATTERNS OF SPREAD

Local invasion

Primary tumors can be exophytic, filling the vagina, but with minimal involvement of the cervical stroma. Endophytic tumors can result in massive expansion of the endocervix, with no visible tumor. Tumor can infiltrate along the uterosacral ligaments and parametrium. The bladder and ureters are immediately adjacent to the cervix. Ureteral obstruction usually occurs along the pelvic sidewall owing to compression by the primary or enlarged lymph nodes. Bladder invasion is uncommon; however, bullous edema of the bladder is a

Table 13.3 Incidence of nodal metastases by stage		
Stage	Positive pelvic nodes (%)	Positive para-aortic nodes (%)
IA$_1$	0	0
IA$_2$ (1–3 mm)	<1.0	0
IA$_2$ (3–5 mm)	4.8	<1.0
IB	16	2
IIA	25	11
III	45	30
IVA	55	40

common cystoscopic finding in patients with advanced-stage disease. Rectal invasion is relatively uncommon.

Lymphatic

The risk of lymphatic spread from the cervix corresponds to the depth of invasion (Table 13.3). In general, it is stated that spread to the pelvic nodes occurs before para-aortic nodal metastases occur. Since the cervix is a midline structure, metastases can occur equally to both the right and left pelvis. Para-aortic metastases can be quite painful. Patients describe back and flank pain that can radiate towards the pelvis. The thoracic duct originates near the abdominal aorta, traverses the chest, and joins the left subclavian vein; accordingly, the supraclavicular nodes can be a site of metastases and should be palpated carefully during the physical examination of all patients with cervical cancer. Treatment for invasive cervical cancer is usually regional and includes the primary nodal basin of the pelvis.

Hematogenous

Hematogenous spread is a late finding in squamous carcinoma of the cervix. The primary is usually quite advanced if liver or lung metastases are present at the time of diagnosis. Hematogenous spread is much more likely in patients with high-grade adenocarcinomas, or neuroendocrine or small-cell tumors. The metastatic workup of patients with small-cell cancer should include a bone scan and a computed tomography (CT) scan of the brain for this reason. Brain and bone metastases are very uncommon in patients with non-small-cell cancers, even late in the natural history of the disease.

Intraperitoneal

Intraperitoneal spread of cervical cancer usually results from erosion of the tumor through the uterosacral ligaments or back wall of the cervix. It is not known how often this occurs in patients with advanced-stage disease, since most do not undergo transperitoneal surgical staging. Actual intraperitoneal metastases indicate a very poor prognosis. Survival following recognition of disease in the abdomen is very rare.

PRESENTATION OF DISEASE

Symptoms

Most patients with early-stage cervical cancer are asymptomatic, and cytologic screening discovers their disease. Patients with more advanced Stage I tumors typically have symptoms related to disruption of the cervical mucosa. These include some type of abnormal vaginal bleeding, including postcoital bleeding or a watery or foul discharge. As the tumor becomes larger and necrotic, the discharge will become fouler and the bleeding heavier. Before the tumor reaches the pelvic sidewall, ureteral obstruction can occur. In most patients, this is asymptomatic, although flank pain can occur. Hip, buttock, and sciatic pain and unilateral leg swelling are signs of pelvic sidewall involvement. The pain is usually described as constant gnawing and is not relieved by positional change.

Bladder invasion is usually accompanied by symptoms of urinary frequency or hematuria. Rectal involvement at presentation is rare, but when it occurs is associated with blood and mucus in the rectum.

Physical examination

Physical examination remains the single most important staging procedure. A speculum exam should always be performed with care so as not to fracture the tumor and initiate bleeding. A single finger in the vagina can help locate the cervix and guide the insertion of the speculum. A sponge can be used to blot the cervix in order to improve visualization, with care being taken not to traumatize the cervix, as indicated above. A Graves speculum is recommended whenever possible to allow better visualization than can be achieved with a Peterson speculum.

When the speculum exam has been completed, a digital exam is performed. Insert both fingers in the vagina and palpate the cervix. Detect if there is spread to the fornices or vagina that was missed on speculum exam. Estimate the diameter of the cervix in centimeters. Try to detect any endocervical expansion. With these findings in mind, perform a rectovaginal examination. Failure to do a rectal exam in a patient with cervical cancer is the mark of an inexperienced or incompetent examiner. Once again, estimate the diameter of the cervix. Palpate the parametrium and, if possible, the uterosacral ligaments for tumor infiltration. These findings can be quite subtle, even for experienced examiners. With the fingers as lateral as possible, sweep along the pelvic sidewall. An examiner using the right hand to do the rectovaginal exam will palpate the patient's right pelvic sidewall with ease, but he/she may have trouble reaching the left sidewall in a patient with a large tumor. In this case, the examiner should examine the left pelvic sidewall with his/her left hand.

Physical findings should be recorded in the medical record immediately. In this regard, an annotated drawing is an excellent method, since it facilitates communication between consultants.

Biopsy, not exfoliative cytology, is the definitive diagnostic test. A Pap smear in a patient with a visible lesion is a waste of time, since blood and inflammatory cells can obscure the situation, and false-negative smears occur in up to 40% of patients in this category. Excessive bleeding from a punch biopsy is rare. When this does occur, ensure that there is adequate visualization, which usually requires a Graves speculum, and apply pressure with a sponge stick for 3–5 minutes. In most cases, the bleeding will have subsided, and a small amount of Monsels solution (ferrous subsulfate) will be adequate to assure hemostasis. In rare cases, an arterial bleeder will be visible. Apply pressure and then Monsels solution as described above. If the bleeding persists, a small but tight pack at the apex of the vagina will stop the bleeding. Remove the pack in 24–36 hours. In rare cases, an exam under anesthesia will be necessary to suture the site and obtain hemostasis.

STAGING

Staging of cervical cancer is based on palpatory findings and some widely available diagnostic tests. Since many patients are never operated on, there is no surgical staging system for cervical cancer. For this reason, nodal status, a powerful prognostic factor, is not included in staging.

Patients with microinvasion, as defined by the Society of Gynecologic Oncologists (SGO), who are to be treated with cone biopsy or hysterectomy do not require staging beyond the routine preoperative testing for these procedures.

All patients with a visible lesion should undergo staging as outlined in the FIGO staging for cervical cancer (see Appendix 3 of this handbook). Patients with more advanced disease should be considered for the studies listed in Table 13.4. Cystoscopy and proctoscopy are required in patients with bulky tumors. Skeletal x-rays, a bone scan, a CT scan of the brain, etc., should be considered only in patients with symptoms.

The best imaging method to identify nodal metastases is a lymphangiography. This technique images the internal structure of the lymph nodes, which is something none of the other noninvasive studies can achieve. Unfortunately, the examination is difficult to perform and is not widely available.

CT depends on nodal size to identify metastases. Since nodes may appear enlarged due to inflammation, it is not as reliable as lymphangiography. On the other hand, CT images the primary tumor (a lymphangiogram does not) and evaluates the renal units for hydronephrosis and hydroureter.

Table 13.4 Workup for patients with visible cervical cancer

All patients
- History and physical examination
- Cervix biopsy
- Complete blood count, serum glucose, liver- and renal-function tests
- Chest x-ray

Common optional studies
- Examination under anesthesia
- CT or MRI of abdomen and pelvis
- Lymphangiogram
- Intravenous pyelogram
- Cystoscopy
- Proctoscopy
- Barium enema
- Skeletal x-rays
- CT or MRI of the brain

Magnetic resonance imaging (MRI) provides the most accurate image of the primary tumor, and it is especially useful in patients with adenocarcinoma about whom there is some question whether they have Stage I cervical cancer or Stage II endometrial cancer. MRI has replaced CT as the single imaging study of choice at the MD Anderson Cancer Center.

A promising new technology for the identification of small nodal metastases is positron emission tomography (PET). Additional, "biologic" imaging studies are in development. Use of these studies remains limited due to cost and availability.

Examination under anesthesia

Prior to widespread availability of CT scanning technology, examination under anesthesia (EUA) was commonly used to stage patients; a cystoscopy and a proctoscopy were commonly performed at the same time. This was an expensive diagnostic procedure – and unnecessary in the case of most patients. Nevertheless, there are patients for whom an EUA will provide very useful information regarding appropriate staging and treatment planning that could not be obtained by other means.

Surgical staging

None of the imaging studies can detect microscopic disease in the lymph nodes, peritoneal cavity, or parametrium. This is the rationale behind surgical staging. Extensive transperitoneal staging combined with extended-field irradiation results in a high incidence of radiation-related bowel injury. A complete retroperitoneal approach will prevent such complications, with the same or better sampling of lymph nodes. Surgical staging may be of greatest significance in patients found, in imaging studies, to have positive pelvic nodes and negative para-aortic nodes. Such patients are at high risk for microscopic para-aortic metastases. Surgical staging can help define the irradiation field for these patients.

Lymphatic mapping

Several small studies have suggested that lymphatic mapping and sentinel-node identification is feasible in radical hysterectomy patients. Laparoscopic sentinel-node identification is possible, expanding the possibilities for less invasive surgical staging. Although promising, lymphatic mapping remains investigational at present.

TREATMENT (Figure 13.1)

Microinvasion

The most practical and clinically useful definition of microinvasion was adopted by the SGO in 1974. Tumors less than 3 mm in depth without lymph-vascular space invasion and negative cone margins are in this category, which overlaps FIGO Stages IA1 and IA2. Although the case series are small, cone biopsy is considered adequate for patients who desire to preserve reproductive options. Hysterectomy – vaginal or abdominal – is the definitive treatment for patients for whom reproductive capability is no longer a desired option.

Stages IB1, IB2, and IIA

Stage IB covers a very wide range of risk categories. This range of risk categories, combined with the complexity of both radical surgery and radical irradiation, makes treatment planning for this group especially challenging. In general, patients with tumor limited to the cervix are candidates for irradiation or surgery. The best candidates for surgery have smaller tumors (Stage IB1), are at low risk for requiring postoperative irradiation (based on physical examination and diagnostic imaging), and are good surgical candidates (based on performance status and body habitus). Patients with larger tumors (Stage IB2) who are treated with radical surgery have a very high risk (up to 80%) of having an indication for postoperative irradiation. In addition, recent trials suggest that patients with tumors 5 cm or larger benefit from chemoradiation compared with irradiation alone.

Laparoscopically assisted radical trachelectomy and pelvic lymphadenectomy is a new option for women with small Stage IB1 tumors who wish to preserve reproductive choices. This procedure is becoming more widely available

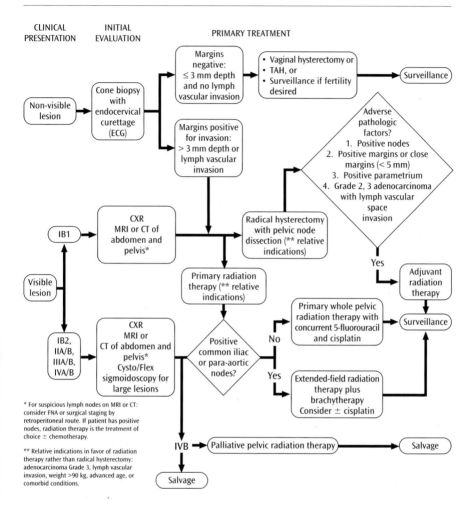

CLINICAL
PRESENTATION

INITIAL
EVALUATION

PRIMARY TREATMENT

Non-visible lesion → Cone biopsy with endocervical curettage (ECG)

Margins negative: ≤ 3 mm depth and no lymph vascular invasion → • Vaginal hysterectomy or • TAH, or • Surveillance if fertility desired → Surveillance

Margins positive for invasion: > 3 mm depth or lymph vascular invasion

Adverse pathologic factors?
1. Positive nodes
2. Positive margins or close margins (< 5 mm)
3. Positive parametrium
4. Grade 2, 3 adenocarcinoma with lymph vascular space invasion

Radical hysterectomy with pelvic node dissection (** relative indications)

Yes → Adjuvant radiation therapy → Surveillance

IB1 → CXR MRI or CT of abdomen and pelvis*

Visible lesion

IB2, IIA/B, IIIA/B, IVA/B → CXR MRI or CT of abdomen and pelvis* Cysto/Flex sigmoidoscopy for large lesions

Primary radiation therapy (** relative indications)

Positive common iliac or para-aortic nodes?

No → Primary whole pelvic radiation therapy with concurrent 5-fluorouracil and cisplatin → Surveillance

Yes → Extended-field radiation therapy plus brachytherapy Consider ± cisplatin

IVB → Palliative pelvic radiation therapy → Salvage

Salvage

* For suspicious lymph nodes on MRI or CT: consider FNA or surgical staging by retroperitoneal route. If patient has positive nodes, radiation therapy is the treatment of choice ± chemotherapy.

** Relative indications in favor of radiation therapy rather than radical hysterectomy: adenocarcinoma Grade 3, lymph vascular invasion, weight >90 kg, advanced age, or comorbid conditions.

Figure 13.1
Treatment guidelines for cervical cancer.

in the USA, although experience in this country is limited. Excellent survival and pregnancy rates have been reported from France and Canada. American gynecologic oncologists are beginning to embrace this procedure.

Pelvic control rates among patients with Stage IB2 tumors receiving optimal radiation therapy are outstanding. Unfortunately, not all patients have access to optimal radiation therapy services. Patterns of Care studies have, over the years, documented the infrequency with which the majority of radiation oncologists in practice perform intracavitary insertions for cervical cancer. In addition, deviations from commonly accepted treatment standards are common among radiation oncologists who treat cervical cancer patients on an infrequent basis. Finally, because of the duration of the treatment, referral to a tertiary-care center is not always practical for radiation therapy; however, it may be practical for radical surgery. Each practice setting is different, and, rightly or wrongly, this will influence treatment planning.

The extent of vaginal involvement usually determines the best option for patients with Stage IIA cancer. Patients with minimal superficial involvement of the vaginal fornix remain candidates for radical surgery, whereas patients with infiltrative vaginal involvement are better suited for radiation therapy. It should be noted that the vaginal fornices generally flatten with age, making it more difficult to get adequate margins in older patients with vaginal involvement.

Some patients with Stage IB disease have lymph-node metastases suspected on diagnostic imaging. Suspicious nodes should be biopsied, usually by CT-guided fine-needle aspiration. If lymph-node metastases are confirmed, then chemoradiation, as described below, should be recommended. Another option is retroperitoneal staging. If there is a positive pelvic node, the risk of microscopic para-aortic disease increases, and this will only be detected surgically. Para-aortic nodal status in patients with known pelvic metastases is vital for appropriate radiation-field design.

What should be done if suspicious lymph nodes are encountered during radical hysterectomy? If a frozen-section analysis confirms metastatic disease, then we recommend completing the staging procedures – in particular with node dissection superior to the site of the positive node – but not proceeding with radical hysterectomy. These patients are candidates for chemoradiation, and further surgery increases the risk of complications and cost without improving survival. On the other hand, Peters et al demonstrated excellent survival for radical hysterectomy patients with positive nodes who received postoperative chemoradiation.

What about radical-hysterectomy patients with negative nodes but high-risk features? Patients with positive or close margins should receive postoperative radiation therapy, possibly with chemotherapy.

What about patients with deep stromal invasion and extensive lymph vascular involvement with negative nodes and margins? A recent Gynecologic Oncology Group (GOG) trial suggested that postoperative radiation therapy improved survival for such patients at the cost of increased complications.

Stages IIB and III

Patients with locally advanced disease are excellent candidates for chemoradiation. Several recent randomized clinical trials have confirmed that the combination of chemotherapy and radiation therapy is superior to pelvic irradiation alone, extended-field irradiation, or hysterectomy plus irradiation. The best chemotherapy regimen has not been determined except that it is platinum-based. Patients with disease limited to the pelvis can receive cisplatin and 5-fluorouracil (5-FU) or weekly cisplatin (Tables 13.5 and 13.6). Chemotherapy

---

Table 13.5 Cisplatin–5-FU treatment schedule

- Place central venous catheter
- Calculated creatinine clearance >50 ml/hr
- Cisplatin 75 mg/m^2 days 1 and 21
- 5-FU 1,000 mg/m^2 per day = 4,000 mg/m^2 over 96 hrs by ambulatory infusion pump (maximum dose 8,000 mg) days 2–5 and 22–25
- Third course of chemotherapy with second intracavitary system if counts and performance permit
- Routine hydration and antiemetics
- 25–50% dose reduction of 5-FU for significant myelosuppression

---

Table 13.6 Weekly cisplatin treatment schedule

- Calculated creatinine clearance >50 ml/hr
- Cisplatin 40 mg/m^2 weekly starting day 1
- Maximum dose 70 mg/week
- Most patients receive 4–6 cycles
- Routine hydration and antiemetics

---

is difficult to combine with extended-field irradiation owing to myelosuppression and nausea. In some patients with a good performance, extended-field irradiation and weekly cisplatin can be given safely.

The cisplatin–5-FU regimen was an arm in the RTOG (Radiation Therapy Oncology Group) 90-01 study. This regimen was based on RTOG experience with this combination in patients with squamous carcinoma of the anus. An important feature is that chemotherapy is given along with the second brachytherapy application. This regimen requires some sort of long-term venous access, a feature that adds expense and some risk of line infections.

The weekly cisplatin regimen was an arm of GOG 120. The GOG had previously shown a benefit to hydroxyurea given with irradiation; however, the results of that study were widely questioned. GOG 120 found that hydroxyurea and adjuvant hysterectomy did not add to the benefit of weekly cisplatin alone. In this protocol, 17.5% of patients received 4 or fewer cycles of cisplatin, 33.5% received 5 cycles, and approximately 49% received 6 or more cycles. Patients did not receive chemotherapy during the brachytherapy.

Management of anemia and total treatment duration are two additional factors that may impact outcomes in patients with advanced cervix cancer. A retrospective Canadian study of patients treated with radiotherapy alone, found improved outcomes for patients with mean average hemoglobin levels greater than 120 g/L, compared with patients with lower levels. The average treatment duration in the Canadian study was 51 days compared with RTOG 90–01 (58 days) and GOG 120 (63 days).

SPECIAL CONSIDERATIONS

Ureteral obstruction

Patients with bulky Stage IIIB tumors may present with ureteral obstruction. Patients with bilateral obstruction require some sort of intervention to preserve renal function. Ureteral stents are ideal, but they can be quite difficult in patients with large tumors. Percutaneous nephrostomy tubes are an alternative. Patients with unilateral obstruction usually do not require either of these procedures, with their associated risks of bleeding and infection, to have adequate renal function in order to receive radiation therapy. Now that many such patients are receiving cisplatin-based chemoradiation, a stent or nephrostomy tube may be appropriate to optimize renal function.

Vaginal bleeding

Vaginal bleeding is a common symptom of cervical cancer; it is usually exacerbated by the several pelvic examinations that occur during the diagnosis and evaluation phases of treatment. Low-energy transvaginal radiation therapy can be used in this situation to control the bleeding. The use of Monsels solution and packing are short-term solutions for urgent situations. In rare cases, a single arterial bleeder can be controlled only by ligation during an examination under anesthesia. More invasive measures, such as arterial embolization, are virtually never appropriate in this situation.

It has been suggested recently that the standard recommendation of maintaining hemoglobin levels at 10 g/dl is inadequate and a better goal is 12 g/dl. Further study is still required to determine if the use of recombinant erythropoietin is a valuable addition to the treatment plan in patients undergoing radiation therapy.

Fistulae

Vesicovaginal or rectovaginal fistulae are rare at the time of diagnosis. They can be very problematic, causing hygiene problems and difficulty packing around the brachytherapy applicator at the time of insertion. Patients with fistulae should receive 40-Gy external-beam therapy along with chemotherapy and then be re-evaluated by a radiation oncologist and gynecologic oncologist. In selected patients, pelvic exenteration is appropriate at this point.

Large uterine fibroids

Occasionally, a patient has uterine fibroids that extend outside the pelvic field. This creates the potential hazard of a partially irradiated uterus. In this situation, external irradiation and one 72-hour low-dose-rate application followed by extrafascial hysterectomy is a useful treatment plan. Patients with a normal-sized uterus do not benefit from hysterectomy as part of the treatment plan, and should receive the standard two low-dose-rate brachytherapy insertions or equivalent.

Palliative treatment

Some patients, particularly the elderly, present with very advanced disease and a very poor performance status. In these patients, the risk of the standard treatments is excessive, however much the patient is suffering with bleeding, foul discharge, and pain. There are several palliative regimens to consider, the simplest of which is two 10-Gy fractions 1 month apart. This regimen is highly effective at controlling symptoms very rapidly and is ideal for patients travelling a long distance for treatment. An alternative for patients close to the treatment center is 3-Gy fractions for 2 weeks.

Neoadjuvant chemotherapy

There was much enthusiasm for this approach in the past few years, prior to the publication of the chemoradiation results discussed above. There were patients who responded in dramatic fashion to neoadjuvant chemotherapy, which allowed reduction in the radicality of the radiation or permitted radical surgery to be performed. Unfortunately, there were also patients who progressed during the neoadjuvant chemotherapy and in whom the required radiation therapy was unnecessarily delayed, with poor consequences. We believe that there is no standard role for neoadjuvant chemotherapy at present.

High-dose-rate brachytherapy

Gynecologic oncologists should be aware of the debate among radiation oncologists concerning the pros and cons of low-dose-rate versus high-dose-rate brachytherapy. Low-dose-rate brachytherapy is the traditional method that requires placement in the operating room and 72 hours of immobilization. Low-dose-rate brachytherapy is more flexible and requires only brief periods of immobilization. Due to the substantial investment this equipment represents, most centers use one or the other.

SURVEILLANCE

The typical surveillance guidelines for patients treated for invasive cervical cancer are shown in Table 13.7. Recent studies suggest that Pap smears rarely identify patients with recurrent disease that would not have been recognized owing to the appearance of a new symptom or detected on a routine pelvic examination. On the other hand, patients who have isolated pulmonary metastases identified on chest x-ray have several treatment options and longer

---

Table 13.7 Cervical cancer post-treatment surveillance

Post cone biopsy
- Pap and ECC every 3–4 months × 2 years
- Pap every 6 months × 3 years
- Annual thereafter

Post TAH or TVH
- Pap every 6 months × 2 years
- Annual thereafter

Post radical surgery or radiation therapy
Year 1
- Exam every 3 months, Pap and chest x-ray annually
Year 2
- Exam every 3 months, chest x-ray biannually, Pap annually
Years 3 and 4
- Exam every 6 months, chest x-ray biannually, Pap annually
Year 5
- Exam every 6 months, chest x-ray and Pap annually

---

survival than patients with recurrences at other locations. This statistical evidence has led to a shift in our surveillance guidelines, with a de-emphasis on Pap smears and an increase in our recommendation of chest x-rays.

RECURRENT DISEASE

Up to 80% of recurrences occur in the first 2 years following primary treatment. Recurrences after 5 years do occur, although they are rare. When a squamous carcinoma appears in the vagina more than 5 years following radiation therapy, it most likely represents a second primary rather that a true recurrence.

Recurrence following radical hysterectomy

Pelvic recurrence following radical hysterectomy should be treated with radiation therapy. This usually includes a combination of external-beam therapy and brachytherapy. The brachytherapy portion can be as simple as a vaginal-dome cylinder or as complicated as an iridium-needle implant. At the very least, patients in this category should be referred to a major center for consultation with a radiation oncologist experienced in this type of treatment.

Central recurrence

An isolated central recurrence or the appearance of a second primary following pelvic irradiation is an indication for pelvic exenteration. This is the only treatment with the potential for long-term survival in this category. Patients with hip or buttock pain, ureteral obstruction, or unilateral lymphedema are poor candidates because of the high risk of unresectability. Nevertheless, because of the poor alternatives, exploration should be considered if there is no obvious contraindication. MRI is especially helpful in the preoperative evaluation of these patients, although the previous pelvic irradiation can make interpretation difficult. We do not perform routine supraclavicular biopsy, although some investigators have recommended this approach. The most important surgical consideration is that an adequate margin is obtained, and partial exenteration should not be done if this will leave a doubtful margin.

The concept of palliative exenteration has been proposed for patients with symptomatic disease and microscopically positive para-aortic lymph nodes or anticipated positive or close margins. We believe that, despite advances in critical care, blood banking, and surgical and anesthetic techniques, pelvic exenteration remains a dangerous operation and should be reserved for patients who can be cured by the operation. Whatever improvement in quality of life is gained by the exenteration, if any, is offset by surgical complications and recurrence following the procedure.

Pelvic-wall recurrence

Pelvic-wall recurrence is devastating. It is painful and frequently results in unilateral lower-extremity edema. In addition, the response rate to any one of a variety of chemotherapeutic compounds is in the single digits. In highly selective cases, some sort of radioactive implant may be appropriate. Some investigators have recommended combined approaches including partial resection and local radiation therapy. This combined approach has not gained acceptance and should be considered investigational.

Extrapelvic recurrence

The treatment options for these patients are much wider than for patients with pelvic-wall recurrence. A common site for recurrence is the para-aortic lymph nodes. This can be confirmed by fine-needle aspiration, and response to chemotherapy is easy to assess with CT. Assuming that the field was not previously irradiated, the pain associated with recurrence at this site can respond well to a short course of external-beam irradiation.

If, following a complete evaluation, an isolated recurrence is found in the lung or brain, consideration should be given to resection. Factors such as interval to recurrence, histology, performance, and initial stage should all be taken into account, since it is a highly selective group of patients for whom this approach is appropriate. Despite the seemingly poor prognosis, there are occasional patients who achieve long-term remission following resection of an isolated metastasis with or without regional radiation therapy or chemotherapy.

Chemotherapy

There are over 60 compounds that have been studied in Phase II trials in patients with recurrent cervical cancer. Despite this exhaustive search, there are no drugs whose profiles show them to be clearly superior. Most investigators and clinicians have identified cisplatin as the single most active drug in this category of patients. Up to 50% of patients receiving cisplatin as a single agent derive some benefit. Perhaps 10% have a complete response, 20% have a partial response, and perhaps an additional 20% have a minor response or stabilization of disease. With dosing in the 50–75 mg/m^2 range and with modern hydration and antiemetic regimens, the complications of cisplatin are manageable. Most clinicians consider carboplatin interchangeable with cisplatin, although this has not been fully established in patients with recurrent squamous carcinoma. There have been many efforts to combine cisplatin with a second agent in order to increase response rates (Table 13.8). For the most part, a second agent adds toxicity without making a significant contribution to improving survival. Multiagent chemotherapy in this patient population should be reserved for clinical trials.

Paclitaxel is an attractive drug in the treatment of recurrent adenocarcinomas of the cervix given its favorable profile in patients with adenocarcinomas of the ovary and breast. Despite this superficial similarity, however, paclitaxel has not proved a major advance in the treatment of recurrent cervical cancer.

Table 13.8 Selected chemotherapy agents studied in Phase II trials for cervical cancer with response rates over 20%

Cisplatin
Ifosfamide
Bleomycin
Vincristine
5-Fluorouracil
Irinotecan (CPT-11)
Vinorelbine
Melphalan

Table 13.9 Steps for breaking bad news

1. Get setting right
2. Find out how much the patient knows
3. Find out what the patient wants to know
4. Sharing the information, educating
5. Respond to the patient's feelings
6. Planning and follow-through

BREAKING BAD NEWS

The American Society of Clinical Oncologists (ASCO) and others have recently focused energy on an often overlooked aspect of clinical training: communicating bad news to patients. Recurrent cervical cancer can occur in the most heartbreaking situations. There are simple steps that can help even inexperienced clinicians communicate bad news in the most caring and sensitive way possible (Table 13.9). Sensitive communication is the first step in discussing advanced-care planning with patients. Over a series of visits, patient preferences regarding DNR ("Do Not Resuscitate") status and hospice care can be discussed. This allows the patient, if she desires, to have an active role in planning her care, and it affords her the opportunity to prioritize her activities while her health permits.

SELECTED READING

Averette HE, Nguyen HN, Donato DM et al, Radical hysterectomy for invasive cervical cancer. A 25-year prospective experience with the Miami technique. *Cancer* 1993; **71**: 1422.

Brader KR, Morris M, Levenback C et al, Chemotherapy for cervical carcinoma: factors determining response and implications for clinical trial design. *J Clin Oncol* 1998; **16**: 1879.

Dargent D, Brun JL, Roy M et al, Pregnancies following radical trachelectomy for invasive cervical cancer. *Gynecol Oncol* 1994; **52**:105.

Delgado G, Bundy BN, Fowler WC Jr et al, Prospective surgical pathological study of stage I squamous carcinoma of the cervix: a Gynecologic Oncology Group study. *Gynecol Oncol* 1989; **36**: 314.

Eifel PJ, Morris M, Irradiation alone or combined with surgery in carcinoma of the cervix: When will we know the answer? *Int J Radiat Oncol Biol Phys* 1995; **31**: 1007.

Grogan M, Thomas GM, Melamed I et al, The importance of hemoglobin levels during radiotherapy for carcinoma of the cervix. *Cancer* 1999; **86**: 1528.

Heller PB, Maletano JH, Bundy BN et al, Clinical–pathologic study of stage IIB, III, and IVA carcinoma of the cervix: extended diagnostic evaluation for paraaortic node metastasis. Gynecologic Oncology Group study. *Gynecol Oncol* 1990; **38**: 425.

Levenback C, Coleman RC, Burke TW et al, Lymphatic mapping and sentinel node identification in patients with cervix cancer undergoing radical hysterectomy and pelvic lymphadenectomy. *J Clin Oncol* 2002; **20**: 688–93.

Morris M, Eifel PJ, Lu J et al, Pelvic radiation with concurrent chemotherapy compared with pelvic and paraaortic radiation for high-risk cervical cancer. *N Engl J Med* 1999; **340**: 1137.

Peters WA, III, Liu PY, Barret RJ et al, Concurrent chemotherapy and pelvic radiation therapy compared with pelvic radiation therapy alone as adjuvant therapy after radical surgery in high-risk early-stage cancer of the cervix. *J Clin Oncol* 2000; **18**: 1606.

Potish RA, Downey GO, Adcock LL et al, The role of surgical debulking in cancer of the uterine cervix. *Int J Radiat Oncol Biol Phys* 1989; **17**: 979.

Rose PG, Bundy BN, Watkins EB et al, Concurrent cisplatin-based chemotherapy and radiotherapy for locally advanced cervical cancer. *N Engl J Med* 1999; **340**: 1144.

Rotman M, Choi K, Guse C et al, Prophylactic irradiation of the para-aortic lymph node chain in Stage IIB and bulky Stage IIB carcinoma of the cervix, initial treatment results of RTOG 7920. *Int J Radiat Oncol Biol Phys* 1990; **19**: 513.

Thigpen JT, Chemotherapy as a palliative treatment in carcinoma of the uterine cervix. *Semin Oncol* 1995; **22**: 16.

Weiser EB, Bundy BN, Hoskins WJ et al, Extraperitoneal versus transperitoneal selective paraaortic lymphadenectomy in the pretreatment surgical staging of advanced cervical carcinoma (a Gynecologic Oncology Group study). *Gynecol Oncol* 1989; **33**: 283.

14
Ovarian and fallopian-tube cancer

Martee L Hensley, Kaled M Alektiar, Dennis S Chi

Epithelial ovarian cancer is the most lethal gynecologic malignancy. It is diagnosed in more than 25,000 women in the USA annually, and accounts for more than 14,000 deaths annually. The incidence of ovarian cancer has increased by 30% over the past decade, while deaths from ovarian cancer have increased by 18%. Fallopian-tube cancer is much rarer, with approximately 300 cases diagnosed annually. Owing to the rarity of fallopian-tube cancer, large studies limited to this cancer are difficult to carry out; furthermore, because fallopian-tube cancer shares many histologic features, chemotherapy-responsiveness, and overall prognosis with epithelial ovarian cancer, these two cancers are frequently managed similarly. For these reasons, they will be discussed together in this chapter. In both fallopian-tube and epithelial ovarian cancers, early-stage disease is frequently curable. A subset of patients with advanced disease may potentially be cured. Approximately 60% of patients present with advanced-stage disease, and while most (approximately 80%) initially respond to chemotherapy, the majority ultimately succumb to their disease. The overall survival rate for ovarian cancer is 38% at 5 years.

EPIDEMIOLOGY

The etiologies of epithelial ovarian and fallopian-tube cancer are not known. Epidemiologic studies have identified certain factors associated with the development of epithelial ovarian cancer. The rarity of fallopian-tube cancer precludes analogous epidemiologic studies. Risk factors for epithelial ovarian cancer may be classified as patient-related risk factors and exposure-related risk factors.

Patient-related factors

Age
The strongest patient-related risk factor for ovarian cancer is increasing age. The mean age at diagnosis is 59 years. The incidence of ovarian cancer

249

increases with each additional year of life, climbing from 15.7 per 100,000 women at age 40 years to 54 per 100,000 at age 79 years. Overall, it is estimated that one woman in 70 in the USA will develop ovarian cancer. Although largely a disease of postmenopausal women, women with a family history of breast and ovarian cancers may be diagnosed with ovarian cancer up to 10 years earlier than the average age at diagnosis within the general population.

Family history

The next strongest risk factor for ovarian cancer is family history. A woman with a single first-degree relative with ovarian cancer has a relative risk (RR) of approximately 3.6 for developing ovarian cancer compared with the general population. Her lifetime risk for ovarian cancer is estimated to be approximately 5%. From 5–10% of ovarian cancers are linked to identifiable, inherited mutations in certain genes. Women who are carriers of a gene with such a cancer-susceptibility mutation are at substantially increased risk for developing ovarian cancer. Families in which three or more first-degree relatives have ovarian or ovarian plus breast cancer are likely to have a cancer-susceptibility genetic mutation that is transmitted in an autosomal-dominant inheritance pattern.

Three familial ovarian cancer syndromes have been defined. The site-specific ovarian cancer syndrome, in which only ovarian cancer is seen, accounts for 10–15% of hereditary ovarian cancers. The hereditary breast/ovarian cancer syndrome is associated with 65–75% of hereditary ovarian cancers. In the hereditary nonpolyposis colorectal cancer syndrome (HNPCC), affected individuals may have colon, endometrial, breast, ovarian, or other cancers. Members of HNPCC kindreds account for an additional 10–15% of hereditary ovarian cancers.

The hereditary breast/ovarian cancer syndrome and, perhaps less frequently, the site-specific ovarian cancer syndrome are linked to mutations in the *BRCA1* and *BRCA2* genes. Women who are heterozygotes for mutations in either *BRCA1* or *BRCA2* have an estimated lifetime risk of 16–60% for developing ovarian cancer, with the higher risks seen among *BRCA1* carriers who have strong family histories of ovarian cancer.

Ethnicity

The incidence of ovarian cancer is higher among white women than among African–American women in the USA. Overall rates of ovarian cancer are higher in North America and northern Europe than in Japan. These differences may be related to genetics, diet, or environmental exposures, or a combination of these potential influences. For example, mutations in the *BRCA1* and *BRCA2* genes are more common among white women of Ashkenazi descent, and are rarely found in African–American women; the incidence of ovarian cancer is higher in countries with higher per capita consumption of animal fat, perhaps partly explaining the lower risk observed among Japanese women.

Reproductive factors

Women who are nulliparous or who have their first childbirth after age 35 years, who have involuntary infertility, or who have late menopause and early menarche have an increased risk of epithelial ovarian cancer. The relative risks associated with these reproductive factors range from approximately 2.0 for nulligravity to 5.0 for a history of infertility, with considerable variability among studies in relative risk estimates. These women have prolonged periods of uninterrupted ovulation, perhaps increasing the probability of genetic errors occurring during epithelial surface repair, with subsequent malignant transformation of the ovarian surface epithelium.

Exposures

Exogenous hormones

Oral contraceptive use has been associated with a decreased risk of epithelial ovarian cancer, particularly among long-term users, in multiple case–control studies. The protective effect persists for some years following discontinuation of use. The relative risk of ovarian cancer is approximately 0.5 among women with 5 or more years of use, compared with never-users. Whether long-term exposure to hormone replacement therapy increases ovarian cancer mortality requires further study.

Treatment of infertile women with ovulation-stimulating drugs may increase the risk of ovarian cancer, although the risk of fertility drug use is confounded by the inherent infertility of the women seeking these agents. Case–control studies in which ovarian cancer rates in women with exposure to fertility drugs were compared with rates among infertile women who had never used fertility drugs have shown a small increased risk, although confidence intervals around the odds-ratio estimates are wide.

Hysterectomy

Women who have undergone hysterectomy for benign disease have been reported to have a reduced risk of ovarian cancer, even when the ovaries are left in place. This observation, however, may be confounded by the fact that hysterectomy allows visualization of the ovaries, and so only normal ovaries are left intact. Consistent with this interpretation of the observed decreased risk, women who had hysterectomies more than 5 years prior to evaluation were as likely to develop ovarian cancer as women who had not undergone hysterectomy.

Smoking

In most studies, smoking has not been related to an increased risk of ovarian cancer.

Screening for ovarian cancer

General population

Transvaginal sonography and serum CA-125 assays have been proposed as screening tests for the detection of early-stage ovarian cancer. Unfortunately, a decrease in mortality with these screening approaches has not been demonstrated in any clinical trial of ovarian cancer screening in the general population. Although sensitivity levels of 90–96% and specificity levels of 98–99% have been reported for detection of an ovarian mass with transvaginal sonography, because of low disease prevalence, the positive predictive value of an abnormal transvaginal sonogram is only approximately 7% for ovarian cancer. The combination of an abnormal transvaginal sonography and an elevated CA-125 level increases the positive predictive value to 26.8% for all ovarian cancers; however, the positive predictive value of these tests for Stage I and II cancers is only 9.8%. High false-positive rates may lead to adverse events in the general population, since laparotomy or laparoscopy is frequently required to rule out ovarian cancer. A decision analysis model showed that the use of transvaginal sonography and CA-125 measurement to screen asymptomatic 40-year-old women would increase life expectancy by only one day. Published guidelines state that ovarian cancer screening for the general population is not currently recommended.

High-risk women

Ovarian cancer screening with periodic transvaginal sonography and serum CA-125 tests is recommended for women who are known to be heterozygote carriers of mutations in either the BRCA1 or BRCA2 genes, or who have been identified as members of an HNPCC kindred. These recommendations are based on expert opinions in published guidelines, owing to the high lifetime risk of ovarian cancer in these groups of women. It is not yet known, however, whether screening high-risk women successfully detects ovarian cancers in early stages, or whether screening decreases mortality. Women with strong family histories consistent with hereditary breast/ovarian cancer syndromes are also reasonable candidates for ovarian cancer screening, regardless of whether genetic mutations have been detected. All women undergoing ovarian cancer screening should understand that false-positive tests are relatively likely, especially with serial screening over a number of years.

Prophylactic oophorectomy to reduce ovarian cancer risk

Prophylactic salpingo-oophorectomy may be recommended for women from families with hereditary ovarian cancer syndromes. Since BRCA-linked hereditary ovarian cancer is rarely diagnosed under the age of 40 years, prophylactic salpingo-oophorectomy may be delayed until childbearing is complete or after the age of 40. Prophylactic salpingo-oophorectomy may be performed laparoscopically. The ovaries should be submitted for histologic evaluation, since occult ovarian cancers have been reported among prophylactic oophorectomy specimens from high-risk women. Women who elect prophylactic oophorectomy should understand that a small risk of intra-abdominal carcinomatosis, histologically indistinguishable from ovarian cancer, persists despite oophorectomy. The best explanation for the phenomenon is that peritoneal mesothelium derives from the same embryologic tissue as the ovaries, and this Müllerian tissue may still undergo malignant transformation in women at risk for ovarian cancer. Women considering prophylactic oophorectomy should be counseled regarding the risks of menopausal symptoms and osteoporosis.

HISTOLOGIC TYPES/TUMOR GRADE

Histology

Epithelial ovarian malignancies are adenocarcinomas that can have a variety of histologic appearances, including serous, mucinous, endometrioid, transitional-cell, and clear-cell carcinomas. Serous carcinomas are the most common, representing 46% of all common epithelial ovarian cancers. Mucinous tumors represent approximately 36% of ovarian cancers, endometrioid 8%, and clear-cell 3%. Fallopian-tube cancers exhibit similar histologies, with serous carcinoma seen most frequently. In general, histologic type does not have an important, independent impact on prognosis, except for clear-cell carcinoma. Women with well- and moderately well-differentiated, non-clear-cell, Stage I cancers have a greater than 90% 5-year survival rate, compared with an approximately 60% 5-year survival rate for those with clear-cell histologies. Whether clear-cell histology conveys an adverse impact on prognosis in advanced-stage disease compared with other histologic types is less clear.

Approximately 25% of epithelial ovarian cancers are borderline malignancies (low-malignant-potential tumors). The differentiation of borderline tumors from frank malignancy requires careful evaluation of the histologic architecture for identification of destructive invasion versus pushing borders. The recognition of borderline histology is important, since women with this histologic diagnosis generally have an excellent prognosis, with more than 85% of women alive 5 years after diagnosis. Initial treatment of low-malignant-potential tumors seldom requires chemotherapy, even when the tumor has spread beyond the ovaries.

Tumor grade

Epithelial ovarian cancers are graded according to their degree of differentiation. Well-differentiated tumors maintain their glandular appearance and are classified as grade 1. Poorly differentiated tumors lose their glandular features, showing sheets of cells, and are classified as grade 3. Grade 2 tumors are those with both glandular features and sheets of cells. All clear-cell carcinomas are considered grade 3. Histologic grade is particularly important in early-stage tumors, impacting both prognosis and treatment.

PATTERNS OF SPREAD OF DISEASE

Ovarian and fallopian-tube cancers have three primary methods of spread: (1) by direct extension to adjacent organs such as the uterus, rectum, and bladder; (2) by exfoliation and dissemination of clonogenic tumor cells throughout the peritoneal cavity; (3) via the lymphatic system that drains the adnexae. Cancer cells metastasize to the lymph nodes by three main routes: (1) via the lymphatics that accompany the ovarian vessels to the para-aortic lymph nodes; (2) following the drainage in the broad ligament to the external and internal iliac lymph nodes; (3) via the lymphatics in the round ligament to the inguinal lymph nodes.

PRESENTATION OF DISEASE

Symptoms and signs of disease

Early-stage disease may remain asymptomatic until ovarian masses are quite large, more than 10–12 cm in some cases. With more advanced disease, women complain of bloating, abdominal discomfort, pelvic pressure, and, occasionally, urinary or rectal symptoms. Ascites-related increased abdominal girth and pleural effusion-related shortness of breath may be presenting symptoms in some patients.

Fallopian-tube cancer differs from ovarian cancer by causing early symptomatology. The most common presenting symptoms in women with early-stage fallopian-tube cancer are abnormal vaginal bleeding, leukorrhea, and pelvic pain. Fallopian-tube carcinomas may cause symptoms earlier than ovarian cancers because of distention of the tube by cancer cells, blood, and increased luminal secretions. Advanced-stage fallopian-tube cancers have signs and symptoms similar to those seen in advanced-stage ovarian cancer.

Detection of cancer

Occasionally, an adnexal mass is detected on routine pelvic examination. Suspicion of a mass is easily confirmed with transvaginal sonography or magnetic resonance imaging (MRI). Large adnexal masses can be imaged by computed tomography (CT) scan. Although the presence of a mass can be confirmed radiographically, these techniques cannot determine whether the mass is malignant or benign. A serum CA-125 test may be helpful; however, CA-125 is elevated in less than 50% of patients with early-stage ovarian cancer and, in some cases, may be elevated in the presence of benign disease, particularly in premenopausal women.

Women with more advanced disease may have abdominal and pelvic tumor masses, ascites, and, less frequently, pleural effusions. These may be imaged with CT scan. In some patients with advanced ovarian cancer, the size of the ovaries may not be increased on radiographic imaging; thus, normal-size ovaries in a woman with abdominal carcinomatosis does not rule out ovarian cancer. CA-125 is elevated in over 90% of women with advanced ovarian cancer.

Method of diagnosis

Whether diagnosing early cancer in a patient with an adnexal mass, or confirming cell type and site of origin in a patient with ascites and carcinomatosis, the definitive diagnosis of ovarian or fallopian-tube cancer is best made by surgical exploration.

Paracentesis for the purpose of obtaining a diagnosis via cell block and cytologic smear is generally not recommended. If the patient has a large malignant cyst, paracentesis can result in spillage of malignant cells into the peritoneal cavity. Furthermore, up to 50% of ascitic fluid samples obtained from patients with true ovarian malignancies will be negative for malignant cells on cell block analysis.

STAGING OF DISEASE AND PROGNOSTIC FACTORS

Staging

Epithelial ovarian cancer and fallopian-tube cancer are surgically staged diseases. An internationally accepted staging system is utilized, according to the International Federation of Gynecology and Obstetrics (FIGO). (See Appendix 3 of this handbook for FIGO staging definitions for ovarian cancer and fallopian-tube cancer.) Appropriate staging for both cancers requires a properly performed laparotomy.

Prognostic factors

Disease stage

The most important prognostic factor for survival in epithelial ovarian cancer and fallopian-tube cancer is disease stage. In ovarian cancer, approximately 26% of patients present with Stage I disease, 15% with Stage II, 42% with Stage III, and 17% with Stage IV. More patients with fallopian-tube cancer are diagnosed with early-stage disease: 33% in Stage I, 33% in Stage II, and 34% in Stages III or IV. The overall survival estimates by disease stage for ovarian cancer are given in Table 14.1.

Suboptimal versus optimal debulking

The volume of residual tumor that remains after initial debulking surgery for both ovarian and fallopian-tube cancers is consistently associated with survival. Patients in whom bulky residual disease persists have 5-year survival rates of approximately 10–20%, compared with 30–50% for patients with no or

Table 14.1 Ovarian cancer survival by stage at diagnosis	
Stage	5-year survival rate (%)
I	85–90
II	80
III	20–30
IV	10–20

minimal (≤1cm) disease after debulking surgery. The observed survival bene-fit among optimally debulked patients is unlikely to be explained by the debulking procedure alone. It is probable that as-yet-unidentified biologic fea-tures of ovarian cancer correlate with residual volume of disease. Possible con-tributing factors in patients with high-volume residual disease that could decrease overall survival include decreased chemotherapy sensitivity in high-volume disease, greater probability for acquired somatic mutations in residual cancer cells leading to drug resistance, unrecognized tumor factors that make better-prognosis tumors more debulkable, and poor-risk tumors that are inher-ently undebulkable.

Histology and tumor grade

Tumor grade and specifically the clear-cell carcinoma histology subtype are important prognostic factors in early-stage ovarian cancer. Patients with poorly differentiated and clear-cell Stage I carcinomas have significantly worse overall survival rates (60% at 5 years) than patients with Stage I, well- or moderately well-differentiated cancers (90% at 5 years), and these patients (with Stage I, poorly differentiated or clear-cell carcinomas) require postoperative chemo-therapy. It is not clear, however, whether clear-cell histology and tumor grade carry independent prognostic information in advanced-stage ovarian cancers.

In fallopian-tube cancer, high tumor grade has been correlated with advanced-stage disease. To date, in this rare cancer, grade and histologic sub-type have not been shown to independently affect prognosis.

Serum and molecular markers

The level of CA-125 at the time of diagnosis correlates with volume of disease, and therefore does not convey independent prognostic information. However, a high postoperative CA-125 level, a slow rate of decline of CA-125 with post-operative chemotherapy, and failure to achieve a normal CA-125 value after 3 cycles of chemotherapy have been shown to be independent adverse prognos-tic factors in several studies. The application of these data to treatment deci-sions for individual patients requires further study.

Molecular and genetic abnormalities in ovarian cancer are under active investigation to determine their roles in carcinogenesis and their clinical implications for treatment and prognosis. Overexpression of p53, and epidermal growth factor receptor (EGFR) expression have been associated with poorer prognosis in some studies. Increased understanding of the molecular mechanisms of chemotherapy resistance will be important for future drug development.

In vitro chemotherapy sensitivity

Assays are commercially available to test panels of chemotherapy agents against tumor tissue obtained from individual patients at the time of surgery. Although, theoretically, this is a rational mechanism for choosing chemotherapy for patients, there are no data demonstrating that assay-directed therapy improves chemotherapy response rates or survival. The utility of such testing requires further study, and its routine use to direct therapy in individual patients is not considered standard.

MANAGEMENT OF OVARIAN AND FALLOPIAN-TUBE CANCER

Early-stage disease

Role of surgery

The surgical staging of ovarian and fallopian-tube cancer involves a thorough search of the peritoneal cavity for metastatic disease based on their known patterns of spread. Several studies have shown that after total abdominal hysterectomy and bilateral salpingo-oophorectomy for apparent Stage I ovarian cancer, approximately 30% of patients will be found to have more advanced disease if a subsequent comprehensive surgical staging procedure is performed.

Although the staging laparotomy is generally acknowledged as the single most important source of information available to the physician determining the appropriate management of early-stage disease, many patients continue to be explored for adnexal masses in community hospitals by general obstetrician–gynecologists; in up to 90% of such cases, an inadequate staging procedure is performed. In contrast, when the primary surgeon is a gynecologic oncologist, the appropriate staging procedure is performed in over 95% of cases.

Table 14.2 outlines the recommended surgical staging procedure for ovarian and/or fallopian-tube cancer that appears confined to the adnexa. Microscopic tumor implants tend to lead to the formation of adhesions, and therefore biopsy of all intraperitoneal adhesions is recommended.

Role of chemotherapy: ovarian cancer

Women with early-stage epithelial ovarian cancer can be divided into favorable

Table 14.2 Recommended surgical staging procedure for patients with apparent early-stage ovarian or fallopian-tube cancer

- Peritoneal washings
- Total abdominal hysterectomy and bilateral salpingo-oophorectomy
  (Unilateral salpingo-oophorectomy may be appropriate for selected patients with Stage IA disease who desire to defer definitive surgery until completion of childbearing.)
- Infracolic omentectomy
- Pelvic and para-aortic lymph-node sampling
- Peritoneal biopsies from:
    cul-de-sac
    rectal and bladder serosa
    right and left pelvic sidewalls
    right and left paracolic gutters
    right and left diaphragms
    any adhesions

and less-favorable prognostic groups, according to the specific stage and histology of the tumor. Patients with Stage IA or Stage IB, and well- or moderately well-differentiated tumors (grades 1 and 2) have a very favorable prognosis, with 5-year disease-free survival rates of greater than 90%. In this favorable-prognosis group, two early, randomized trials did not demonstrate a significant disease-free or overall survival benefit to adjuvant chemotherapy. Women who, after careful surgical staging, are in this favorable-prognosis group do not require postoperative chemotherapy and can be spared its associated toxicities.

Women with Stage IA or Stage IB, poorly differentiated (grade 3) or clear-cell histology tumors, all women with Stage IC tumors, and all women with Stage II tumors have a less-favorable prognosis, with 5-year disease-free survival rates of approximately 80%. In the USA, these patients generally receive adjuvant, platinum-based chemotherapy; however, it should be noted that randomized trials comparing the outcomes of patients receiving adjuvant therapy with those of patients in a no-treatment control arm have not yet shown a clear survival benefit to adjuvant therapy in this higher-risk group. An Italian study did, however, demonstrate superior disease-free survival among patients with Stage IA or IB, grade 2 or 3 tumors who received cisplatin, compared with those who received no adjuvant treatment.

In the USA, randomized trials in these patients with less-favorable-prognosis, early-stage disease have compared intravenous cisplatin with intraperitoneal phosphorus-32 (^{32}P). Patients receiving intravenous cisplatin had longer disease-free survival, and generally less toxicity, compared with patients treated with ^{32}P. Overall survival has not differed significantly between these two treatments; however, the potential survival advantage of adjuvant cisplatin may be obscured by the fact that patients who fail ^{32}P treatment may be salvaged effectively by cisplatin treatment at the time of relapse. The Gyneco-logic Oncology Group (GOG) compared intravenous cisplatin plus cyclophos-phamide given for three cycles with intraperitoneal ^{32}P. This trial demonstrated a disease-free survival advantage to cisplatin-based adjuvant therapy in patients with Stage IA grade 3, Stage IB grade 3, Stage IC, and Stage II ovarian cancer.

Success in advanced-stage ovarian cancer with paclitaxel combined with cis-platin, or its analogue carboplatin, prompted the adoption of these combina-tions for further study in early-stage, unfavorable-prognosis ovarian cancer. A trial of six cycles of paclitaxel and carboplatin versus 3 cycles of these agents has recently been completed. In the current GOG study, women with Stage IA grade 3, Stage IB grade 3, Stage IC, and Stage II ovarian cancer receive three cycles of paclitaxel plus carboplatin followed by standard surveillance or by weekly treatment with paclitaxel for 24 weeks.

Role of chemotherapy: fallopian-tube cancer
The activity of chemotherapy in fallopian-tube cancer appears similar to the activity seen in ovarian cancer. The clinical trials of adjuvant treatment in early-stage epithelial ovarian cancer described above did not include patients with primary fallopian-tube cancer. The rarity of early-stage fallopian-tube cancer makes it unlikely that randomized trials of adjuvant treatment versus observation will be performed. Treatment decisions have often been extrapo-lated from the ovarian experience. Patients with high-grade Stage I cancers and patients with Stage II cancers are frequently treated with platinum- and pacli-taxel-based chemotherapy.

Role of irradiation: ovarian cancer
In early-stage ovarian cancer, postoperative irradiation could be considered instead of chemotherapy. There are two radiation modalities that have been used for ovarian cancer: ^{32}P and whole-abdomen radiation (WAR). Intraperi-toneal ^{32}P represents an attractive treatment approach for patients with ovarian cancer. This radioactive isotope is a pure beta-emitter with a mean energy of 0.69 MeV and an average tissue penetration of 1.4–3.0 mm. These properties allow the delivery of high doses of radiation to the peritoneal surface, while sparing the underlying normal tissue. Prospective randomized trials comparing ^{32}P with chemotherapy have shown equivalent survival rates. The GOG ran-domized 141 patients with poorly differentiated Stage I and Stage II tumors to melphalan or 15 mCi of intraperitoneal ^{32}P. With a median follow-up of greater than 6 years, the outcomes for the two treatment groups were similar with respect to 5-year disease-free survival rates (80% in both groups) and overall survival rates (81% with melphalan versus 78% with ^{32}P, $p = 0.4$). In the ^{32}P arm, 6% of patients required laparotomy for bowel obstruction, while 3% of patients in the melphalan arm developed leukemia. The critics of this study point out the fact that ^{32}P was not compared with cisplatin-based chemo-therapy, which represents the standard chemotherapy approach. The GOG recently reported a second trial of 205 patients with Stage I–IIA (high-risk)

disease randomized to 15 mCi intraperitoneal ^{32}P versus three cycles of cyclophosphamide and cisplatin. With a median follow-up of 6 years, there was no statistically significant difference in overall 5-year survival rates (84% for the chemotherapy arm versus 76% for the ^{32}P arm). The authors concluded that chemotherapy is preferred because of the longer progression-free interval.

WAR represents another option for patients with early-stage disease. Unlike ^{32}P, WAR treats not only the peritoneal surface, but also the pelvic and para-aortic lymph nodes. Several randomized trials have compared WAR with chemotherapy, including two trials in which cisplatin-based chemotherapy was used. Most of these trials showed no statistically significant difference in survival, but some did show a trend toward improvement in disease-free survival with chemotherapy. Furthermore, some trials show a superior therapeutic ratio, since the complication rate with chemotherapy is lower than with WAR; however, it must be noted that the overlap of abutting fields with the moving-strip technique used in the reported studies may have contributed significantly to the high incidence of gastrointestinal damage among patients treated with WAR. In a randomized trial from Canada, 125 patients with optimally debulked Stage I, II, and III disease were randomized to two different doses of WAR. The rate of any grade 3 complication in that trial was 4%. Most investigators now use the open-field technique with appropriate shielding of the kidneys. The total dose is usually 25–30 Gy given at 10–15 Gy per fraction.

In summary, intraperitoneal ^{32}P or WAR as adjuvant therapy for high-risk early-stage patients seems to offer a similar survival rate to chemotherapy. Therefore, it should at least be considered as an alternative to chemotherapy for patients who refuse or are not good candidates for chemotherapy. Special attention, however, must be paid to ensure adequate distribution of ^{32}P throughout the peritoneal cavity and, in the case of WAR, to ensure the selection of optimal treatment techniques.

Role of irradiation: fallopian-tube cancer
The data in the literature are very scant on the role of radiation therapy in the management of this rare disease. Certain assumptions, however, can be made about its potential role. In patients with Stage I–II disease, pelvic irradiation may be indicated to reduce the local-regional relapse. Some authors recommend using pelvic and para-aortic irradiation or WAR due to the high failure rate in the upper abdomen. For patients with more advanced disease, the recommendations are similar to those for ovarian cancer.

Advanced-stage disease

Role of surgery
When advanced-stage ovarian or fallopian-tube cancer is encountered at surgical evaluation, the operative goal changes from adequate staging to aggressive surgical cytoreduction, or "debulking." Surgical cytoreduction refers to the removal of as much tumor as possible. For many solid tumors, aggressive sur-

gical resection is justified only if all known tumor can be removed, rendering the operation potentially curative. For ovarian and fallopian-tube cancers, however, numerous studies, including those by the GOG, have demonstrated higher response rates to chemotherapy, prolonged progression-free intervals, and improved median survivals when patients are "optimally" versus "suboptimally" cytoreduced.

The terms "optimal" and "suboptimal" refer to the diameter of the largest residual tumor nodule that remains after debulking surgery. Authors have used maximal tumor diameters varying from 0.5–3.0 cm when defining optimal and suboptimal cytoreduction. The GOG has shown that surgical debulking to 2 cm or less of residual disease resulted in a significant survival benefit; however, all residual diameters greater than 2 cm had equivalent survival. Therefore, unless patients with advanced-stage ovarian or fallopian-tube cancer can be surgically cytoreduced to optimal residual disease status, aggressive surgical debulking provides no survival benefit. The GOG studies analyzing survival and residual disease status included a small number of patients with residual tumor diameters between 1–2 cm, and consequently, the GOG currently defines optimal residual disease status as that which measures 1 cm or less. A recent study from our institution of 282 patients with advanced ovarian carcinoma supports the current GOG definition.

The percentage of patients with advanced-stage ovarian or fallopian-tube cancer that can be successfully debulked to optimal residual disease status varies widely within the literature, but averages 40–50%, which means that the majority of patients are suboptimally cytoreduced. The European Organization for Research and Treatment of Cancer (EORTC) performed a prospective, randomized trial in patients with suboptimal disease that evaluated the benefit of a brief course of chemotherapy, followed by a second attempt at "interval" cytoreduction, before completing a prescribed chemotherapy regimen. After 3 cycles of cyclophosphamide and cisplatin, patients without disease progression were randomly assigned to undergo either interval debulking surgery or no surgery, followed by 3 more cycles of the same chemotherapy. Patients who underwent interval cytoreduction demonstrated a significant improvement in both progression-free survival (18 versus 13 months) and overall survival (26 versus 20 months). The GOG is currently performing a confirmatory prospective, randomized trial evaluating interval cytoreduction. The schema of the GOG trial is the same as that of the EORTC trial except that patients will receive paclitaxel and cisplatin instead of cyclophosphamide and cisplatin.

Role of chemotherapy

Following cytoreductive surgery, patients with advanced-stage epithelial ovarian cancer should receive systemic chemotherapy. Cisplatin-based therapy has been shown to be superior to alkylating agent-based treatment, and has remained the backbone of systemic therapy for ovarian cancer. Paclitaxel was identified as having significant activity in patients with platinum-resistant disease, and was therefore adopted for testing in the post-cytoreductive-surgery setting. Two seminal trials (GOG 111 and OV10), showing that paclitaxel plus cisplatin improved response rates, progression-free survival, and overall survival compared with cyclophosphamide plus cisplatin, established paclitaxel-plus-platinum therapy as standard therapy for advanced-stage disease.

The cisplatin analogue carboplatin is associated with less neurotoxicity, less nephrotoxicity, and less nausea than cisplatin. Two large, randomized trials have compared paclitaxel plus cisplatin with paclitaxel plus carboplatin. Results of these studies show that these regimens are equivalent in terms of response rates and progression-free survival, and that the carboplatin/paclitaxel combination is easier to administer and is associated with less toxicity. These results make paclitaxel 175 mg/m^2 over 3 hours plus carboplatin dosed at an AUC (area under the curve) of 5–7.5, with both drugs delivered by vein every 3 weeks for a total of 6 cycles, a reasonable standard approach for most patients with advanced-stage epithelial ovarian cancer following cytoreductive surgery. Preliminary data from a recent randomized trial suggests that more prolonged treatment with paclitaxel may confer additional survival benefit. Among patients with advanced-stage disease, the clinical response rate to paclitaxel/platinum chemotherapy is approximately 80%, and the median survival is approximately 35 months.

The tendency of ovarian cancer to spread within the peritoneal cavity, the standard employment of initial cytoreductive surgery, and the ability to achieve high intraperitoneal drug concentrations have made intraperitoneal (i.p.) chemotherapy a rational treatment modality in ovarian cancer. Prior to the availability of paclitaxel, a randomized trial compared intravenous (i.v.) cyclophosphamide plus i.v. cisplatin with i.v. cyclophosphamide plus i.p. cisplatin in patients with optimally debulked, Stage III cancers. Median survival was 8 months longer, and neurotoxicity was less in the i.p. arm compared with the i.v. arm. An intergroup study compared i.v. cisplatin plus paclitaxel to carboplatin (AUC 9) followed by i.v. paclitaxel plus i.p. cisplatin. This study also demonstrated a survival advantage for patients receiving i.p. cisplatin. The current GOG study for optimally debulked ovarian cancer incorporates the survival advantage seen with i.p. cisplatin compared with i.v. cisplatin, and the survival advantage seen with paclitaxel compared with cyclophosphamide. In this study, patients are randomized to i.v. paclitaxel plus i.v. cisplatin versus i.v. paclitaxel plus i.p. cisplatin and i.p. paclitaxel. This study should further clarify the role of i.p. therapy for the subset of ovarian cancer patients with Stage III disease and minimal volume of cancer at the end of cytoreductive surgery.

The role of high-dose chemotherapy with stem-cell support has been investigated in ovarian cancer. Thus far, these trials have not shown high-dose therapy to be superior to standard-dose therapy in terms of disease-free survival. Prior randomized trials of high-dose versus standard-dose carboplatin have not shown superiority to the higher-dose regimens. High-dose chemotherapy with stem-cell support has a treatment-associated mortality rate of 1–5%. Treatment of ovarian and fallopian-tube cancer with high-dose therapy should be done only as part of a clinical trial carried out by experienced investigators.

Treatment with standard-dose paclitaxel and carboplatin is relatively well tolerated. Alopecia is seen in essentially all patients during treatment. Paclitaxel can cause an anaphylactoid reaction in up to 10% of patients. The risk of this reaction is dramatically decreased by premedicating patients with dexamethasone, diphenhydramine, and an H_2-receptor antagonist (ranitidine, cimetidine, or other). Paclitaxel may cause muscle and joint discomfort, and, particularly with cumulative doses, neurotoxicity. Both paclitaxel and carboplatin cause myelosuppression, with neutropenia more common than thrombocytopenia. Most often, neutropenia is asymptomatic, but febrile neutropenia may occur. Nausea and vomiting are generally easily controlled with serotonin-receptor (5-HT$_3$) antagonist-type antiemetics. Carboplatin may cause potentially severe hypersensitivity reactions. These types of reactions are generally seen in patients who have received an extended number of carboplatin courses previously.

Response rates and survival times in patients with advanced-stage fallopiantube cancer treated with platinum-based chemotherapy are similar to those seen in patients with advanced-stage epithelial ovarian cancer. Patients with either ovarian or fallopian-tube primary adenocarcinomas are eligible for more recent clinical trials of chemotherapy. Patients with advanced-stage fallopiantube cancer who are not enrolled on clinical treatment trials should receive platinum and paclitaxel-containing chemotherapy, with potential toxicities and expected responses similar to those discussed for ovarian cancer.

Role of irradiation

There are at least five prospective, randomized trials that have investigated the value of consolidation treatment following chemotherapy with WAR or further chemotherapy. Two of these trials had such small sample sizes that no meaningful conclusions could be drawn from them. The other three trials had more than 50 patients in each arm, and all showed no statistically significant difference in overall survival between WAR and further chemotherapy. In one of these studies, patients with complete pathologic response were randomized to further chemotherapy versus WAR versus observation. There was improvement in disease-free survival in favor of WAR or chemotherapy, compared with observation, but no improvement in overall survival. With regard to ^{32}P as consolidation treatment, the GOG has completed a prospective, randomized trial in patients with negative second-look laparotomy. The patients were randomized to observation versus ^{32}P. The results of this trial are eagerly awaited. In summary, consolidation with WAR seems to be equivalent to further chemotherapy. Attention to dose and technique in this subset of patients is very important, since most of them have had multiple laparotomies and many cycles of chemotherapy, increasing the probability of abdominal complications of radiation therapy.

Second-look surgery and intraperitoneal chemotherapy

Currently, the term *second-look surgery* refers to a systematic surgical exploration performed in patients with advanced-stage ovarian or fallopian-tube

Table 14.3 Summary of initial treatment recommendations for ovarian cancer by stage at presentation

After initial staging procedure/ cytoreductive surgery	Recommendation
Stage IA, grade 1 or 2[a]	Observation
Stage IB, grade 1 or 2[a]	Observation
Stage IA or IB, grade 3; Stage IC; Stage II	Paclitaxel + carboplatin, 3–6 cycles or participation in a GOG clinical trial
Stage III, optimally debulked	Paclitaxel + carboplatin, 6 cycles or participation in a GOG clinical trial
Stage III, suboptimally debulked; Stage IV	Paclitaxel + carboplatin, 6 cycles, or participation in a clinical trial

[a]Chemotherapy may be considered for grade 2 tumors.

cancer who have completed a planned course of chemotherapy and are in a complete clinical remission. The surgery is performed via laparotomy or laparoscopy. In patients with no gross evidence of tumor, multiple biopsies are obtained from the same locations as a staging procedure. Approximately 50% of patients with a complete clinical response to cytoreductive surgery and primary chemotherapy (no evidence of disease on CT scan, and CA-125 ≤ 35 U/ml) will have a negative second-look operation. However, even among this group of patients, with a pathologic complete remission, half will develop recurrent disease. A study of intraperitoneal cisplatin consolidation chemotherapy in patients with a negative second-look procedure showed that disease-free survival is prolonged in patients who receive intraperitoneal cisplatin consolidation compared with a cohort of historical control patients in clinical complete remission who did not receive intraperitoneal consolidation.

Patients with a microscopically positive second-look procedure are offered salvage therapy. Treatment options for this group of patients include both intraperitoneal and systemic therapy. There are no trials showing that one approach is superior to the other, and there is no standard chemotherapy agent for this situation. As discussed above, in relation to primary therapy, patients with very small-volume disease may be excellent candidates for intraperitoneal chemotherapy, since high intratumoral concentrations of drug may be achieved, perhaps overcoming drug resistance. Options for patients with microscopic disease at second look therefore include: i.p. cisplatin as a single agent, i.p. cisplatin combined with other agents as part of a clinical trial, additional systemic therapy with weekly paclitaxel, or other systemic salvage agent (see the "Recurrent disease" section below). Clinical-trial participation should be encouraged for this group of patients.

For those patients who have gross disease at the time of second look, several authors have demonstrated that there is a survival benefit if most or all of the disease can be resected at the time of the second-look procedure. Therefore, those patients who are found to have gross disease that is potentially resectable at second-look laparoscopy will benefit from converting the procedure to a full laparotomy in order to perform a "secondary cytoreduction."

Recurrent disease

Role of surgery

Although no prospective, randomized trials have been performed, it appears that in patients whose tumors remain sensitive to chemotherapy, surgical cytoreduction to small-volume disease prior to secondary chemotherapy may be of benefit. For the majority of women with ovarian cancer, the disease eventually progresses within the peritoneal cavity, leading to intestinal obstruction in some patients. If conservative measures fail to result in relief of the obstruction, surgical exploration is the only management option that may restore intestinal function. Approximately 80% of patients who undergo exploration will have their obstruction relieved. However, about half of those patients who are unable to undergo a definitive surgical procedure develop enterocutaneous fistulae and/or further progression of disease.

Role of chemotherapy

Women with ovarian or fallopian-tube cancer who fail to achieve a complete response to primary surgery and chemotherapy and women whose disease recurs after completion of primary therapy are unlikely to be cured. Although a number of agents that may induce objective tumor responses in patients with persistent and recurrent ovarian cancer have been identified, it is not clear whether tumor response correlates with prolonged survival among patients receiving second-line chemotherapy. There are no randomized trials comparing second-line chemotherapy with best supportive care in ovarian cancer. When making decisions about employing second-line chemotherapy, the patient should be aware that, while cure is unlikely, the goal of continued treatment is to control tumor-related symptoms, limit disease progression if possible, and improve or maintain quality of life.

Attempts have been made using retrospective evaluations to determine which patients with refractory or relapsed ovarian cancer may respond again to platinum-based therapy, and which patients require agents that are non-cross-resistant with platinum. Patients who initially responded to platinum-based therapy and recur 6 or more months after completion of treatment are generally considered "platinum-sensitive." Patients who do not have a complete response to primary platinum-based chemotherapy or who relapse less than 6 months after treatment are unlikely to respond to further platinum therapy and are considered "platinum-refractory."

Patients with platinum-sensitive disease may be retreated with platinum

Table 14.4 Chemotherapy options for patients with recurrent ovarian cancer

Initial response to platinum, relapse >6 months after completion of treatment	No complete response to platinum, or relapse <6 months after completion of treatment
Carboplatin, or cisplatin ±paclitaxel	Oral etoposide Topotecan Liposomal doxorubicin Gemcitabine Tamoxifen Ifosfamide Vinorelbine Docetaxel Paclitaxel

agents (carboplatin or cisplatin). Response rates of 20–60% may be expected, with the probability of responding correlating directly with the duration of the initial remission.

A number of chemotherapy agents have been identified that may be non-cross-resistant with platinum-based therapy, and treatment with one of these may be reasonable in patients with platinum-refractory disease who have a good performance status. Objective response rates for most agents are 20–30% and are mostly reported from Phase II trials. In some studies, not all patients were truly platinum-refractory. There are no studies showing improved progression-free survival or improved quality of life compared with best supportive care in the platinum-refractory population. Patient performance status, patient preferences, costs, potential toxicities, and effects on quality of life should be considered when choosing management strategies for the platinum-refractory patient. Clinical-trial participation should be encouraged, since none of the currently available agents is curative in this high-risk group of ovarian cancer patients.

Table 14.4 shows treatment options for salvage therapy of ovarian cancer. In the platinum-refractory patient, no trials have demonstrated any one agent to be superior to another. Choice among the agents is frequently based on drug delivery schedule, side-effect profile, and the patient's underlying organ function.

Role of irradiation

Palliation of symptoms, especially in patients with recurrent pelvic disease, may have significant impact on the quality of life of patients in their final months of life. Several investigators have reported 50–70% complete resolution of symptoms after palliative radiation. The duration of palliation could be up to 1 year in about one-third of patients. The recommended dose range is usually 35–45 Gy, depending on the patient's performance status and the types of treatments received in the past.

FUTURE TREATMENTS

The role of clinical research in improving the outcomes of ovarian and fallopian-tube cancer cannot be overemphasized. Research efforts are needed at all points in the natural history of ovarian cancer. Clinical-trial participation is critical, since ovarian cancer is relatively rare, and studies that can truly change the standard of care require large numbers of patients.

Screening

New technologies for screening need to be identified and evaluated with the hope of diagnosing more patients with early-stage disease. Ongoing studies will determine the impact of screening and prophylactic oophorectomy in high-risk women in terms of ability to detect early-stage cancers, the frequency of false-positive tests, costs of screening, and effects on quality of life.

First-line treatment

An ongoing European study will assess whether delaying debulking surgery until three cycles of paclitaxel/carboplatin chemotherapy have been administered results in similar outcomes in newly diagnosed patients as the current standard of initial debulking surgery followed by chemotherapy. Substantial research is being focused on attempts to improve primary chemotherapy in order that an increased percentage of women achieve complete clinical remission. It is hoped that increased numbers of patients achieving complete clinical remission with primary chemotherapy will lead to improved overall survival. Primary chemotherapy studies are testing three-drug regimens (adding non-cross-resistant agents to paclitaxel/platinum combinations), sequential two-drug regimens (using non-cross-resistant agents in rapid sequence with paclitaxel/platinum combinations), alternative treatment schedules, and high-dose chemotherapy regimens. The role of consolidation therapy is being investigated in trials using long-term systemic therapy, and in trials using intraperitoneal chemotherapy for patients with minimal residual disease at second-look evaluation surgery. Molecularly targeted agents are being developed and tested as novel anti-cancer therapies.

Treatment of recurrent disease

Many trials are underway to identify new agents for platinum-resistant ovarian cancer. Identifying new agents for this population will serve two purposes: (1) if a new agent is well tolerated and has high response rates, it may offer better palliation and preservation of quality of life compared with other salvage choices; (2) a highly active drug in the platinum-refractory population may then be tested as part of initial chemotherapy.

Novel anti-cancer therapies

Trials are underway to evaluate the ability of vaccine treatments given to patients in clinical remission to prolong their disease-free survival. Monoclonal antibodies directed against CA-125 are being tested. With increased understanding of the molecular biology of ovarian cancer, abnormal genes may be targeted by specific treatments, or "replaced" with gene therapy. The relatively unique limited peritoneal involvement seen with ovarian cancer makes intraperitoneal gene-therapy delivery particularly attractive. Research aimed at defining the molecular mechanisms of platinum resistance is likely to lead to valuable therapeutic interventions for the platinum-refractory population of ovarian cancer patients.

SELECTED READING

Alberts DS, Liu PY, Hannigan EV et al, Intraperitoneal cisplatin plus intravenous cyclophosphamide versus intravenous cisplatin plus intravenous cyclophosphamide for stage III ovarian cancer. N Engl J Med 1996; 335: 1950.

Barakat RR, Almadrones L, Venkatraman ES et al, A phase II trial of intraperitoneal cisplatin and etoposide as consolidation therapy in patients with stage II–IV epithelial ovarian cancer following negative surgical assessment. Gynecol Oncol 1998; 69: 17.

Boyd J, Sonoda Y, Federici M et al, Clinical and pathologic features of hereditary ovarian cancers associated with germline mutations in BRCA1 or BRCA2. Gynecol Oncol 1999; 72: 444 (Abst).

Burke W, Daly M, Garber J et al, Recommendations for follow-up care of individuals with inherited predisposition to cancer II. BRCA1 and BRCA2. JAMA 1997; 277: 997.

Chi DS, Liao JB, Leon LF et al, Identification of prognostic factors in advanced epithelial ovarian carcinoma. Gynecol Oncol 2001; 82: 532.

DuBois A, Lueck HJ, Meier W et al, Cisplatin/paclitaxel vs carboplatin/paclitaxel in ovarian cancer: update of an Arbeitgemeinschaft Gynaekologische Oncologie (AGO) Study Group trial. Proc Am Soc Clin Oncol 1999; 18: 356a (Abst 1374).

Eisenkop SM, Friedman RL, Spirtos NM, The role of secondary cytoreductive surgery in the treatment of patients with recurrent epithelial ovarian carcinoma. Cancer 2000; 88: 144.

Ford D, Easton DF, Bishop DT et al, Risk of cancer in BRCA1 mutation carriers. Lancet 1994; 343: 692.

Gemignani ML, Hensley ML, Cohen R et al, Paclitaxel-based chemotherapy in carcinoma of the fallopian tube. Gynecol Oncol 2000; 80: 16.

Hoskins WJ, McGuire WP, Brady MF et al, The effect of diameter of largest residual disease on survival after primary cytoreductive surgery patients with suboptimal residual epithelial ovarian carcinoma. Am J Obstet Gynecol 1994; 170: 974.

Hoskins WJ, Rubin RC, Dulaney E et al, Influence of cytoreductive surgery at the time of second-look laparotomy on the survival of patients with epithelial ovarian carcinoma. *Gynecol Oncol* 1989; **34**: 365.

Landis SH, Murray T, Bolden S, Wingo PA, Cancer statistics, 1999. *CA Cancer J Clin* 1999; **49**: 8.

McGuire WP, Hoskins WJ, Brady MF et al, Cyclophosphamide and cisplatin compared with paclitaxel and cisplatin in patients with stage III and stage IV ovarian cancer. *N Engl J Med* 1996; **334**: 1.

Mackey SE, Creasman WT, Ovarian cancer screening. *J Clin Oncol* 1995; **13**: 783.

Markman M, Bundy BN, Alberts DS et al, Phase III trial of standard-dose intravenous cisplatin plus paclitaxel versus moderately high-dose carboplatin followed by intravenous paclitaxel and intraperitoneal cisplatin in small-volume stage III ovarian carcinoma: An intergroup study of the Gynecologic Oncology Group, Southwestern Oncology Group, and Eastern Oncology Group. *J Clin Oncol* 2001; **19**: 1001.

Markman M, Rothman R, Hakes T et al, Second-line platinum therapy in patients with ovarian cancer previously treated with cisplatin. *J Clin Oncol* 1991; **9**: 383.

Munoz KA, Harlan LC, Trimble EL, Patterns of care for women with ovarian cancer in the United States. *J Clin Oncol* 1997; **15**: 3408.

NIH Consensus Development Conference Panel, Ovarian cancer: screening, treatment, and follow-up. Washington, DC, National Institutes of Health, April 5–7, 1994. NIH Consensus Statement 12.

Ozols RF, Bundy BN, Fowler J et al, Randomized phase III study of cisplatin (CIS)/paclitaxel (PAC) versus carboplatin (CARBO)/PAC in optimal stage III epithelial ovarian cancer (OC): a Gynecologic Oncology Group trial (GOG 158). *Proc Am Soc Clin Oncol* 1999; **18**: 356a (Abst 1373).

Piccart MJ, Bertelson K, James K et al, Randomized intergroup trial of cisplatin-paclitaxel versus cisplatin-cyclophosphamide in women with advanced epithelial ovarian cancer: Three-year results. *J Natl Cancer Inst* 2000; **92**: 699.

van der Burg MEL, van Lent M, Buyse M et al, The effect of debulking surgery after induction chemotherapy on the prognosis in advanced epithelial ovarian cancer. *N Engl J Med* 1996; **332**: 629.

Van Nagell JR Jr, DePriest PD, Gallion HH, Pavlik EJ, Ovarian cancer screening. *Cancer* 1993; **71**: 1523.

Young RC, Walton LA, Ellenberg SS et al, Adjuvant therapy in Stage I and II epithelial ovarian cancer. Results of two prospective randomized trials. *N Engl J Med* 1990; **322**: 1021.

Zanetta G, Rota S, Chiari S et al, Behavior of borderline tumors with particular interest to persistence, recurrence, and progression to Invasive carcinoma: a prospective study. *J Clin Oncol* 2001; **19**: 2658.

15
Germ-cell and ovarian sex cord–stromal tumors

Karen H Lu, David M Gershenson,
Elizabeth A Poynor, Paul J Sabbatini

GERM-CELL TUMORS

Malignant germ-cell tumors occur primarily in adolescents and young women. Over the last several decades, we have refined treatment regimens and emphasized preservation of fertility in the management of patients with these tumors. Germ-cell tumors are derived from the primordial germ cells of the ovary. Although rare, the diagnosis of a malignant germ-cell tumor must be considered in the workup of an adolescent or young woman with a pelvic mass. Appropriate intraoperative decision making is crucial in order to adequately treat and stage the cancer without compromising future fertility. Histopathologic classification of the tumor and extent of disease determines whether postoperative chemotherapy is indicated.

Epidemiology

Malignant germ-cell tumors account for fewer than 5% of all ovarian cancers in the USA. In Asian countries, however, they represent up to 15% of all ovarian cancers. The mean age of women diagnosed with a malignant germ-cell tumor is between 16 and 20 years, and the range is from 6 to 46 years. Because of this age distribution, germ-cell tumors are occasionally diagnosed in pregnancy.

Histologic types of germ-cell tumors

Germ-cell tumors are classified based on histologic similarity to embryonic and extraembryonic structures and level of differentiation (Table 15.1). Appropriate pathologic diagnosis is crucial for surgical and postoperative management, since the different germ-cell tumors have important differences in natural history. Dysgerminomas are the most common malignant germ-cell tumor, accounting for 50% of all malignant germ-cell tumors in women. Dysgerminomas are the histologic equivalent of the seminoma, the most common germ-cell tumor in men. In 20% of women with dysgerminomas, there will be

Table 15.1 Classification of germ-cell tumors
Dysgerminoma
Yolk-sac tumor (endodermal sinus tumor)
Embryonal carcinoma
Polyembryoma
Choriocarcinoma
Teratoma: Immature Mature Monodermal (struma ovarii, carcinoid)
Mixed forms

disease bilaterally: 10% are seen grossly, and 10% are noted microscopically. They do not characteristically secrete serum markers, although human chorionic gonadotropin (hCG) may be elevated due to the occasional presence of syncytiotrophoblasts. Dysgerminomas may arise in a dysgenetic gonad. If known preoperatively, removal of the contralateral dysgenetic gonad is indicated. Endodermal sinus tumors, also called yolk-sac tumors, are the second most common germ-cell tumor and account for 20% of all malignant germ-cell tumors. They are characterized by the secretion of α-fetoprotein (AFP). They are rarely bilateral, and are characterized histologically by Schiller–Duval bodies, which are papillary structures surrounding a central vessel. Endodermal sinus tumors have a propensity for distant hematogenous dissemination to the lungs. Immature teratomas account for 20% of malignant germ-cell tumors. While rarely bilateral, a mature teratoma may be seen in the contralateral ovary in 10% of cases. Immature teratomas are graded as low-grade or high-grade based on the amount of immature neural tissue they contain. While the majority of patients with immature teratomas will not secrete tumor markers, approximately one-third of patients with immature teratomas will secrete AFP.

Embryonal tumors and nongestational choriocarcinomas are uncommon. Embryonal tumors classically occur in younger adolescents, with a mean age of 15 years. Adolescents with embryonal tumors can develop hormonal abnormalities, including irregular vaginal bleeding, precocious puberty, and hirsutism. Embryonal tumors can secrete both AFP and hCG. Nongestational choriocarcinoma also occurs in young girls, and is associated with precocious puberty. Patients with nongestational choriocarcinoma will have elevated serum hCG. Polyembryoma is an extremely rare, highly malignant germ-cell tumor. Polyembryoma may be seen mixed with immature teratoma, and serum AFP may be elevated in these patients.

Approximately 10% of malignant germ-cell tumors will be mixed, and will contain at least two germ-cell elements. Dysgerminoma is the most common component and is often seen with endodermal sinus tumor or immature teratoma. Elevated serum AFP in a patient with dysgerminoma should prompt further pathologic review of the specimen. Importantly, treatment and prognosis should be based on the nondysgerminomatous component.

Presentation of disease

Although nonspecific, subacute abdominal pain and a palpable pelvic mass are the most common symptom and sign of a woman presenting with a germ-cell tumor. In 10% of cases, acute abdominal pain may also occur as a result of rupture, torsion, or hemorrhage. Germ-cell tumors grow rapidly and are frequently large at the time of diagnosis, ranging in size from 7–40 cm, with a median of 16 cm. Other symptoms may include fever, abnormal vaginal bleeding, and abdominal distention.

Serum tumor markers, as discussed above, can aid in the preoperative diagnosis of malignant germ-cell tumors. Table 15.2 shows the characteristic tumor markers for the different germ-cell tumors. Lactate dehydrogenase (LDH), while nonspecific, may be elevated in patients with dysgerminoma or other germ-cell tumors.

Of women with germ-cell tumors, 70% present with Stage I disease, while 25–30% of women will have Stage III disease. Spread of disease can occur intraperitoneally, via lymphatics, or hematogenously.

Table 15.2 Serum tumor markers in malignant germ-cell tumors of the ovary[a]		
Histology	AFP	hCG
Dysgerminoma	–	±
Endodermal sinus tumor	+	–
Immature teratoma	±	–
Choriocarcinoma	–	+
Embryonal carcinoma	+	+
Mixed germ-cell tumor	±	±
Polyembryoma	±	±

[a]AFP, α-fetoprotein; hCG, human chorionic gonadotropin.

Surgical management

The initial approach to a woman suspected of having a malignant germ-cell tumor is an exploratory laparotomy. An adequate incision is necessary for removal of the mass and to properly determine the extent of disease. The surgeon should begin with a thorough and systematic exploration of the abdomen and pelvis. The subsequent operative procedure should take into consideration the patient's desire for fertility. For a woman who has completed childbearing, a total abdominal hysterectomy with bilateral salpingo-oophorectomy is reasonable. In a patient who desires to retain fertility, a unilateral salpingo-oophorectomy may be sufficient. Bilateral ovarian involvement is exceedingly rare, except in the case of dysgerminoma. Bilateral involvement occurs in approximately 10–15% of dysgerminomas. Mature cystic teratomas may also occur in 5–10% of women with dysgerminomas. Inspection of the contralateral ovary should be performed. If there is suspicion of contralateral ovarian involvement, a biopsy or ovarian cystectomy can be performed. If the contralateral ovary appears normal, biopsy is unnecessary. After removal, the mass should be given to the pathologist for frozen-section diagnosis.

Surgical staging should be performed to determine the extent of disease and to guide therapeutic decision making. Staging should consist of obtaining peritoneal fluid if present, or performing cytologic washings of the pelvis and paracolic gutters. Inspection and palpation should be performed in a methodical way. If disease is limited, random staging biopsies should be performed. Pelvic and para-aortic nodes should be carefully palpated and suspicious nodes removed. Sampling of the pelvic and para-aortic nodes should occur. When metastatic disease is encountered at initial surgery, resection of as much tumor as is possible is recommended. In women with bilateral ovarian involvement who desire future fertility, consideration can be given to performing ovarian cystectomy and preserving a portion of uninvolved ovary.

A significant portion of women with germ-cell tumors will have their initial surgery in community hospitals and may have inadequate surgical staging. In these cases, a chest x-ray and an abdominal–pelvic computed tomography (CT) scan should be obtained, as well as baseline tumor-marker studies. An experienced pathologist should review the case to confirm the diagnosis. In general, a repeat laparotomy for staging purposes is not recommended.

Chemotherapy

Early-stage disease

Whether adjuvant chemotherapy is recommended or not depends on histologic type of germ-cell tumor (Table 15.3). For well-staged, Stage I patients with dysgerminoma and low-grade immature teratoma, careful observation and follow-up is sufficient. The 10-year survival rate for patients with Stage IA dysgerminoma patients is 90%.

Historically, a high percentage of patients with early-stage, completely

Table 15.3 Treatment by germ-cell tumor stage/type

Dysgerminoma

Stage I	Surgery[a]
Stage II–IV	Surgery[a] and chemotherapy[b]

Endodermal sinus tumor

Stage I	Surgery[a] and chemotherapy[b]
Stage II–IV	Surgery[a] and chemotherapy[b]

Immature teratoma

Stage I – low-grade	Surgery[a]
Stage I – high-grade	Surgery[a] and chemotherapy[b]
Stage II–IV	Surgery[a] and chemotherapy[c]

[a]Surgery includes resection of primary tumor and surgical staging. Specific surgical procedures for patients desiring preservation of fertility are discussed in the text.
[b] 3–4 cycles of bleomycin – etoposide – cisplatin (BEP: see Table 15.4).
[c] 4–6 cycles of BEP.

Table 15.4 The BEP regimen

Cisplatin	20 mg/m^2, days 1–5
Etoposide	100 mg/m^2, days 1–5
Bleomycin	30 units i.v. weekly or 10–15 units q day $\times$ 3 days by continuous infusion

Courses are given at 21-day intervals.

resected endodermal sinus tumors and embryonal carcinomas relapsed and died from disease. Therefore, patients with Stage I endodermal sinus tumor and embryonal carcinomas, or mixed tumors containing these elements, require adjuvant chemotherapy. In addition, patients with Stage I, nongestational ovarian choriocarcinoma and Stage I, high-grade immature teratoma should receive adjuvant chemotherapy. In these patients, 3 or 4 cycles of BEP (bleomycin, etoposide, and cisplatin) given every 21 days is recommended (Table 15.4). Discussion of side effects of the chemotherapy drugs is important, including cisplatin-induced neuro- and nephrotoxicities, and the rarer bleomycin-induced pulmonary fibrosis and etoposide-related acute leukemia. Baseline creatinine-clearance and pulmonary-function tests should be obtained. During treatment, tumor markers that were elevated preoperatively can be serially obtained to follow response to chemotherapy. Overall, patients with endodermal sinus tumors, embryonal carcinomas, and mixed tumors confined to the ovaries who receive adjuvant BEP have long-term cure rates of greater than 90%.

Late-stage disease

In contrast to epithelial ovarian cancer, women with advanced-stage germ-cell tumors can often be cured with combination chemotherapy. Patients with metastatic germ-cell tumors of all histologies should receive combination chemotherapy with BEP. Earlier regimens with vincristine, dactinomycin (actinomycin-D), and cyclophosphamide (VAC) or cisplatin, vinblastine, and bleomycin (PVB) have been replaced by BEP. Four to six courses given every 21 days should be planned, and physicians can follow tumor markers if elevated. Full doses of medication and strict adherence to schedule are important. Granulocyte colony-stimulating factor (G-CSF) may be used in order to continue full dosing and adherence to schedule. In general, carboplatin should not be substituted for cisplatin. Cure rates for Stage III disease treated with combination chemotherapy are 60–80%.

Recurrent disease

Of the germ-cell patients who recur, 90% do so in the first 2 years after initial therapy. Patients who have completed therapy are generally seen every 3 months for the first 2 years. Patients who had elevated serum tumor markers will have serum tumor-marker studies performed monthly for the first 2 years. In women with Stage I dysgerminoma treated with surgery alone, relapse rates are approximately 15–25%. Patients who relapse are given combination chemotherapy with BEP for 3–4 cycles. Virtually all of these women will be salvaged.

Patients who have previously received combination chemotherapy and have persistent or recurrent disease present physicians with more challenging management issues. Prognosis is usually better for patients who are platinum-sensitive (i.e., who showed a response to platinum and progressed later than 6 weeks off treatment). Options for treatment include standard-dose therapy with cisplatin, vinblastine, and ifosfamide, or high-dose chemotherapy with stem-cell rescue. These patients should also be considered for clinical trials.

Late effects

In the last two decades, refinement of combination chemotherapy has resulted in the cure of the majority of patients with germ-cell tumors. We have subsequently been faced with new issues surrounding the late effects of our initial surgical and medical treatment of these patients. Use of etoposide has been associated with the development of acute leukemia. The risk of developing this second malignancy is low, and depends on the cumulative dose of etoposide given. In the largest published study, none of 67 patients who received three courses of etoposide developed acute leukemia, while 2 of 348 patients who received more than three courses did. While physicians and patients should be aware of the risk, the benefits of etoposide should be considered along with the risks.

While young women treated for malignant germ-cell tumors are at risk for infertility, the majority should be able to conceive and bear children. Appropriate surgical management and minimizing procedures that contribute to adhesion formation is crucial. BEP combination chemotherapy has not been shown to have adverse effects on ovarian function, and the majority of patients can expect resumption of menses and ovulation after chemotherapy.

OVARIAN SEX CORD–STROMAL TUMORS

Epidemiology and classification

The World Health Organization (WHO) has divided ovarian neoplasms according to presumed sites of origin: (1) surface epithelium; (2) germ cells (migrating to the ovary from the yolk sac); (3) ovarian stroma (include the sex cords and are the beginnings of the endocrine apparatus). Sex cord–stromal tumors account for 90% of *functioning* ovarian neoplasms, but only 7% of all ovarian tumors, with 1,800 new cases diagnosed in the USA each year.

Sex cord–stromal tumors can be classified as in Table 15.5.

In general, these tumors are of low malignant potential with a favorable long-term prognosis. Some tumors are diagnosed at an earlier age, and added morbidity comes from estrogen (granulosa, theca, or Sertoli cell) or androgen (Sertoli–Leydig or steroid cell) production, including precocious puberty, abnormal menstrual bleeding, and increased risks of breast or uterine cancer.

Although these tumors can be detected at any age, the peak incidence is in the perimenopausal years, with the average age of diagnosis at 52 years. The exception to this is the juvenile granulosa-cell tumor. Approximately one-half of juvenile granulosa-cell tumors will occur below the age of 10 years, and rarely occur after the third decade of life. Thecomas occur at later ages, with the vast majority being diagnosed during and after the sixth decade of life (although luteinized thecomas may occur in younger women). Sertoli–Leydig-cell tumors are very uncommon and usually present at a young age, with the

---

Table 15.5 Classification of sex cord–stromal tumors

I.   Sex cord–stromal tumors
    A.   Granulosa–stromal-cell tumors
        1.   Granulosa-cell tumor
            a.   Adult type
            b.   Juvenile type
        2.   Thecoma, fibroma, or sclerosing stromal tumor
II.   Sertoli–stromal-cell tumors
    A.   Sertoli-cell tumor
    B.   Leydig-cell tumor
    C.   Sertoli–Leydig-cell tumor
III. Sex cord tumors with annular tubules (SCTAT)
IV.   Gynandroblastoma
V.   Steroid-cell tumors
VI.   Unclassified

majority presenting in the second and third decades of life. Fibromas, the most common form of sex cord–stromal tumor, may occur at any age. Fibromas are also associated with Gorlin syndrome, characterized by an inherited predisposition to ovarian fibromas along with basal-cell nevi. Sex cord tumors with annular tubules are associated with Peutz–Jeghers syndrome (PJS) in 35% of cases. It is also important to note that approximately 15% of patients with PJS and SCTAT will develop the highly aggressive form of cervical cancer known as "adenoma malignum."

Presentation of disease

The sex cord–stromal tumors account for the vast majority of ovarian tumors that are active for hormonal production. Thus, the clinical presentation of these tumors is not infrequently via their endocrinologic manifestations. The results of these endocrinologic manifestations are dependent on the age of the individual, and may range from precocious puberty to menstrual abnormalities and postmenopausal bleeding.

Granulosa-cell tumors may present with a pelvic mass, severe pain secondary to ovarian torsion, rupture or hemorrhage into the tumor, or estrogenic endocrine manifestations. Many women will present with menstrual abnormalities ranging from amenorrhea, oligomenorrhea, or menometrorrhagia in the premenopausal woman, to postmenopausal bleeding in older patients. Due to the excess estrogen production of these tumors, it is not uncommon for women to have concurrent endometrial pathology, ranging from endometrial hyperplasia to frank endometrial cancer. These tumors may also produce progesterone, so that decidual changes of the endometrial stroma may be seen, along with secretory changes in the glands.

As with adult granulosa-cell tumors, the patient with a juvenile granulosa-cell tumor may present with a pelvic mass, severe abdominal pain, increased abdominal girth, or endocrinologic manifestations such as isosexual precocious puberty. These patients often have breast enlargement, development of pubic hair, increased vaginal secretions, and other secondary sexual characteristics.

Thecomas are considered to be the most hormonally active tumors, and the vast majority of patients present with signs and symptoms of excess estrogen production, similar to granulosa-cell tumors. Luteinized granulosa-cell tumors may produce androgens, and women may present with masculinization.

Sertoli-cell tumors are associated with excess estrogen production and the aforementioned manifestations, but also may be associated with excess rennin production resulting in refractory hypertension and hypokalemia. Women with Sertoli–Leydig-cell tumors will often have symptoms related to a pelvic mass and, approximately 50% of the time, present with signs of excess androgen production. The most common triad is amenorrhea, voice deepening, and hirsutism. Other signs of masculinization may also occur, such as clitoromegaly, breast atrophy, and temporal hair loss. These patients may also have signs of excess estrogen production due to peripheral conversion of androgens and also production by the tumor. Laboratory abnormalities in virilized women with a Sertoli–Leydig-cell tumor are usually notable for both elevated testosterone and testosterone/androstenedione levels, with normal urinary 17-ketosteroids.

Other sex cord–stromal tumors that are rare and associated with hormone production include the SCTAT, which may present with menstrual irregularities and postmenopausal bleeding. Gynandroblastomas present most commonly with hyperandrogenic manifestations, but excess estrogen production may be present.

Fibromas are the most common of the sex cord–stromal tumors, and they do not produce any hormonal substances. These tumors usually present as a solid adnexal mass, and may reach quite large sizes. They may also be associated with ascites, and occasionally with a pleural effusion (Meigs syndrome).

Pathology/prognostic factors

In general, granulosa cells and Sertoli cells are thought to derive from sex cord cells, while theca cells, Leydig cells, and fibroblasts derive from pluripotent mesenchymal cells. Granulosa-cell tumors account for 70% of malignant sex cord tumors, and those occurring in patients less than age 30 years (juvenile type) differ from the 95% of granulosa-cell tumors that occur after age 30 (adult type).

The majority of adult granulosa-cell tumors exceed 10–15 cm in diameter and are unilateral in 95% of cases. Associated symptoms are a combination of physical ones related to size (pain, distention) and those caused by estrogen excess, as discussed above. Histologically, adult granulosa-cell tumors are cystic, with areas filled with blood or fluid, and consist almost exclusively of a population of granulosa cells. Mitotic figures are numerous, but generally not atypical. Stage is the most important prognostic factor. Other factors, such as rupture, size, histologic subtype, ploidy, and nuclear atypia, have all been correlated with survival, and controversy exists regarding the importance of each factor. A variety of serum markers have been evaluated, and serum inhibin levels have been shown to be elevated at diagnosis, to normalize following surgery, and in some cases, to be elevated several months prior to clinical detection of recurrent disease.

Juvenile granulosa-cell tumors generally occur in prepubertal patients presenting with symptoms of precocious puberty or virilization. Tumors are large, and are also unilateral in 95% of cases. Histologically, they are similar to adult granulosa-cell tumors, with the exception of more rounded hyperchromatic nuclei without grooves, and they have abundant eosinophilic cytoplasm. Survival is good for patients with Stage IA or IB disease (97% at 3.5 years), but the course of juvenile granulosa-cell tumors is more aggressive than that of the adult variety if diagnosed in the advanced stage, based on data on a small number of patients in the literature. Stage at presentation remains the most important prognostic factor, although tumor size, mitotic activity, and nuclear atypia have been reported as significant when considered without regard to stage. In addition, unlike the adult variety, late relapse (after 3 years) in juvenile forms is uncommon.

Theca-cell tumors account for only 1% of sex cord–stromal tumors, and sizes of up to 40 cm have been reported with lipid-filled stromal cells.

Fibromas are the most common sex cord–stromal tumor, and are characterized by increasing edema as their size increases, resulting in ascites in 10–15% of tumors that grow larger than 10 cm. Fibromas are generally considered benign lesions, although variants with increased cellular density and atypia can be considered tumors of low malignant potential. In contrast, fibrosarcomas are highly vascular tumors with hemorrhage, and have increased mitotic figures and marked pleomorphism.

Sertoli–Leydig-cell tumors are extremely uncommon, with most ranging from 5 to 15 cm in diameter. Many are solid and cystic, and may range from well- to poorly differentiated. Heterologous elements occur in approximately 20%. Stage remains the most important prognostic factor, and despite size, Sertoli–Leydig-cell tumors rarely have extra-ovarian spread.

Sex cord tumors with annular tubules (SCTAT) are distinguished by simple or complex ring-shaped tubules ("annular tubules"). When these tumors are associated with PJS, they are often small and bilateral, with areas of calcification. Non-PJS-associated tumors are more often unilateral.

Surgical management

The surgical management is guided by the malignant potential of sex cord–stromal tumors, their ability for hormone production, and the desire of the patient for future fertility. Granulosa-cell tumors constitute the majority of malignant sex cord–stromal tumors, and 22% may be associated with invasive carcinoma of the endometrium. Since the average age of a person with a granulosa-cell tumor is 52 years, most patients will undergo total abdominal hysterectomy with bilateral salpingo-oophorectomy (TAH–BSO) with staging. In general, surgical staging when required consists of a vertical midline incision (although laparoscopic assessment is under study). Palpation of intra-abdominal organs is performed, with washings from the pelvis, right and left paracolic gutters, and right and left hemidiaphragm. Multiple biopsies of the peritoneal surface are obtained, along with sampling of pelvic and para-aortic nodes. An omentectomy is performed. If the patient is appropriate to consider future fertility, unilateral salpingo-oophorectomy (USO) with uterine curettage and staging may be performed instead. These tumors have a propensity for late recurrence, and women are candidates for subsequent resection of recurrence. In contrast to adult granulosa-cell tumors, the juvenile variety occurs in young women in 78% of cases, and most of these patients will undergo USO with staging. Only 5% will have bilateral involvement, so that only visual inspection of the contralateral ovary is required, without biopsy.

Thecomas, fibromas, sclerosing stromal sarcomas, gynandroblastomas, well-differentiated Sertoli–Leydig-cell tumors, and SCTAT with PJS generally do not require extended staging procedures. A USO in patients desiring future fertility, or TAH–BSO in those who do not, will suffice. As with any tumor with potentially excess estrogen production, curettage must be performed if the uterus is left in place. In contrast, in patients with an intermediate- or high-grade Sertoli–Leydig-cell tumor, or with SCTAT not associated with PJS, and in patients with a steroid tumor not otherwise specified, an extended surgical staging procedure should be performed in addition to USO and dilation and curettage (D&C), or TAH–BSO. In patients with SCTAT and PJS, careful attention must also be paid to the cervix pre- and postoperatively, since these women are at risk to develop adenoma malignum of the cervix.

Chemotherapy/radiation therapy

Surgical management remains the mainstay of treatment of sex cord–stromal tumors. In general, there are no data to support the use of adjuvant chemotherapy or radiation therapy in patients with Stage I disease (the most common finding). The presumed benefit of radiation therapy or chemotherapy in more advanced disease is unclear, and trials are hampered by small numbers and heterogeneous populations. A variety of chemotherapeutic regimens have been reported by the Gynecology Oncology Group (GOG), and show modest responses of limited duration. A regimen of dactinomycin, 5-fluorouracil, and cyclophosphamide showed a response rate of 23% among a total of 13 patients. More recently, the combination of bleomycin, etoposide, and cisplatin (BEP) showed a response rate of 82% in 9 patients with poor-prognosis stromal tumors. This prompted a larger GOG study in 57 patients with incompletely resected Stage II–IV granulosa-cell tumors, Sertoli–Leydig-cell tumors, unclassified sex cord–stromal tumors, thecoma, or recurrent disease who were retreated with BEP using negative second-look laparotomy as the endpoint. Of the 38 patients who had second-look laparotomy to confirm response, 14 (37%) had no residual disease. Toxic deaths in two patients from bleomycin resulted in a dose reduction, leading to the recommended regimen being bleomycin 20 U/m^2 day 1 q 3 weeks × 4, etoposide 75 mg/m^2 days 1–5 q 3 weeks, and cisplatin 20 mg/m^2 days 1–5 q 3 weeks × 4. Platinum remains a mainstay of most regimens, and there have been anecdotal reports of modest responses with other agents such as ifosfamide, paclitaxel, and gemcitabine. Small series have evaluated the use of radiation therapy in patients with either gross residual after attempted resection or recurrent disease, and clinical responses have been seen. In a series of 34 patients, 14 of whom had measurable disease at the start of radiation therapy, 6 of the 14 (43%) had a clinical complete response. The optimal approach for patients with advanced sex cord–stromal tumors, or for patients with recurrent disease, has not been defined, and must be individualized without the benefit of randomized data. In relapsed patients, repeat surgical resection is always of prime consideration if complete resection can be performed. Platinum-based chemotherapy and localized radiation therapy can both be useful in appropriately selected cases.

SELECTED READING

Gershenson DM, Management of early ovarian cancer: germ cell and sex cordstromal tumours. *Gynecol Oncol* 1994; 55: S62.

Williams S, Blessing JA, Liao S et al, Adjuvant therapy of ovarian germ cell tumors with cisplatin, etoposide, and bleomycin: a trial of the Gynecologic Oncology Group. *J Clin Oncol* 1994; 12: 701.

Gershenson DM, Update on malignant ovarian germ cell tumours. *Cancer* 1993; 71: 1581.

Gershenson DM, Morris M, Cangir A et al, Treatment of malignant germ cell tumors of the ovary with bleomycin, etoposide, and cisplatin. *J Clin Oncol* 1990; 8: 715.

Kurman RJ, Norris HJ, Malignant germ cell tumors of the ovary. *Hum Pathol* 1977; 8: 551.

Podratz KC, Young RH, Hartmann LC, Ovarian sex cord–stromal tumors. In: *Principles and Practice of Gynecologic Oncology*, 3rd edn (Hoskins WJ et al, eds) Philadelphia: Lippincott, Williams and Wilkins, 2000: 1075.

Homesley H, Bundy B, Hurteau J et al, Bleomycin, etoposide, and cisplatin combination therapy of ovarian granulosa cell tumors and other stromal malignancies: a Gynecology Oncology Group study. *Gynecol Oncol* 1999; 72: 131.

Wolf JK, Mullen J, Eifel PJ et al, Radiation treatment of advanced or recurrent granulosa cell tumors of the ovary. *Gynecol Oncol* 1999; 73: 35.

16
Endometrial cancer

Paul J Sabbatini, Kaled M Alektiar, Richard R Barakat

Carcinoma of the uterine corpus remains the most common pelvic malignancy affecting women worldwide, and the fourth most common cancer in women, following breast, colon, and lung cancers. It is estimated that 38,300 cases will occur in the USA in 2001. Fortunately, endometrial cancers are often detected at an earlier stage than other malignancies, such as ovarian cancer, since patients often present with abnormal vaginal bleeding. The mainstays of therapy remain surgical resection and staging, followed in most instances by radiation therapy. Currently available chemotherapy and endocrine therapy offer limited responses in the recurrent setting. Clinical investigation is aimed at identifying new agents with improved activity, and evaluating the role of chemotherapy applied earlier in the disease course. New treatments are needed for patients with advanced and recurrent disease.

EPIDEMIOLOGY AND RISK FACTORS

Endometrial cancer occurs most commonly in postmenopausal women, although 25% of cases occur before menopause and 5% in patients less than 40 years of age. The incidence of endometrial cancer is higher in western countries than eastern ones, and environmental factors are important, since immigrant populations generally assume the risk of native ones. In the USA, Caucasian women have a twofold higher risk of developing this disease than African–American women, and it is more common among urban than rural residents.

Factors for increased risk of endometrial carcinoma include the following: unopposed estrogens (4–15×), obesity (3× if <30 lbs IBW), nulliparity (2×), menopause after age 52 (2.5×), hypertension (1.5×), diabetes mellitus (3×), diet (possible relationship to high fat intake), complex endometrial hyperplasia, and use of tamoxifen. Of note, patients with simple endometrial hyperplasia appear to have only a slightly increased risk, while up to 29% of those with complex hyperplasia will develop invasive adenocarcinoma. The risk for tamoxifen is the subject of many recent studies given the data supporting its use in the prevention of breast cancer. Risk estimates vary between 2.5 and 9 times but are consistently linked to duration of treatment. It is notable that in the National Surgical Adjuvant Breast and Bowel Project's prevention trial, NSABP-P1, with 13,000 patients, all of the endometrial cancers were discovered at an early stage.

Smoking actually decreases the risk of endometrial cancer, most likely through an antiestrogenic mechanism. Combination oral contraceptives also decrease risk.

HISTOLOGY

Endometroid adenocarcinoma is present in 75–80% of cases. Grade (1 = well differentiated, 2 = moderately differentiated, and 3 = poorly differentiated) is an important variable for determining prognosis and potential treatment. Squamous differentiation is present in 30–50% of cases. Clear-cell carcinomas may occur, often in older women, and, as in cervix, vaginal, or ovarian sites, confer a poor prognosis. Papillary serous differentiation occurs in less than 10% of cases. As in ovarian cancers, these tumors tend to have a propensity for early intraperitoneal spread rather than localized recurrence, and are considered to be quite aggressive.

In general, tumors of endometroid histology fail locally, although metastasis to pulmonary, bone, brain, or other distant sites may occur. Serous and clear-cell cancers tend to fail more diffusely in the peritoneal cavity, in keeping with the failure pattern of this histology from other primary sites.

PRESENTATION

Fortunately, the most common presenting symptom for early-stage endometrial cancer in postmenopausal women is vaginal bleeding or abnormal discharge. In the general population, 15% of postmenopausal women presenting with abnormal bleeding will have endometrial carcinoma. Of the patients with endometrial carcinoma, 80–90% will have noted an abnormal discharge prior to diagnosis. The diagnosis is obviously more difficult in premenopausal women, and endometrial sampling must be performed in all women noting a change in menstrual habits, including menorrhagia or metrorrhagia. No data exist to support screening in the general population in those patients not receiving unopposed estrogen hormone replacement or tamoxifen.

DIAGNOSIS

The gold standard for assessing abnormal uterine bleeding and diagnosing uterine carcinoma remains fractional dilatation and curettage. This procedure entails curetting the endocervix, followed by sounding of the uterus. The cervix is then dilated, and systematic curetting of the entire endometrial cavity is performed. Outpatient endometrial biopsy or aspiration curettage that avoids general anesthesia may be performed prior to formal dilatation and curettage, but these are definitive only if positive for cancer.

STAGING

Cancer of the uterus is surgically staged. See Appendix 2 of this handbook for the FIGO staging system.

THERAPY BY STAGE

Primary management currently consists of surgery followed, in selected instances, by radiation therapy. There is no role for chemotherapy as part of definitive primary treatment (except in Stage IV disease) pending the results of randomized clinical trials.

Surgery

To appropriately stage by the FIGO criteria, the surgical procedure should minimally include an adequate abdominal incision, usually vertical, sampling of peritoneal fluid for cytologic evaluation (intraperitoneal cell washings), and abdominal and pelvic exploration with biopsy or excision of any extrauterine lesions suspicious for tumor. Total abdominal hysterectomy and bilateral salpingo-oophorectomy (TAH–BSO) are the standard operative procedures for carcinoma of the endometrium. The plane of excision lies outside the pubocervical fascia and does not require unroofing of the ureters. The ovarian and fallopian tubes are removed en bloc with the uterus. In some cases, pelvic lymph-node sampling is indicated. This consists of a sample of lymph nodes taken from the distal common iliac and from the superior iliac artery and vein. A third sample of lymphatics is obtained from the group of nodes that lie along the obturator nerve. In a lymph-node sampling procedure, it is important to try to achieve an adequate sample of nodes from each anatomic site, but no attempt is made to perform a complete lymphadenectomy. Since lymph-node sampling is not routinely performed by the general gynecologist, it is important to identify the subset of patients who will benefit from selective lymphadenectomy; this subset of patients may require the further surgical expertise of a gynecologic oncologist. If there is no gross intraperitoneal tumor noted at the time of laparotomy, pelvic and para-aortic lymph nodes should be sampled for the following indications: myometrial invasion greater than one-half (outer half of myometrium); tumor presence in the isthmus–cervix or adnexa, or other extrauterine metastases, regardless of tumor grade; presence of serous, clear-cell, undifferentiated, or squamous types; and lymph nodes that are visibly or palpably enlarged.

For patients in whom para-aortic node sampling is indicated, sampling can be performed through a midline peritoneal incision over the common iliac arteries and aorta. Node sampling can also be performed on the right by mobilizing the right colon medially and on the left by mobilizing the left colon medially. In each case, a sample of lymphatics and lymph nodes is resected along the upper common iliac vessels on either side and from the lower portion of the aorta and vena cava. On the left side, the lymph nodes and lymphatics are slightly posterior to the aorta, and on the right side, they lie primarily in the vena caval fat bed. After these procedures, the patient is surgically staged according to the FIGO criteria (see Appendix 2). The overall surgical complication rate after this type of staging is approximately 20%, with a serious complication rate of 6%.

In the Gynecologic Oncology Group (GOG) study 33, 46% of the positive para-aortic lymph nodes were enlarged, and 98% of the cases with aortic node metastases came from patients with positive pelvic nodes, adnexal or intra-abdominal metastases, or outer one-third myometrial invasion. These risk factors affected only 25% of the patients, yet they yielded most of the positive para-aortic node patients. Overall, 5–6% of patients with clinical Stage I and II (occult) endometrial carcinoma have tumor spread to these lymph nodes. The key to the surgical management of patients with endometrial cancer is identifying patients at risk for retroperitoneal nodal metastasis, since both patients with pelvic and aortic disease can be salvaged with adjuvant radiation therapy. Postoperative irradiation to the pelvis and aortic area appears to be effective, since approximately 36% will remain tumor-free at 5 years. Although accounting for only 5–6% of patients with early-stage endometrial cancer, it is important that patients with metastatic spread to the para-aortic nodes be identified, since approximately 40% will be salvaged with extended-field radiation therapy.

Lymph nodes need not be sampled for tumor limited to the endometrium, regardless of grade, because less than 1% of these patients have disease spread to pelvic or para-aortic lymph nodes. Patients whose only risk factor is inner-one-half myometrial invasion, particularly if the grade is 2 or 3, fall within a gray zone regarding lymph-node sampling. This group has 5% or less chance of node positivity. Lymph-node sampling should be performed in these instances if there seems to be any question about the degree of myometrial invasion. This includes invasion that approaches one-half of the myometrial thickness in patients who are medically fit to undergo the sampling procedures.

The depth of myometrial invasion can be assessed easily at the time of surgery. The excised uterus is opened, preferably away from the operating table, and the depth of myometrial penetration and presence or absence of endocervix involvement is determined by clinical observation or by microscopic frozen section. The reported accuracy rate for determining the depth of myometrial invasion by gross visual examination of the cut uterine surface is 91%.

Nine percent of patients with endometrial carcinoma have positive pelvic lymph nodes (Stage IIIC). The incidence is increased to 51%, 32%, and 25%, respectively, in patients with extrauterine metastases, adnexal involvement, and deep myometrial invasion. Patients with this as their only high-risk factor should be treated with postoperative whole-pelvic irradiation. In the GOG study 33, 13 (72%) of 18 patients were disease-free at 5 years after treatment.

Laparoscopic surgery

An alternative method of surgically staging patients with clinical Stage I endometrial cancer is gaining in popularity. This approach combines laparoscopically assisted vaginal hysterectomy with laparoscopic lymphadenectomy. Childers and colleagues described their experience with this procedure in 59 patients with clinical Stage I endometrial carcinoma. The laparoscopic procedure included a thorough inspection of the peritoneal cavity, obtaining intraperitoneal washings, and performing a laparoscopically assisted vaginal hysterectomy. Laparoscopic pelvic and aortic lymph-node sampling were performed in all patients with grade 2 or 3 lesions, as well as those patients with grade 1 lesions who were found to have greater than 50% myometrial invasion on frozen section. In two patients, laparoscopic lymphadenectomy was precluded by obesity.

Six patients who were noted to have intraperitoneal disease at laparoscopy underwent exploratory laparotomy. Two additional patients required laparotomy for complications including a transected ureter and a cystotomy. The mean hospital stay was 2.9 days.

Laparoscopically assisted surgical staging is feasible in select groups of patients. It is not known, however, whether it is applicable to all patients with clinical Stage I disease. In particular, two groups of patients may not be ideal candidates, the first owing to the presence of intra-abdominal adhesions and the second because of their weight. Para-aortic lymphadenectomy is technically more difficult through the laparoscope; to obtain adequate exposure, it is necessary to elevate the mesentery of the small bowel into the upper abdomen, which becomes increasingly difficult as the patient's weight increases, especially for patients whose weight exceeds 180 lbs.

Although laparoscopically assisted vaginal hysterectomy with surgical staging may provide an alternative approach to the management of endometrial cancer, its equivalency to the standard laparotomy approach remains unproven with respect to cancer outcome. The GOG is conducting a randomized trial of these two approaches to help answer this question.

Radiation therapy

Radiation therapy plays a central role in the management of endometrial cancer. It is often used as an adjuvant treatment before or after surgery for patients with Stage I–III disease. Under certain circumstances, it is also used as a definitive treatment for those patients who are resectable but medically inoperable.

Adnexal or serosal involvement
These patients have a 5-year survival rate of 75% following pelvic radiation therapy. Usually, the pelvis is treated to a total dose of 50.4 Gy at 1.8 Gy per fraction.

Vaginal involvement
This substage represents a very small group of patients, and the amount of available data with which to guide treatment is very limited. Depending on the location of the vaginal involvement, the nature of irradiation can range from adjuvant, if the upper vagina is involved, to definitive, if the lower vagina is involved. In the former group, the patients could be treated with pelvic irradiation followed by intravaginal brachytherapy; for the latter, the brachytherapy component is usually done with a Syed implant in order to treat the uterus and the whole length of the vagina. In addition, the pelvic irradiation field should extend to include the inguinal lymph nodes.

Positive pelvic nodes
The standard treatment approach for this substage is postoperative pelvic irradiation to a total dose of 50.4 Gy. The 5-year survival rate is usually 70%. Some authors recommend WAR or chemotherapy. The latter approach is warranted in patients with positive cytology as well as positive pelvic lymph nodes.

Positive para-aortic nodes
These patients are generally treated with extended-field irradiation that includes the pelvis and para-aortic lymph nodes. The dose is usually limited to 45 Gy at 1.8 Gy per fraction in order to limit the dose to the bowel. Alternatively, patients could be treated with WAR or chemotherapy. The 5-year survival rate is 35%.

Stage IV disease and rare histology
If the patient is resectable with minimal gross residual disease (<2 cm), WAR is indicated, with a reported 3-year progression-free survival rate of 30%. If the tumor is unresectable, neoadjuvant chemotherapy followed by definitive or preoperative irradiation, depending on the response, could be considered. Tumors with papillary serous or clear-cell histologies behave more like ovarian cancer, with a high rate of failure in the upper abdomen. Therefore, many patients with these types of tumors are treated with WAR or chemotherapy, except for those with very early-stage tumors. For patients with uterine sarcomas, postoperative irradiation is usually recommended for mixed Müllerian tumor (MMT) and stromal sarcomas in order to reduce the rate of local failure. For patients with leiomyosarcoma, the predominant form of relapse is distant; therefore, any improvement in local control will have little impact on the outcome. At MSKCC, local irradiation is considered in the case of leiomyosarcoma if an incomplete local resection of the primary tumor occurs and no extrapelvic disease is identified. When irradiation is given, the dose is usually 50.4 Gy to the whole pelvis.

Radiation treatment techniques

Intravaginal brachytherapy

The goal of treatment is to deliver the highest dose of radiation to the vaginal mucosa while limiting the dose to the surrounding normal structures such as the bladder or bowel. Intravaginal brachytherapy can be delivered with *low-dose-rate* cesium-137 (^{137}Cs) sources, which require admission to the hospital. The dose is usually 60 Gy prescribed to the vaginal mucosa. The treatment is generally delivered by the two ovoids from a Fletcher–Suit applicator, where only the vaginal cuff is irradiated. Alternatively, a cylinder could be used to treat one-half to two-thirds of the length of the vagina. Occasionally, the whole length of the vagina needs to be treated, especially in patients with grade 3 tumors, which have a tendency to relapse in the distal periurethral region. More recently, *high-dose-rate brachytherapy* using iridium-192 (^{192}Ir) sources has been shown to be an attractive alternative to low-dose-rate brachytherapy. The treatment is given on an outpatient basis without the need for anesthesia and without radiation exposure to medical personnel. At MSKCC, patients start treatment 4–6 weeks after surgery. The treatment is given in three fractions of 7 Gy to a total dose of 21 Gy. The dose is prescribed to 0.5 cm depth from the mucosal surface. The treatment is usually delivered using a 3-cm diameter cylinder to treat one-half to two-thirds of the length of the vagina, or the whole vagina in the case of grade 3 tumors. The toxicity associated with intravaginal brachytherapy when used alone has been very low. The 5-year actuarial complication rate for grade 2, 3, and 4 disease is about 4%. The dose per fraction is lowered to 4–5 Gy when pelvic irradiation is added.

Pelvic irradiation

The goal of this approach is to treat the vagina as well as the pelvic lymph nodes. The treatment is usually delivered with high-energy photons (15 MeV) to spare the skin and subcutaneous tissue. The standard field arrangement is a four-field box technique that allows some sparing of bowel in the lateral fields. The toxicity of postoperative pelvic irradiation is higher than that of intravaginal brachytherapy. The reported rates in the literature range from 5–20%, depending on the sequence of irradiation and surgery and on whether or not patients had lymph-node dissection. When pelvic irradiation is used alone, the dose is usually 50.4 Gy at 1.8 Gy per fraction. When used in addition to intravaginal brachytherapy, the dose is lowered to 45 Gy in order to decrease the dose to the surrounding normal structures. If pelvic irradiation is indicated, it is unclear whether intravaginal brachytherapy is still needed. At MSKCC, this combined approach is routinely used with excellent local control (96%) and minimal toxicity (2–5%). Other investigators, however, have shown equivalent results with pelvic irradiation alone. In GOG study 99, for example, the vaginal/pelvic local control rate was 98.5% with pelvic irradiation alone. Most authors, however, agree on a combined approach for patients with Stage IIB disease.

Locally recurrent disease
The treatment approach depends on whether or not the patient has had prior irradiation.

Previously irradiated patients
These patients generally have limited therapeutic options. The reported 5-year local control and overall survival rates are 33% and 16%, respectively. If radiation is to be given, an interstitial implant to a dose of 35–40 Gy could be considered. This approach should be used with caution, however, owing to the potential increase in late complications. Isolated pelvic central recurrence after irradiation is rare. If it does occur, selected patients may benefit from pelvic exenterative surgery. There are no large published series, but some long-term survivors have been reported. The MSKCC reported its experience with 44 patients who underwent pelvic exenteration for recurrent endometrial cancer between 1947 and 1994. Primary therapy usually consisted of TAH–BSO, with most receiving either pre- or postoperative radiation therapy. Prior to exenteration, 10 of 44 (23%) patients had never received any form of radiation therapy. The median interval between initial surgery and exenteration was 28 months (range 2–189 months). Exenteration was total in 23 patients (52%), anterior in 20 patients (46%), and limited to posterior in one patient. One vascular injury led to the only intraoperative death. Major postoperative complications occurred in 35 (80%) patients, and included intestinal/urinary tract fistulas, pelvic abscess, septicemia, pulmonary embolism, and cerebrovascular accident. The median survival for the entire group of patients was 7.36 months, with nine (20%) patients achieving long-term survival (>5 years). Although only 20% of patients achieved long-term survival, this procedure remains the only potentially curative option for the few patients with central recurrence of endometrial cancer who have failed standard surgery and radiation therapy.

Radiation-naive patients
These patients should be staged like those with primary vaginal cancer because of prognostic and therapeutic implications. If the patient has Stage I disease with very minimal disease in the vaginal cuff, they could be treated with intravaginal irradiation and pelvic irradiation. For higher stages, the patient should be treated with pelvic irradiation and an interstitial implant to improve the dose distribution in the paravaginal region. The reported 5-year local control and overall survival rates are 56% and 48%, respectively.

THERAPY FOR RECURRENT DISEASE

Options for the treatment of recurrent disease include endocrine therapy, standard chemotherapy, and inclusion in clinical trials.

Endocrine therapy

In general, the best response rates for endocrine therapy correlate with well-differentiated histology, a long disease-free interval following primary treatment (approaching 12 months), and increased progesterone-receptor concentrations. The rate of receptor positivity is tightly correlated with and increases with well-differentiated histology, and receptor status generally does not need to be determined for routine clinical management.

Progestational agents are the most well studied, although a variety of hormonal manipulations have been attempted. The overall response rate for progestin therapy is 25%, with overall progression-free survival of 4 months, and overall survival remains unchanged at 10–12 months. Partial responses are the rule, but a minority of patients may have complete responses that can last for years. Hormonal therapy can be considered first line in patients with well-differentiated or moderately differentiated histology, reserving cytotoxic chemotherapy for progression. (See Table 16.1.)

A study by the GOG has shown that doses of medroxyprogesterone higher than 200 mg/day are not beneficial, and that response remains highly correlated with histology (37%, grade 1; 23%, grade 2; and 9%, grade 3) when comparing well-differentiated with moderately or poorly differentiated tumors. The most common adverse effects of megestrol acetate, the most commonly used agent, are fluid retention, increased appetite with weight gain, and a possible increased risk of thrombosis, although this is debatable.

Chemotherapy

Currently, chemotherapy for patients with recurrent advanced endometrial cancer remains palliative. Responses are generally partial in 20–40% of patients. Progression-free intervals are generally 4–5 months, and overall survival remains at 10–12 months. The small number of patients who achieve complete remissions may have responses lasting several years. Chemotherapy regimens with single agents usually have lower response rates than combination approaches, but progression-free survival and overall survival for combination regimens are not significantly increased, and the toxicity of combination therapies is greater. No advantage has been seen for combinations of chemotherapy with endocrine therapy. (See Table 16.2.)

Table 16.1 Common endocrine-therapy regimens in advanced endometrial cancer

Agent	Dose/schedule	Response rate [range] (%)
Megestrol acetate	40 mg orally q.i.d.	20 [11–56]
Medroxyprogesterone	200 mg orally daily	25 [14–53]
Tamoxifen	20 mg orally b.i.d.	18 [0–53]

Table 16.2 Common chemotherapy regimens in advanced endometrial cancer

Single agents			
Regimen	Dose (mg/m^2)	Schedule (wks)	Approximate response rate (%)
Cisplatin	50	q 3	21
Carboplatin	AUC 4–5	q 4	28
Doxorubicin	60	q 3	26
Ifosfamide	1,500 (3–5 day)	q 3–4	24
Paclitaxel	175 (3 hr)	q 3–4	36
Combination regimens			
Regimen	Dose (mg/m^2)	Schedule (wks)	Approximate response rate (%)
Doxorubicin +cisplatin	60 50	q 3–4	42
Paclitaxel +cisplatin	135 (24 hr) 75	q 3–4	67[a]
Paclitaxel +carboplatin	175 (3 hr) AUC 5	q 3–4	63
Cyclophosphamide +doxorubicin +cisplatin	400–600 50 50	q 3–4	45

[a]Progression-free survival 8 months.

General treatment strategy for recurrent disease

Combination endocrine therapy with chemotherapy, including sequential or alternating therapies, has not been shown to be superior to either modality alone. In general, endocrine therapies should be initially applied to patients with well-differentiated or moderately well-differentiated tumors, and cytotoxic chemotherapy should be reserved for progression. Single-agent chemotherapy is preferable, and combinations are generally considered only if the higher response rate is needed because of major symptoms or life-threatening disease, recognizing that an impact on overall survival has not been shown.

FOLLOW-UP

Based on surveillance data that have been correlated with outcome, and on consensus opinion at MSKCC and other institutions, the following recommendations for follow-up can be proposed:

For patients with Stage I or II disease, office visits are scheduled every 6 months for the first 3 years and annually thereafter. Pap tests are performed annually. No routine chest radiographs are required. CA-125 levels are followed if elevated at diagnosis.

For patients with Stage III and IV disease, office visits are scheduled more frequently, at 3-month intervals for the first 2 years, at 6-month intervals for years 3–5, and then annually thereafter. Pap tests are performed every 6 months. Chest radiographs are obtained yearly. CA-125 levels are followed if elevated at diagnosis.

Routine health maintenance is performed in all patients according to standard guidelines (blood pressure, lipid profile, mammogram, immunizations, stool guaiac ± endoscopy, etc.). Further evaluation is based on symptoms.

FUTURE THERAPY

Using previously tested regimens, no benefit for adjuvant treatment with either chemotherapy or hormonal therapy has been proven. Clinical trials are attempting to answer the question of whether radiation therapy and chemotherapy are equivalent in terms of improving outcome in the adjuvant setting. For example, a Phase III protocol has been completed by the GOG comparing WAR therapy with combination cisplatin–doxorubicin chemotherapy in patients with Stage III–IV disease. The results are pending. If these approaches are equivalent, the chemotherapy arm may have fewer long-term complications than the radiation-therapy arm in this setting. The next step is to move regimens with higher response rates (perhaps paclitaxel with carboplatin) forward and compare these combinations with radiation treatment. A randomized trial by the GOG comparing doxorubicin and cisplatin (the current standard) with doxorubicin and paclitaxel to determine if the paclitaxel-containing regimen is superior has been accrued; results are not yet available. Whether chemotherapy is beneficial in addition to radiation therapy is unknown, and these clinical trials are currently underway. New agents with improved response rates are needed, and Phase I trials are reasonable in patients who have had progression on at least one standard chemotherapy agent.

SELECTED READING

Barakat RR, Goldman NA, Patel DA et al, Pelvic exenteration for recurrent endometrial cancer. *Gynecol Oncol* 1999; 75: 99.

Barakat R, Greven K, Muss H, Endometrial cancer. In: *Cancer Management: A Multidisciplinary Approach* (Coia LR, Hoskins WJ, Pazdur R, Wagman LD, eds). Mellville, NY: PPR, 1999: 269.

Creutzberg CL, van Putten WL, Koper PC et al, Surgery and postoperative radiotherapy versus surgery alone for patients with stage-1 endometrial carcinoma: multicentre randomised trial: PORTEC Study Group. Post Operative Radiation Therapy in Endometrial Carcinoma. *Lancet* 2000; **355**: 1404.

Gemignani ML, Curtin JP, Zelmanovich J et al, Laparoscopic-assisted vaginal hysterectomy for endometrial cancer: clinical outcomes and hospital charges. *Gynecol Oncol* 1999; 73: 5.

Lentz SS, Advanced and recurrent endometrial carcinoma: hormonal therapy. *Semin Oncol* 1994; **21**: 100.

Markman M, Kennedy A, Webster K et al, Persistent chemosensitivity to platinum and/or paclitaxel in metastatic endometrial cancer. *Gynecol Oncol* 1999; **73**: 422.

Morrow CP, Bundy BN, Kumar RJ et al, Relationship between surgical–pathological risk factors and outcome in clinical stages I and II carcinoma of the endometrium. A Gynecologic Oncology Group study. *Gynecol Oncol* 1991; **40**: 55.

Thigpen JT, Brady MF, Alvarez RD et al, Oral medroxyprogesterone acetate in the treatment of advanced or recurrent endometrial carcinoma: a dose response study by the Gynecologic Oncology Group. *J Clin Oncol* 1999; **17**: 1736.

17
Breast cancer

Mary L Gemignani

Breast cancer remains the most common cancer in women, and is second only to lung cancer as the leading cause of cancer-related death. It is estimated that in the USA, 192,200 new cases will be diagnosed in 2001, with 40,200 cancer deaths in women. The lifetime risk among women in the USA of being diagnosed with breast cancer is 12% (1 in 8); the lifetime risk of dying from breast cancer is 3.6% (1 in 28). Although breast cancer remains a serious health concern in the USA as well as in other countries, breast cancer mortality is declining in the USA and in other industrialized countries. This is thought to be due to increased utilization of mammographic screening, early detection of disease, and the availability of improved therapies.

EPIDEMIOLOGY

The incidence of breast cancer increases with age. Early menarche, late menopause, and nulliparity are thought to be risk factors for breast cancer. Atypical lobular or ductal hyperplasia also increases the risk. Other risk factors are early exposure to ionizing radiation, long-term postmenopausal estrogen replacement therapy, and, possibly, alcohol consumption. The most important risk factor is family history of breast cancer. It is currently estimated that 5–10% of all breast cancers are attributable to highly penetrant mutations in breast cancer susceptibility genes. Two such tumor suppressor genes, *BRCA1* and *BRCA2*, have been well characterized.

Breast cancer has also been noted to occur in association with other cancers. The association between breast and ovarian carcinoma was first reported by Lynch in 1971. Other associated syndromes include Li–Fraumeni syndrome, Cowden syndrome, and the breast–ovarian cancer syndrome.

BRCA1 AND *BRCA2*

The identification and successful cloning of these breast cancer susceptibility genes have expanded our knowledge of familial breast cancer. The initial investigations in families with a high incidence of breast cancer only or of breast and ovarian cancers led to the discovery of a single autosomal-dominant cancer susceptibility gene, *BRCA1*. Linkage studies done in 1990 in early-onset breast cancer families led to cloning of the *BRCA1* gene at the University of Utah in Salt Lake City in 1994. The *BRCA1* gene consists of 22 coding exons distributed over approximately 100 kb of genomic DNA on chromosome 17q21. It is thought to be responsible for approximately 45% of early-onset hereditary breast cancers, and nearly 90% of hereditary ovarian cancers in families with a high incidence of breast and ovarian cancers. Two specific mutations, 185delAG and 5382insC, are present in approximately 1% and 0.25% of the Ashkenazi Jewish population, respectively. They are thought to be founder mutations (i.e., an altered gene or genes seen with a high frequency in a population originating from a small ancestral group, one or more of the founders of which was a carrier of the mutant gene).

BRCA2 was isolated on chromosome 13q12–13 in 1995. The *BRCA2* gene is composed of 26 coding exons distributed over approximately 70 kb of genomic DNA. This gene appears to account for 35% of families with early-onset breast cancer. It confers a lower risk of ovarian cancer compared with breast cancer. A single mutation, 6174delT, is found in approximately 1.4% of the Ashkenazi Jewish population. Together, both *BRCA1* and *BRCA2* mutations are found in approximately 1 in 40 Ashkenazi Jewish individuals.

Initial estimates of the penetrance of *BRCA1* and *BRCA2* used large pedigrees with many cases of cancer. For both genes, the point estimate for penetrance of all disease-associated alleles seemed to be 70–90% for breast cancer by age 70 years, but the risk of breast cancer by age 50 may be lower for *BRCA2* mutations.

ANATOMY

The adult breast lies between the second and sixth ribs in the vertical plane and between the sternal edge medially and midaxillary line laterally. The average breast measures 10–12 cm in diameter and 5–7 cm centrally. It is concentric, with a projection into the axilla that is called the *axillary tail of Spence*. The glandular breast is divided into 15–20 segments (lobes) that converge at the nipple in a radial arrangement. These lobes are made up of 20–40 lobules. Each lobule is made up of 10–100 alveoli (tubulo-saccular secretory units). Collecting milk ducts drain each segment. There is subcutaneous connective tissue between the lobes of glandular tissue.

The breast lies on the pectoralis muscle and is enveloped by a superficial pectoral fascia that is continuous with the superficial abdominal fascia of Camper. The blood supply of the breast is mostly from superficial vessels. The principal blood supply is derived from the internal thoracic artery and lateral thoracic artery. The superficial veins follow the arteries and drain through perforating branches of the internal thoracic vein that are tributaries of the axillary vein and perforating branches of posterior intercostal veins.

The axilla is a pyramidal space between the arm and thoracic wall. It contains the axillary vessels and their branches, the brachial plexus and its branches, and lymph nodes embedded in fatty tissue. The axilla has an axillary fascia that is an investing layer extending from the pectoralis major to the latissimus dorsi. The clavipectoral fascia is a condensation of the fascia extending from the clavicle to the axillary fascia in the floor of the axilla. Halsted's ligament is a dense condensation of this fascia. The axillary artery may be divided into three parts based on location in relation to the pectoralis minor.

The primary route of lymphatic drainage of the breast is through the axillary lymph nodes. The lymph nodes are also divided into levels based on location relative to the pectoralis minor. Level 1 lymph nodes lie lateral to the lateral border of the pectoralis minor muscle. Level 2 nodes lie behind the pectoralis minor muscle, and Level 3 nodes are medial to the medial border of this muscle.

In dissection of the axilla, nerve branches of the brachial plexus are encountered. The lateral pectoral nerve supplies the pectoralis major and gives a branch that communicates with the medial pectoral nerve. The medial pectoral nerve passes between the axillary artery and vein to enter the deep surface of the pectoralis minor and continue into the pectoralis major. It is the main nerve innervation to the pectoralis minor. The thoracodorsal nerve runs downward, crossing the lateral border of the scapula and the teres major to enter the costal surface of the latissimus dorsi. The long thoracic nerve is located on the medial wall of the axilla on the serratus anterior. It arises from the C5–C7 roots and enters the axilla through the cervicoaxillary canal. Injury to this nerve results in paralysis to part or all of the serratus anterior. The functional deficit is inability to raise the arm above the level of the shoulder. The intercostobrachial nerve innervates the medial aspect of the upper arm, and disruption will cause numbness.

HISTOPATHOLOGIC CHARACTERISTICS

Noninvasive breast cancer

Ductal carcinoma in situ (DCIS)

Ductal carcinoma in situ is an abnormal proliferation of malignant epithelial cells within the mammary ductal–lobular system without invasion into the surrounding stroma. It is classified as a heterogenous group of lesions with different growth patterns and cytologic features. Classification of DCIS has traditionally been based on architectural pattern. The most common types are comedo, cribriform, micropapillary, papillary, and solid.

Comedo-type DCIS is characterized by the presence of abundant necrosis. Microscopically, the cells are large, with pleomorphic nuclei, and have numerous mitotic figures. *Cribriform*-type DCIS is characterized by a fenestrated, sieve-like growth pattern. Cells are small to medium in size and have uniform hyperchromatic nuclei with rare mitoses. *Micropapillary* DCIS has small tufts of cells that project into the lumen of involved spaces and do not have fibrovascular cores. The cells are small to medium in size, with hyperchromatic nuclei and rare mitoses. *Papillary* DCIS is also characterized by intraluminal projection of cells. In contrast to micropapillary DCIS, however, these cells have true fibrovascular cores and thus constitute true papillae. *Intracystic papillary* carcinoma is a variant of papillary DCIS in which the cells are primarily in a single cystically dilated space. *Solid*-type DCIS is characterized by tumor cells that fill and distend involved spaces without a specific architectural pattern.

Lobular carcinoma in situ (LCIS)

Foote and Stewart initially described lobular carcinoma in situ in 1941 as a noninvasive lesion arising from the lobules and terminal ducts of the breast. Their initial report identifies three important features of LCIS: (1) it is usually an incidental microscopic finding that is not detected clinically or by gross pathologic examination; (2) it is multicentric, and the associated cancer may be ductal or lobular; (3) the risk for subsequent cancer is the same for both breasts. LCIS is characterized by a solid proliferation of small cells, with round to oval nuclei, that distorts the involved spaces in the terminal ductal–lobular units.

Invasive carcinoma

Invasive duct carcinoma

Invasive duct carcinoma is the most common group of malignant mammary tumors, and comprises 65–80% of all mammary carcinomas. Included in this group are tubular, medullary, metaplastic, mucinous (colloid), papillary, and adenoid cystic carcinoma. *Invasive duct carcinoma not otherwise specified (NOS)* is a generic term that includes tumors that may express elements of more than one of the specific forms of duct carcinoma.

Subtypes of invasive duct carcinoma

- *Tubular (well-differentiated) carcinoma* is a form of mammary carcinoma in which the lesion is characterized by elements resembling normal breast ductules. Although these elements may be seen in invasive duct carcinoma NOS, 75% of the tumor must be tubular to be designated a tubular carcinoma. It comprises less than 2% of all breast carcinomas in most series.
- *Medullary carcinomas* are usually large circumscribed tumors that have a tendency to cystic degeneration. Tumors form large, broad sheets that are circumscribed and have an intense lymphoplasmacytic reaction around and within the tumor. Medullary carcinomas comprise 7% of all breast carcinomas.
- *Metaplastic carcinomas* refer to tumors that have glandular epithelium with a nonglandular differentiation. The mechanism by which this metaplasia occurs is not well understood. These tumors are characterized by the presence of homologous (epithelial) or heterologous (mesenchymal) elements. Two types have been described: squamous and pseudosarcomatous metaplasia. They constitute less than 1% of all mammary carcinomas.

- *Mucinous (colloid) carcinomas* are characterized by the presence of abundant extracellular mucin around clusters of tumor cells. However, gland formation is uncommon. In their pure form, these tumors constitute 1–2% of breast carcinomas.
- *Papillary carcinoma* is applied to carcinomas that form a mass in which there is a predominantly a frond-forming growth pattern. They constitute 1–2% of breast carcinomas.
- *Adenoid cystic carcinomas* constitute less than 0.1% of mammary carcinoma. They are characterized by a mixture of glandular (adenoid) and stromal components. The histopathologic appearance is similar to that of tumors that arise in the salivary glands.

Infiltrating lobular carcinoma

Infiltrating lobular carcinomas have been reported to constitute 10–14% of invasive carcinomas. They are characterized by uniform cells with small, round nuclei and limited cytoplasm. The presence of intracytoplasmic mucin vacuoles often give the cells the appearance of signet-ring cells. The cells tend to grow circumferentially around ducts and lobules with a linear arrangement. This pattern is referred to as "Indian-file" or targetoid growth. There is often an associated desmoplastic stromal reaction.

Inflammatory carcinoma

Inflammatory carcinoma is characterized by the cutaneous finding present with an underlying invasive carcinoma. Usually, the invasive tumor is a poorly differentiated infiltrating duct carcinoma. Upon microscopic evaluation, skin involvement often reveals tumor emboli in dermal lymphatics with an associated lymphocytic reaction in the dermis.

Metastases from extramammary tumors

The most common primary site of an occult extramammary tumor is the lung. Other primary sites include the ovaries, the uterus, the kidneys, and the stomach. In those previously diagnosed, melanoma, prostate, cervix, uterus, and urinary bladder are the most common. Metastatic ovarian cancer may simulate papillary or mucinous carcinoma of the breast. A workup and history are often helpful in difficult cases. Often, identification of an in situ component helps to provide definitive evidence of a mammary origin.

CLINICAL PRESENTATION/DIAGNOSIS

The widespread use of screening mammography has resulted in a significant increase in the detection rate of DCIS as well as nonpalpable invasive breast cancer. Classically, however, the initial presentation of breast cancer is a breast mass.

Physical examination

Obtaining a thorough history, including a family history, is the initial step in a breast examination. Breast examination should be done with the patient in both the sitting and supine position. The steps of breast examination are illustrated in Figures 17.1–17.5. Multipositional examination is important, since breast retraction and subtle changes may be missed if the patient is examined in only one position. Symmetry, retraction, and changes in the skin, as well as the nipple, should be noted. If lymph nodes are palpable, their size and character should also be noted.

Mammography

The primary role of mammography is to screen women with no symptoms and to detect breast cancer at an early stage. It is often used in conjunction with the physical examination if a mass is found. Because some palpable cancers are invisible mammographically, the study cannot be used to exclude cancer. If the clinical examination is suspicious, a negative mammogram should not delay further investigation.

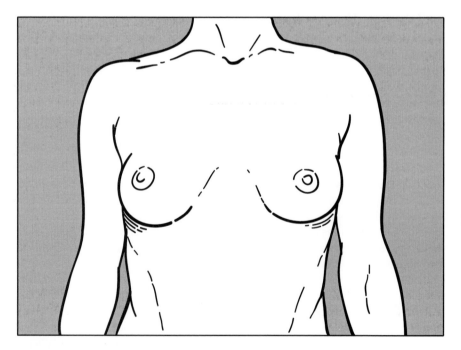

Figure 17.1

Inspection of patient with arms at sides.

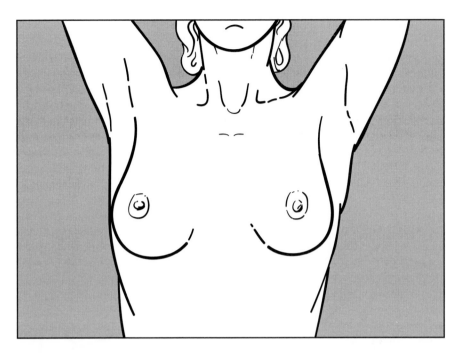

Figure 17.2
Inspection of patient with both arms raised.

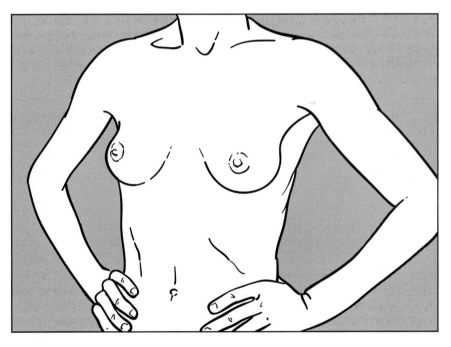

Figure 17.3
Hands at waist, pectoral muscles contracted.

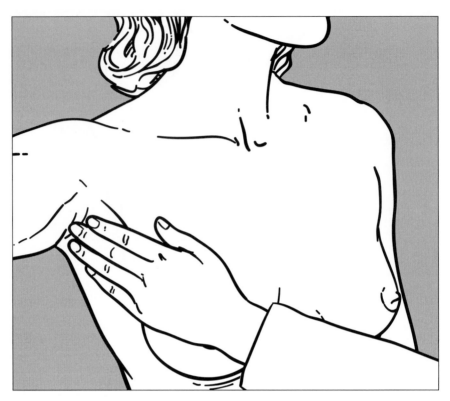

Figure 17.4
Palpation with patient upright, with support of ipsilateral elbow; axillary nodes and also supraclavicular nodes examined.

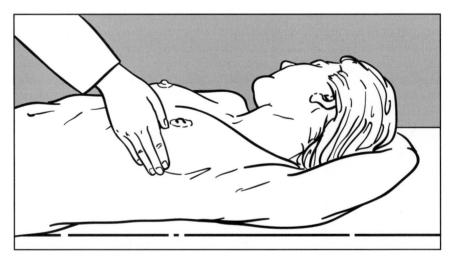

Figure 17.5
Palpation of breast in supine position.

Table 17.1 American College of Radiology (ACR) BI-RADS™ assessment categories[a]	
BI-RADS™ categories	Assessment
0	Need additional imaging evaluation – assessment is *incomplete*
1	Negative
2	Benign finding
3	Probably benign finding – short interval follow-up suggested
4	Suspicious abnormality – biopsy should be considered
5	Highly suggestive of malignancy – appropriate action should be taken

[a]American College of Radiology (ACR), *Illustrated Breast Imaging Reporting and Data System (BI-RADS™)*, 3rd edn. Reston, VA: American College of Radiology, 1998.

Mammographic screening in women 40 years or older has reduced mortality by 20–30%. The accuracy of the mammogram depends on the density of the breast and could vary between 70% and 98%. In 1994, the *Mammography Quality Standards Act* was passed by the US Congress and is administered by the Food and Drug Administration. It requires that mammography facilities monitor the results of their breast cancer detection programs, including the number of recommended biopsies, and the size, number, and stage of cancers detected. The American College of Radiology (ACR) Breast Imaging Reporting and Data System uses a terminology and lexicon system called *BI-RADS™* for reporting abnormalities seen on mammography (Table 17.1).

Microcalcifications seen on mammography are due to cellular secretions and calcifications of necrotic cancer cells. They can occur in a linear or clustered pattern. Suspicion of malignancy is increased when microcalcifications are associated with a mass or asymmetry, or when they are pleomorphic or numerous (greater than five in number).

The incidence of biopsies performed based on the first mammogram is 2–3%, and 1–2% per subsequent screen. Approximately 30% of cancers detected are DCIS. Among the invasive cancers, approximately one-half are less than 1 cm in size, and less than 20% have positive nodes.

Screening interval

In 1997, The American Cancer Society (ACS) and the National Cancer Institute (NCI) modified the guidelines for mammographic screening for women aged 40–49 years, recommending regular mammograms for women in this age group. The recommended intervals differ; ACS recommends a yearly mammogram starting at age 40, while NCI recommends a mammogram every 1 or 2 years.

Ultrasound and magnetic resonance imaging (MRI)

Ultrasound can be used to determine whether a mass is solid or cystic, and can be used in conjunction with aspiration biopsies. Because of its low specificity, it is not a good screening modality. Presently, magnetic resonance imaging (MRI) also has no role in breast cancer screening. It is currently used in evaluation of suspected breast implant ruptures and to evaluate worrisome postlumpectomy bed fibrosis and suspected pectoralis involvement. Its role in evaluating palpable abnormalities in mammographically negative/ultrasound negative dense breasts is currently under investigation. Future uses may also include evaluation of occult breast cancers and evaluation of multifocal disease in patients who are interested in breast conservation.

Biopsy techniques

Triple diagnosis refers to the use of three evaluation steps in diagnosing a breast lesion: clinical assessment by palpation, results of mammography, and results of fine-needle aspiration biopsy.

Fine-needle aspiration (FNA)/fine-needle aspiration biopsy (FNAB)

The diagnostic approach to a breast mass depends on the age and menopausal status of the patient. In premenopausal patients, breast cancer should be included in the differential of a breast lump. There is a role for evaluating a breast abnormality when ovarian hormones exert the least influence, 3–10 days after the onset of menstruation. If a mass proves on aspiration to be a cyst, the fluid can be discarded unless it is grossly bloody. Excisional biopsy should be performed if bloody fluid is noted, if the cyst reaccumulates in the same position 4–6 weeks after initial aspiration, or if there is a mass palpable after aspiration.

A *fine-needle aspiration (FNA)* may be performed on a solid mass (see Figure 17.6). Usually, a 21-gauge or 25-gauge needle on a 10-cc syringe is used. Approximately 3 cc of air is aspirated into the syringe to facilitate expulsion of the contents onto the slide following the procedure. The needle is introduced into the lesion, and suction is applied on the syringe. It is necessary to perform multiple – between 10 and 15 – passes through the lesion, with changes in direction of the needle to allow extensive sampling and evaluation of the consistency of the mass. Carcinomas will feel hard and gritty. Sampling should be continued until material can be seen in the hub of the needle. It is important to fill the needle, not the syringe, and to take care to release the suction before withdrawing the needle from the lesion so as to prevent aspiration of the material into the syringe. The sample is then ejected onto a glass slide, gently smeared with another slide, and placed in a sterile jar containing 95% ethanol for transport to the cytology lab.

An FNA requires a skilled cytopathologist to interpret the results. It has been reported to have a false-positive rate of less than 1%. Most surgeons,

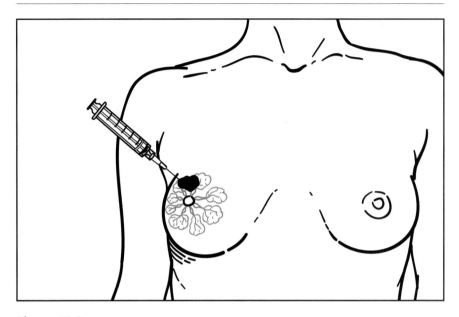

Figure 17.6
Aspiration biopsy.

however, will not perform definitive surgery (i.e., a mastectomy or axillary dissection) without a prior surgical biopsy, core-needle biopsy or frozen-section diagnosis at the time of surgery. An FNA that is positive for adenocarcinoma provides a preliminary diagnosis and helps to guide subsequent management. The false-negative rate is reported to be between 0.4% to 35% and is often due to inadequate sampling. It also depends on the cytopathologist, the size of the lesion (more common in tumors smaller than 1 cm), location within the breast, and the cellular composition of the lesion. As with any other biopsy, reported atypical changes should be followed by excision. Negative findings of an FNA in the presence of a suspicious mass must not preclude further diagnostic evaluation and follow-up.

Stereotactic core biopsy

A stereotactic core biopsy is a biopsy done under mammographic guidance. The core biopsy equipment is added to a standard upright mammogram unit or designated specific stereotactic prone unit. Using a 14-gauge core needle, and with removal of at least five cores/lesion, the concordance rate is 71–99%. The advantages of a core biopsy include the potential to eliminate a surgical biopsy if the biopsy is benign. Different quadrants may be sampled, and if a patient desires or requires a mastectomy, a surgical biopsy may be eliminated. Possible disadvantages include hematoma and tumor seeding. The locations of some lesions are not amenable to stereotactic biopsy (i.e., if close to the chest wall).

Surgical biopsy

Incisional biopsy is a diagnostic procedure that removes a portion of a mass for diagnosis. Usually, this can be accomplished by FNAB or core biopsy. Excisional biopsy is the complete removal of a lesion with or without a margin of normal surrounding tissue. Although it is important to place the incision so as to yield the best cosmetic result, consideration should also be given to further surgical management should the mass be malignant. Curvilinear incisions placed along the Langer's lines in the upper half of the breast and radial incisions in the lower half of the breast give the best cosmetic results (see Figure 17.7). Incisions should be placed over the palpable mass; in younger women with a suspected fibroadenoma, a periareolar incision may be appropriate even if the lesion is a considerable distance from the areola.

Preoperative needle localization

Using mammography and sometimes ultrasound, nonpalpable abnormalities can be localized for subsequent surgical excision. With this approach, the volume of tissue removed may be minimized. A hookwire system is used, which allows the wire to be placed either through the lesion or no more than 5 mm away from it. A radiograph of the specimen, postexcision, is performed to ensure that the lesion has been surgically removed.

STAGING

Staging refers to grouping of patients according to the extent of their disease. Currently, staging is determined by the American Joint Committee on Cancer (AJCC). It is a clinical and pathologic staging system based on the TNM system (T refers to tumor, N to nodes, and M to metastasis). The 1992 AJCC version allows for the inclusion of all information available prior to first definitive treatment, including operative findings and pathologic information.

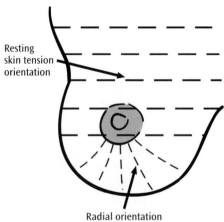

Resting skin tension orientation

Radial orientation

Figure 17.7
Optimal orientation of biopsy incisions.

TNM classification

The primary tumor is classified according to size. The clinical measurement is the one judged to be most accurate (physical examination or mammogram). Pathologically, the tumor size is a measurement of the invasive component. Paget's disease of the nipple without an associated tumor mass or invasive carcinoma on pathologic interpretation is classified as Tis; associated with a tumor, it is classified according to the tumor size. Inflammatory carcinoma is a clinical diagnosis characterized by skin changes and is classified as T4d. (See Tables 17.2–17.5.)

The presence or absence of metastatic involvement in the axillary lymph nodes is the most important prognostic factor. Most clinical trials group patients based on nodal status. Patients are grouped into the following

Table 17.2 Primary tumor (T)	
T classification	Description
TX	Primary tumor cannot be assessed
T0	No evidence of primary tumor
Tis	Carcinoma in situ
T1	Tumor 2 cm or less:
	T1a 0.5 cm or less
	T1b >0.5 cm and <1 cm
	T1c >1 cm, but not >2 cm
T2	Tumor >2 cm, but <5 cm
T3	Tumor >5 cm
T4	Tumor of any size with direct extension to chest wall or skin:
	T4a extension to chest wall
	T4b edema (including peau d'orange), ulceration of the skin of the breast, or satellite skin nodules confined to the same breast
	T4c (both T4a and T4b)
	T4d inflammatory carcinoma

Table 17.3 Regional lymph nodes (N)	
N classification	Description
NX	Regional lymph nodes cannot be assessed
N0	No regional lymph node status
N1	Metastasis to movable ipsilateral axillary lymph node(s)
N2	Metastasis to ipsilateral axillary lymph node(s) fixed to one another or to other structures
N3	Metastasis to ipsilateral internal mammary lymph node(s)

Table 17.4 Distant metastasis (M)	
M classification	Description
MX	Presence of distant metastasis cannot be assessed
M0	No distant metastasis
M1	Distant metastasis (include metastasis to ipsilateral supraclavicular node[s])

Table 17.5 Stage grouping	
Stage	TNM grouping
Stage 0	Tis N0 M0
Stage I	T1 N0 M0
Stage IIA	T0 N1 M0
	T1 N1 M0
	T2 N0 M0
Stage IIB	T2 N1 M0
	T3 N0 M0
Stage IIIA	T0 N2 M0
	T1 N2 M0
	T3 N1 M0
	T3 N2 M0
Stage IIIB	T4 Any N M0
	Any T N3 M0
Stage IV	Any T Any N M1

categories: those with negative nodes, those with 1–3 positive nodes, and those with 4 or more positive nodes.

TREATMENT OF BREAST CANCER

Historical perspective

William Halsted popularized the radical mastectomy in 1894. The treatment of invasive breast cancer was based on the theory that breast cancer spreads in a local fashion, with direct extension of cancer cells, particularly through the lymphatics. Radical mastectomy involved the removal of the breast with overlying skin, pectoral muscles, and all axillary contents. The failure of this technique to cure some patients was thought to be due to the inability to clear all the surrounding lymphatics, and in the 1950s, the extended radical mastectomy was developed. The extended radical mastectomy included the en bloc removal of ipsilateral internal mammary lymph nodes. The failure of this procedure to improve survival eventually cast doubts on the established Halstedian principles as well as the need for the radical mastectomy. The change to a modified radical mastectomy occurred when it became apparent that failure after surgery was due to systemic failure rather than the surgical procedure employed. A modified radical mastectomy includes removal of the breast, the underlying pectoral fascia, and some of the axillary lymph nodes. A total mastectomy involves the removal of the breast and underlying pectoral fascia without an axillary lymph-node dissection. One of the most important roles for surgery in the treatment of breast cancer remains local-regional control.

Breast-conservation therapy

Randomized trials have established that breast-conservation therapy and mastectomy yield equivalent survival outcomes. Most women with early breast cancer in the USA are treated with breast-conservation therapy, the strategy of which is to remove the bulk of disease and to use radiation to eradicate any residual cancer cells. Clinical trials to evaluate and compare lumpectomy and irradiation with mastectomy were initiated by Veronesi at the National Cancer Institute of Italy in Milan and by Bernard Fisher at the National Surgical Adjuvant Breast and Bowel Project (NSABP B-06 trial).

Breast-conservation therapy entails removal of the mass with a rim of normal breast tissue; this procedure is called a *lumpectomy*. A *quadrantectomy* involves removal of the quadrant of the breast containing the cancer. Increasing the volume of resection of breast tissue has been associated with a decrease in local recurrence, but often yields a poor cosmetic outcome. Patient selection is an important component of breast-conservation therapy. Classic absolute contraindications to breast-conservation therapy include pregnancy, two or more tumors in separate quadrants of the breast, history of prior irradiation, and diffuse microcalcifications on mammography. Relative contraindications are related to obtaining a poor cosmetic result and include a large tumor-to-breast ratio and tumor location under the nipple. A history of connective-tissue disease or collagen vascular disease is also a relative contraindication. Young age and the presence of an extensive intraductal component have also been reported to yield higher local recurrence rates with breast-conservation therapy.

Axillary dissection/sentinel lymph-node biopsy

The status of the axillary lymph nodes is the most important prognostic indicator in breast cancer. Metastatic involvement of nodes progresses in a stepwise manner. Skip metastases occur in less than 2% of cases. Axillary lymph-node dissection provides prognostic information, but has minimal or no therapeutic benefit in women with clinically negative lymph nodes and is

beneficial in intermediate-risk patients – those with negative nodes and tumors greater than 1 cm in size with some adverse features.

The combination of cyclophosphamide, methotrexate, and 5-fluorouracil (5-FU) (CMF) is widely used as adjuvant treatment for premenopausal breast cancer patients. A doxorubicin-based regimen (5-FU, doxorubicin [Adriamycin®], and cyclophosphamide: FAC) has been shown to be more effective as adjuvant therapy in patients with positive nodes.

Preliminary results on high-dose chemotherapy have not shown better results than standard treatment regimens. To date, five randomized trials of high-dose chemotherapy with bone-marrow or stem-cell transplantation have been reported in advanced breast cancer. The first, reported in 1995 by Bezwoda et al, conducted in South Africa, showed that the high-dose chemotherapy arm had fewer deaths and a lower rate of relapse. The investigators ultimately admitted to fraud after review of a separate trial of high-dose therapy in patients with high-risk primary breast cancer (see Weiss et al (2000) in 'Selected reading'). The study in the metastatic patients has also been formally reviewed, and reviewers were unable to verify the reported data (Weiss et al, 2001). The other four trials did not demonstrate an increase in overall survival.

Premenopausal women with node-positive and estrogen-receptor-positive (ER-positive) tumors are treated with adjuvant chemotherapy. Those with node-negative, ER-positive tumors are candidates for hormonal therapy, unless other factors such as tumor size or adverse histologic features are present.

In postmenopausal women with ER-positive tumors and positive nodes, tamoxifen alone and CMF-type chemotherapy have almost equivalent survival benefits. Postmenopausal women with ER-negative tumors are treated similarly to premenopausal women.

Breast reconstruction

Immediate versus delayed reconstruction

Breast reconstruction represents a major advance in cancer rehabilitation for patients undergoing a mastectomy. Traditionally, a 2-year waiting period was initiated after surgery for surveillance and detection of local recurrence. With early, operable breast cancers, Stage I and II disease, reconstruction has not interfered with detection or treatment of local recurrence. Immediate reconstruction has the advantage of combining the two procedures into one, thus requiring only one hospitalization and one anesthesia. Furthermore, if an immediate reconstruction is planned, a greater amount of skin can be saved at the time of the mastectomy, thereby facilitating the reconstruction. Also, when done in combination with mastectomy, scar tissue, which would be encountered at a delayed date, is avoided.

Delayed reconstruction can be performed if the patient is ambiguous about the reconstruction, or if operative risk is increased with prolonged anesthesia. Also to be considered in the case of patients with locally advanced disease is

Table 17.6 Autologous tissue transfer
• Latissimus dorsi myocutaneous flap • Transverse rectus abdominous musculocutaneous flap (pedicle flap or free flap) • Gluteal musculocutaneous free flap

whether reconstruction will considerably delay adjuvant irradiation or chemotherapy.

Options for reconstruction

Reconstruction options include expandable breast prostheses (implants) and autologous tissue transfer. Tissue-transfer operations may yield the greatest symmetry between breasts, especially with larger breasts; however, they take longer, require greater surgical expertise, involve a longer recovery, and mean another scar (at the donor site). Table 17.6 lists the types of autologous tissue transfers.

Therapy by stage

Stage 0

Treatment of noninvasive breast cancer is surgical. Ductal carcinoma in situ is the most common type of noninvasive breast cancer. Mammography has led to a striking increase in DCIS diagnosis. The clinical spectrum of DCIS is broad, and the size and subtype of DCIS govern its biological behavior. The comedo subtype is the most common and the most aggressive, with the highest local-recurrence rates.

Total mastectomy remains the gold standard for treatment, with or without immediate breast reconstruction. Axillary metastases from pure DCIS (i.e., those without an invasive component) are rare; thus, an axillary dissection is not required. Breast conservation is also a treatment option. The NSABP B-17 trial is the only trial comparing lumpectomy and radiation therapy with lumpectomy alone in patients with DCIS. This trial randomized 818 women with DCIS detected as either a palpable lump or by mammography. The recurrence rate was 16.4% in the lumpectomy-alone group and 7% in the group receiving radiation therapy. In addition, this reduction was most apparent for invasive carcinomas. Fifty percent of the local relapses in the patients who had not received irradiation were invasive, compared with 28% in the irradiation group. Problems with the study included the fact that no subset analysis was performed. Thus, it is not clear which group would benefit from irradiation and lumpectomy and which group would be candidates for lumpectomy alone. An update of the NSABP B-17 study found that margin status and presence of comedo necrosis were independent predictors for local recurrence. Further study into breast-conservation treatment without irradiation is presently underway.

Stage I and II disease

Modern surgery for early breast cancer aims to ensure accuracy of diagnosis, complete removal of all local disease, optimal cosmetic results, and an effective multidisciplinary approach. Assessment of axillary lymph nodes remains important for assessment of the risk for systemic disease and the need for systemic therapy. The choice between breast-conservation therapy (lumpectomy and irradiation) and mastectomy is dictated by the size of the primary tumor, considerations related to cosmetic result, the presence of any contraindications to breast conservation, and patient preference. The axillary nodal status may be determined by sentinel-node biopsy, in those patients who are candidates, or through formal axillary dissection. An axillary dissection is usually performed for clinically positive nodes, for suspicious nodes, and in cases where the sentinel node yields evidence of metastases by either routine pathology (hematoxylin and eosin, H & E) or immunohistochemical analysis. Adjuvant postoperative chemotherapy is usually given, but may be avoided in low-risk groups, such as those with tumors smaller than 1 cm and negative nodes.

With high-risk groups who have four or more positive nodes, there is a role for chest-wall irradiation (after mastectomy) as well as irradiation of the supraclavicular nodes. Some Stage I and II patients may also be candidates for tamoxifen therapy.

Locally advanced breast cancer (Stage III)

Treatment of locally advanced breast cancer can include preoperative chemotherapy. With this approach, previously inoperable tumors become operable and may be amenable to breast-conservation treatment. Data are available that show that adjuvant chemotherapy and hormonal therapy may be beneficial after preoperative chemotherapy and regional treatment (surgery, irradiation). Inflammatory cancers may also benefit from this treatment approach.

Stage IV/recurrent disease

Metastatic breast cancer can be treated with chemotherapy, hormonal therapy, radiation therapy, and limited surgery. Most patients will succumb to their disease, and the goal of therapy is palliation and prolonging quality of life. Treatment is based on age of the patient, hormone-receptor status, extent of disease, and disease-free interval in those with recurrent disease. Hormonal manipulation is often the first course in patients with ER-positive tumors. These include antiestrogens, aromatase inhibitors, gonadotropin-releasing hormone analogues, and progestins. Patients who respond to one hormonal agent will respond to another agent once one becomes ineffective.

Antiestrogens are first-line agents and have 20–35% objective response rates. Chemotherapy should be given to patients with metastatic breast cancer refractory to hormonal treatment. The CMF and FAC combinations are first-line chemotherapy regimens with 40–80% rates. Combinations of taxanes and anthracyclines have similar response rates. Bone is the most common site of metastasis in breast cancer. Bisphosphonates (pamidronate and clodronate) added to hormonal therapy or chemotherapy greatly reduce pain and incidence of bone-related complications. (See Tables 17.7 and 17.8.)

Table 17.7 Therapy by stage

Stage	Surgery	Adjuvant treatment
Stage 0	TM versus BCT	
Stage I	TM versus BCT ±SLN/ALN MRM	Chemo T > 1 cm ±TAM
Stage II	MRM versus BCT/ALN	Chemo ± TAM RT supraclavicular nodes ± CW if >4 positive nodes
Stage III	MRM versus BCT/ALN	Chemo ± neoadjuvant chemotherapy ± TAM RT supraclavicular nodes ± CW RT breast (inflammatory breast cancer)
Stage IV	Surgery for local control	± Chemo ± hormonal agents

TM, total mastectomy; BCT, breast-conservation therapy (includes lumpectomy and breast irradiation); SLN, sentinel-node biopsy; MRM, modified radical mastectomy; ALN, axillary lymph-node dissection; Chemo, chemotherapy; TAM, tamoxifen; RT, radiation therapy; CW, chest wall, if mastectomy performed.

Table 17.8 Prognosis by stage/10-year survival based on the National Cancer Data Base (NCDB)[a]

Stage	10-year survival rate (%)
Stage 0	95
Stage I	88
Stage II	66
Stage III	36
Stage IV	7

[a]The NCDB is a joint project of the Commission on Cancer of the American College of Surgeons and the American Cancer Society. It collects and analyzes data from a wide variety of sources throughout the USA, including small community hospitals.

Chemoprevention

The use of tamoxifen in an adjuvant setting in patients with invasive breast cancer significantly reduces the rate of contralateral breast cancer, by 40–50%. A large-scale, double-blind trial (NSABP-P1 trial) examined the use of tamoxifen as a chemopreventive agent. The trial randomized 13,388 women with a 1.66% or greater predicted risk of cancer within 5 years to tamoxifen versus placebo. The Gail mathematical model, based on age, nulliparity, history of benign breast disease, and family history, was used to determine the risk. A 49% reduction in the incidence of invasive cancer was found ($p < 0.00001$), along with a 69% reduction in ER-positive tumors. No statistically significant effect was noted on ER-negative tumors. The mean follow-up time was 4 years. Cancer risk was reduced among all age and risk groups.

This reduction in risk led an independent committee to unblind the NSABP-P1 trial more than 1 year earlier than planned; as a result, there are questions about the optimal dose and duration of treatment. The reduction in risk occurred mainly with ER-positive tumors; thus, it is unclear whether the tamoxifen treats microscopic/subclinical disease rather than preventing the progression of premalignant disease.

The adverse effects were seen in women over the age of 50 years. Thirty-six cases of endometrial cancers were seen in the tamoxifen group versus 15 in the placebo group. All of the endometrial cancers were Stage I cancers. There was also an increase in cases of thromboembolic disease, including pulmonary emboli.

Ongoing trials include the STAR/P2 trial comparing tamoxifen versus raloxifene in postmenopausal women.

Future therapy

Understanding the biology of breast cancer may help in the identification of new therapies. For example the HER2/*neu* oncogene is overexpressed in 20–30% of breast cancers. It is associated with more aggressive tumors and with resistance to some chemotherapeutic agents. Monoclonal antibodies against the extracellular domain of the HER2/Neu oncoprotein have been developed (Herceptin® [trastuzumab] is a humanized anti-HER2 antibody). The addition of Herceptin to first-line chemotherapy for HER2-overexpressing metastatic breast cancers has been shown in a randomized trial to increase response rate and to prolong disease-free and overall survival.

Future therapy will encompass integration of molecular genetics into treatment strategies. Further investigation into the biology of breast cancer and further development in understanding of the molecular basis of breast cancer are needed.

SELECTED READING

Blackwood MM, Petrek JA, Axillary dissection: current practice and technique. *Curr Prob Surg* 1995; **32**: 257.

Bland KI, Copeland EM (eds), *The Breast: Comprehensive Management of Benign and Malignant Diseases,* 2nd edn. Philadelphia: WB Saunders, 1998.

Borgen PI, Moore MP, Heerdt AS, Petrek JA, Breast-conservation therapy for invasive carcinoma of the breast. *Curr Prob Surg* 1995; **32**: 191.

Fisher B, Highlights from recent National Surgical Adjuvant Breast and Bowel Project studies in the treatment and prevention of breast cancer. *CA Cancer J Clin* 1999; **49**: 159.

Fremgen AM, Bland KI, McGinnis LS et al, Clinical highlights from the National Cancer Data Base, 1999. *CA Cancer J Clin* 1999; **49**: 145.

Greenlee RT, Hill-Harmon MB, Murray T, Thun M, Cancer statistics, 2001. *CA Cancer J Clin* 2001; **51**: 15.

Harris JR, Lippman ME, Morrow M, Hellman S (eds), *Diseases of the Breast.* Philadelphia: Lippincott-Raven, 1996.

Weiss RB, Rifkin RM, Stewart FM et al, High-dose chemotherapy for high-risk primary breast cancer: an on-site review of the Bezwoda study. *Lancet* 2000; **355**: 999.

Weiss RB, Gill GG, Hudis CA, An on-site audit of the South African trial of high-dose chemotherapy for metastatic breast cancer and associated publications. *J Clin Oncol* 2001; **19**: 2771.

18
Colorectal cancer

Harvey G Moore, José G Guillem

INCIDENCE

Colorectal cancer (CRC) is the most common cancer of the gastrointestinal tract. Approximately 135,000 new cases were predicted for the year 2001, with over 57,000 anticipated deaths from the disease. In women, CRC is the third leading cause of cancer-related deaths, after lung and breast cancer. In men, it is also third, following cancer of the lung and prostate. An American has an approximately 5% chance of developing colorectal cancer during a 70-year life span. Most cases are diagnosed after the age of 50 years. Approximately 6–8% of cases, however, are diagnosed in patients under the age of 40.

Populations in Western Europe, North America, Australia, and New Zealand have the highest incidence of colonic polyps and cancers. In general, there is a strong correlation between geographic prevalence of adenomas and colorectal cancers. When populations migrate from low-risk to high-risk areas, both adenoma and cancer frequencies increase.

In individuals with one or more first-degree relatives diagnosed with colorectal cancer, the risk increases three- to nine-fold. This risk is considerably higher in families with hereditary syndromes, including *familial adenomatous polyposis (FAP)*, which occurs in between 1 in 8,000 to 1 in 29,000 individuals. The risk is also significantly increased in individuals with a family history of *hereditary nonpolyposis colorectal cancer (HNPCC)*. (See further discussion below.)

Previous primary colorectal cancer increases an individual's risk of developing *metachronous* polyps and cancers.

DIET

There is a direct correlation between mortality from colorectal cancer and per-capita consumption of calories, meat protein, and dietary fat and oil, as well as elevations in serum cholesterol. It has been proposed that ingestion of animal fats leads to an increased proportion of anaerobes in the gut microflora, resulting in conversion of bile acids to carcinogens. This is supported by the finding of increased fecal anaerobes in the stool of patients with CRC. Any geographic variation in incidence does not appear to be genetic, since migrant groups tend to assume the CRC incidence rates of their adopted countries.

HEREDITARY SYNDROMES

A summary of hereditary syndromes is outlined in Table 18.1.

Familial adenomatous polyposis

Familial Adenomatous Polyposis (FAP) is caused by a mutation of the adenomatous polyposis coli (*APC*) gene on chromosome 5 and is characterized by the development of many (>100) adenomatous polyps throughout the colon and rectum. Polyposis may also involve the upper gastrointestinal tract, especially the duodenum. In addition, a number of extraintestinal manifestations are associated with FAP (Table 18.1.)

Familial adenomatous polyposis is inherited in an autosomal-dominant pattern, with close to 100% penetrance. Although most patients have germline mutations in the *APC* gene, approximately 10–30% of cases represent new mutations. Familial adenomatous polyposis occurs in approximately 1 in 10,000 births and accounts for less than 1% of all CRCs. Virtually all affected individuals will develop CRC by age 40 unless a prophylactic colectomy is performed. The incidence of CRC is proportional to the number of polyps. The majority of FAP patients present with left-sided or distal CRC and have a high frequency of synchronous or metachronous cancers. Currently, genetic testing is available for at-risk individuals with a protein truncation test (PTT), which detects mutations in the *APC* gene.

Hereditary nonpolyposis colorectal cancer (HNPCC)

Hereditary nonpolyposis colorectal cancer (HNPCC) is a syndrome predisposing affected individuals to various cancers, most commonly CRC. Hereditary nonpolyposis colorectal cancer is not generally associated with multiple polyps. In fact, the incidence of adenoma is similar to that of patients with sporadic CRC. Patients with HNPCC have a predilection for right-sided colon cancer, and there is a higher incidence of mucinous, signet-ring, and poorly differentiated cancers among these individuals.

Although CRC is the most common cancer in these patients, other cancers may be associated with HNPCC. The Amsterdam criteria I and II are the most commonly used diagnostic criteria. The Amsterdam I criteria include only colorectal cancer, while the Amsterdam II criteria include other cancers such as endometrial, small-bowel, ureter, and renal pelvis. The Amsterdam criteria, I and II, are summarized in Table 18.2. Currently, genetic testing may be performed in at-risk individuals by testing DNA obtained from peripheral blood leukocytes for mutations in mismatch-repair (MMR) genes.

Table 18.1 Summary of hereditary syndromes

Characteristic	FAP	HNPCC
Incidence	1 in 10,000 births	Similar to sporadic CRC development
Number of polyps	Many, often >100	Similar to sporadic CRC development
Inheritance pattern	Autosomal-dominant	Autosomal-dominant
Prognosis	CRC, unless colectomy	CRC in 60% by age 60; Cumulative lifetime risk almost 80%
Treatment	Prophylactic colectomy	Subtotal colectomy
Most common region of colon involvement	Left-sided	Right-sided
Average age of CRC development	35 years	40–45 years
Genetic testing	Adenomatous Polyposis Coli (APC) gene testing	Mismatch repair (MMR) gene testing

Extraintestinal manifestations	• Gardner's syndrome:
	  (1) Desmoid tumors in abdomen
	  (2) Osteomas
	  (3) Sebaceous cysts
	• Turcot's syndrome:
	  Brain tumors
	• Congenital hypertrophy of the retinal pigment epithelium
	• Dental odontomas
	• Other tumors, including:
	  (1) Gastric
	  (2) Small intestine (duodenum)
	  (3) Pancreatic
	  (4) Biliary tree
	  (5) Gastric
	  (6) Thyroid
	  (7) Adrenal
	  (8) Central nervous system
	  (9) Urinary bladder
	  (10) Testicle
	  (11) Embryonal
		• Extracolonic cancers:
		  (1) Endometrial
		  (2) Ovarian
		  (3) Stomach
		  (4) Small intestine
		  (5) Urinary transitional cell
		  (6) Hepatobiliary
		  (7) Skin
		  (8) Pancreas
		  (9) Brain
		  (10) Hematologic
		  (11) Soft tissue
		  (12) Larynx

Table 18.2 Amsterdam criteria (revised)[a]
(1) HNPCC-associated cancer in 3 relatives (CRC, cancer of endometrium, small bowel, ureter, or renal pelvis), one a first-degree relative of the other two
(2) At least two successive generations affected
(3) At least one colorectal cancer diagnosed before age 50
(4) FAP excluded
[a]Modified from Vasen H et al, New clinical criteria for hereditary nonpolyposis colorectal cancer (HNPCC, Lynch syndrome) proposed by the International Collaborative Group on HNPCC. *Gastroenterology* 1999; **116**: 1453.

Other hereditary conditions include Peutz–Jeghers syndrome, juvenile polyposis syndrome, Cowden's disease, Cronkite–Canada syndrome, Ruvalcaba–Myhre–Smith syndrome, and hereditary mixed-polyposis syndrome.

PREMALIGNANT CONDITIONS

Ulcerative colitis (UC)

The overall incidence of CRC in patients with pancolitis is 1% per year after 10 years, such that after 20 years of even quiescent disease, the risk for CRC is 10%. Because of the flat, burrowing, infiltrative characteristics of the lesions, patients often present with locally advanced disease.

Crohn's disease

The increased incidence of CRC in patients with Crohn's disease is not fully appreciated. However, it is higher than that of the general population, yet lower than that of patients with UC.

EPIDEMIOLOGY

Colorectal polyps may be classified as follows: *adenomatous, hyperplastic,* and *miscellaneous.*

Adenomatous polyps

Adenomatous polyps comprise 67% of all colorectal polyps found at initial colonoscopy in the USA. They are true neoplasms with malignant potential. Adenomas rarely occur in average-risk individuals younger than 50 years of age and are more frequent in males.

Hyperplastic polyps

Hyperplastic polyps comprise 11% of all colorectal polyps. Pure hyperplastic polyps are not considered premalignant lesions. However, adenomatous change may be present on histologic evaluation. These "serrated" or mixed polyps have been associated with the development of carcinoma. In addition, hyperplastic polyps may be a marker for the subsequent development of both hyperplastic and adenomatous polyps. Hyperplastic polyps increase in frequency with age. They are usually asymptomatic, unless numerous, when there may be associated rectal bleeding and/or diarrhea. Grossly, these polyps are small (<3 mm), sessile, flat, and tan–pink in color. Because it is impossible to distinguish hyperplastic polyps from adenomatous polyps at endoscopy, they require excision for histologic confirmation.

Miscellaneous polyps

Miscellaneous polyps comprise 22% of all colorectal polyps. Miscellaneous polyps include *inflammatory* and *hamartomatous polyps*.

Inflammatory
Inflammatory polyps are non-neoplastic growths, which arise from mucosal ulceration and repair. They occur most often in conjunction with ulcerative colitis, but may also be seen in Crohn's disease. These polyps are uniform in width from base to head. They often appear inflamed.

Hamartomatous
Hamartomatous polyps arise from smooth muscle in the muscularis mucosa and are generally considered to have no malignant potential. Hamartomatous polyps commonly occur in children between the ages of 4 and 5 years who are affected by *juvenile polyposis syndrome*, but they may also occur in infants and adults. Common symptoms include rectal bleeding, mucous discharge, and abdominal pain. Intussusception or rectal prolapse may also occur. Grossly, the juvenile polyp is pedunculated, bright red to brown, spherical, and about 1–3 cm in size, with a granular surface that bleeds easily upon contact.

Hamartomas also commonly occur in *Peutz–Jeghers syndrome*. This autosomal-dominantly inherited syndrome is characterized by mucocutaneous pigmented lesions of the buccal mucosa, lip and palate, hands, and perianal region, as well as hamartomatous polyps. Polyps are most commonly located in the small bowel, although both gastric and colorectal hamartomas may occur. Grossly, they range in size from 0.1 to 10 mm, but may grow to be 4 cm in diameter. Although hamartomatous polyps are generally considered benign lesions, patients with Peutz–Jeghers syndrome appear to have an increased risk of both gastrointestinal and extraintestinal malignancies. The exact extent of risk is controversial, and has been reported to be between 2% and 40% at 40 years.

HISTOLOGIC TYPES AND CHARACTERISTICS

An adenomatous polyp, or adenoma of the colon, is a benign neoplasm, with unrestricted cell division in a circumscribed area of glandular epithelium within the colonic mucosa. The surface is usually described as flat and velvety, with a shaggy appearance like the texture of a raspberry. Grossly, polyps can have several forms: (1) *pedunculated,* or with a stalk; (2) *sessile,* or flat; (3) *semisessile,* or raised.

Histologically, the architecture of adenomatous polyps can vary from branched tubular glands to elongated, fingerlike villi. Polyps can be classified as (1) *tubular,* (2) *villous,* or (3) *tubulovillous.* Tubular adenomas represent 65–85% of adenomatous polyps, are usually *pedunculated,* and have a 5% risk of harboring cancer. Villous adenomas represent 5–10% of adenomatous polyps, are usually sessile, and may have up to a 40% risk of harboring cancer. Large (>4 cm) villous adenomas of the rectum with areas of induration are at particularly high risk of harboring cancer, and should be completely excised. Patients with large villous adenomas may occasionally present with severe diarrhea and hypokalemia. Tubulovillous adenomas comprise 10–25% of adenomas and have approximately a 20% risk of containing cancer.

Severe atypia, previously designated *carcinoma in situ,* is the term used to describe cancer confined to the epithelium of a polyp that has not yet invaded the muscularis mucosae layer of the bowel wall. With progressive dysplasia, microscopic features such as nuclear atypia, loss of polarity, and mitotic figures become apparent.

Adenomas are significant because of their malignant potential. At the time of diagnosis, approximately 5–8% of adenomas have severe dysplasia, while 3–5% harbor invasive carcinoma. In general, the risk of cancer in an adenoma that is less than 1 cm in diameter is very low, but the risk increases to approximately 50% for adenomas larger than 2 cm in size.

ADENOMA–CARCINOMA SEQUENCE

Most, if not all, CRCs arise from preexisting adenomas. As a cancer grows, it expands on the mucosal surface and replaces previously benign adenomatous tissue. Although the duration of this sequence is variable, it generally takes approximately 8–10 years.

The adenoma–carcinoma sequence suggests that colonic mucosa progresses through multiple stages of carcinogenesis leading to the development of an invasive cancer (Figure 18.1). This sequence appears to be driven by the successive accumulation of somatic mutations within colonic epithelial cells. The earliest change appears to be the formation of aberrant crypt foci that then lead to the formation of microadenomas. Continued proliferation onto the surface epithelium leads to the formation of a raised lesion, or adenoma. As proliferation continues, cells become increasingly dysplastic. Eventually, this uncon-

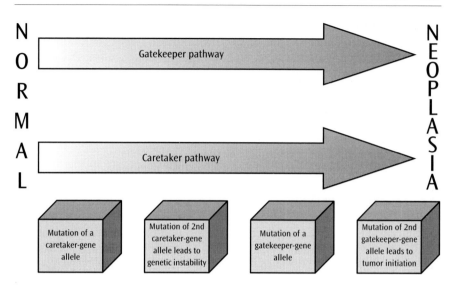

Figure 18.1

Pathways to neoplasia. Adapted from Kinzler KW, Vogestein B, Cancer susceptibility genes. Gatekeepers and caretakers. *Nature* 1997; **386:** 761–3.

trolled growth violates the muscularis mucosal barrier, resulting in an invasive cancer.

Less commonly, some CRCs appear to arise de novo, especially in inflammatory bowel disease (IBD). These flat cancers are usually advanced and seem to begin as intramucosal cancers, with no evidence of a preexisting polyp.

SIGNS AND SYMPTOMS

Most adenomas are asymptomatic and discovered incidentally. Signs and symptoms of CRC are varied and nonspecific.

Subacute presentation includes the following: anemia, change in bowel habits, abdominal pain, mucous discharge, weight loss, fever, and minor bleeding per rectum.

Acute presentation includes the following: more severe bleeding per rectum, perforation, or partial or complete obstruction (inability to pass flatus or feces, cramping abdominal pain, and abdominal distention with tympany on physical exam).

Tumors in the right colon typically do not cause any change in bowel habits – with the exception of large, mucous-secreting tumors, which may cause diarrhea. Although patients may notice tarry stools, more often the bleeding is occult and undetected by the patient. Chronic blood loss may result in anemia and associated weakness, fatigue, dizziness, or palpitations. For this reason, iron-deficiency anemia should always be evaluated, especially in a post-menopausal female or adult male. Because the bleeding associated with colo-rectal cancer may be intermittent, a negative fecal occult blood test does not rule out a diagnosis of CRC.

Tumors in the narrower left colon are commonly associated with lower abdominal pain, described as "crampy" in nature, and relieved by bowel move-ments. These patients are more likely to notice changes in bowel habits, as well as passage of blood per rectum.

Acute presentation

Despite advances in screening for CRC, a significant proportion of patients, par-ticularly the elderly, present with acute symptoms due to obstruction or perfora-tion of the colon. Complete obstruction occurs in less than 10% of patients but represents a surgical emergency requiring immediate diagnosis and treatment. If the obstruction is not relieved, the colon continues to expand, resulting in ischemia of the bowel wall. The patient will complain of severe abdominal pain. On exam, there will be rebound tenderness and decreased or absent bowel sounds. Without immediate treatment, bowel-wall ischemia will progress to necrosis and perforation with fecal peritonitis and sepsis. Signs and symptoms include the following: obstipation/constipation, crampy abdominal pain, abdominal distention, tympanitic abdomen, and palpable abdominal mass.

SCREENING AND DIAGNOSIS

The American Cancer Society guidelines for screening and surveillance of colorectal neoplasms can be found in Table 18.3.

Colonoscopy is the most accurate method for detecting polyps (especially polyps less than 1 cm in size) and provides the most complete examination of the colon. This procedure allows for visualization of the entire colorectal mucosa as well as portions of the terminal ileum. In addition, tissue biopsy and brushings may be performed for diagnosis. A polypectomy may also be performed. Diagnostic colonoscopy is safe. The rate of major complications such as perforation and bleeding is less than 0.2%.

A high-quality *double-contrast barium enema (DCBE) with flexible sigmoid-oscopy* is an alternative to colonoscopy. It is less costly, does not require seda-tion, and is associated with fewer complications. However, DCBE is less sensitive for polyps measuring less than 1 cm in diameter. Since most lesions missed by DCBE are in the sigmoid colon, endoscopic examination of this area with a flexible sigmoidoscope is required. The combination of DCBE and flex-ible sigmoidoscopy is reported to have a sensitivity of 98% for carcinoma and 99% for adenomas.

Table 18.3 American Cancer Society guidelines for screening and surveillance of colorectal neoplasms[a]

Risk category	Recommendation[b,c]	Age to begin	Interval[b,c]
Average risk			
Patients ≥50 years who do not fit in categories below	FOBT + flexible sigmoidoscopy *or* Flexible sigmoidoscopy *or* FOBT *or* Colonoscopy *or* DCBE	50	FOBT every year and flexible sigmoidoscopy every 5 years* Every 5 years* Annually* (multi-sample) Every 10 years* Every 5 years*
Moderate risk			
Patients with single, small (<1 cm) adenomatous polyps	Colonoscopy	At time of initial polyp diagnosis	TCE within 3–6 years after initial polyp removal. If normal, as per average risk recommendations
Patients with large (>1 cm) or multiple adenomas of any size, or high-grade dysplasia or villous change	Colonoscopy	At time of initial polyp diagnosis	TCE within 3 years after initial polyp removal. If normal, repeat 3 years. If still normal, as per average-risk individual
Personal history of CRC s/p curative resection	TCE	Within 1 year after resection	If normal, TCE in 3 years. If still normal, TCE every 5 years

Continued

Table 18.3 Continued

Risk category	Recommendation[b,c]	Age to begin	Interval[b,c]
CRC or adenomatous polyps in first-degree relative younger than age 60 or in two or more first-degree relatives of any age	TCE	Age 40 or 10 years before the youngest case in the family, whichever is earlier	Every 5–10 years
CRC in other relatives	As per average risk recommendations (above); may consider beginning screening before age 50		
High risk			
Family history of FAP	Early surveillance with endoscopy, counseling to consider genetic testing, and referral to specialty center	Age 10–12	If genetic test positive or polyposis confirmed, consider colectomy. Otherwise, endoscopy every 1–2 years
Family history of HNPCC	Colonoscopy and counseling to consider genetic testing	Age 21	If genetic test positive or if patient has not had genetic testing, colonoscopy every 2 years until age 40, then every year
IBD (Chronic ulcerative colitis, Crohn's disease)	Colonoscopy with biopsy for dysplasia	8 years after the start of pancolitis; 12–15 years after the start of left-sided colitis	Every 1–2 years

[a]Modified from Smith RA, von Eschenbach AC, Wender R et al. American Cancer Society guidelines for the early detection of cancer: update of early detection guidelines for prostate, colorectal, and endometrial cancers. Also: update 2001: Testing for early lung cancer detection. *CA Cancer J Clin* 2001: **51**: 38–75.

[b]Digital rectal exam should be performed at the time of each sigmoidoscopy, colonoscopy, or DCBE.

[c]FOBT, fecal occult blood test; TCE, total colorectal examination (includes either colonoscopy or DCBE performed in conjunction with flexible sigmoidoscopy); DCBE, double-contrast barium enema.

[c]All positive results should be followed up with colonoscopy.

In patients with CRC, a complete colon and rectal examination is required to rule out synchronous carcinomas. The presence of a rectosigmoid polyp is predictive of proximal neoplastic disease, because 3–50% will have one or more synchronous neoplasms.

A digital rectal exam is essential to the evaluation of all colon cancer patients. In patients with rectal cancer, a digital rectal exam evaluates size, mobility, whether the lesion is tethered or fixed, extension to adjacent organs, and possibly enlarged lymph nodes. Equally important is the determination of the lowermost edge of the tumor relative to the upper edge of the anorectal ring. Finally, digital rectal exam may detect other intrapelvic deposits.

A rigid sigmoidoscope should be used to visualize the rectal tumor, obtain a biopsy sample, and measure the distance between the distal edge of the tumor and the anal verge. This distance helps determine whether a sphincter-sparing procedure can be performed.

Endorectal ultrasonography is extremely useful in the staging of rectal cancer. Accuracy for determination of depth of tumor invasion (μT) is approximately 82%, and approximately 77% for determining perirectal lymph-node involvement (μN).

A *chest x-ray* and *computed tomography (CT) of the abdomen/pelvis* should be obtained to evaluate for metastatic disease. In addition, an abdominal/pelvic CT may provide useful information about the extent of local-regional disease.

Serum carcinoembryonic antigen (CEA) levels are important in evaluating patients with CRC. Although not useful as a screening test, an elevated preoperative CEA level in a CRC patient suggests a poor prognosis. Carcinoembryonic antigen is a glycoprotein that can be found in embryonic and fetal tissues and in numerous cancers, including CRC, but is absent in normal adult colonic mucosa. Carcinoembryonic antigen levels are also likely to be normal in patients with CRC that has not penetrated the bowel wall. Carcinoembryonic antigen levels are useful to monitor for recurrence of CRC or metastases. Postoperative levels can be used to indicate completeness of surgical resection or presence of occult metastases. A rising CEA level after treatment may indicate a recurrence before clinical disease becomes evident. Elevated CEA levels are, however, somewhat nonspecific, and can be elevated in patients with tumors of the lung, breast, stomach, or pancreas. Levels may also be elevated in smokers, cirrhotics, pancreatitis, renal failure, and ulcerative colitis.

Staging

Factors that correlate with outcome include depth of tumor penetration into the bowel wall, involvement of regional lymph nodes, and the presence of metastatic disease.

The most commonly used staging system is the *tumor–node–metastasis (TNM) system,* which identifies depth of invasion of the tumor (T stage), regional lymph-node involvement (N stage), and presence of metastases

Table 18.4 TNM staging system[a]

Primary tumor (T)	Regional lymph nodes (N)	Distant metastases (M)
TX: Primary tumor cannot be assessed	NX: Regional lymph nodes cannot be assessed	MX: Presence of distal metastasis cannot be assessed
T0: No evidence of primary tumor	N0: No regional lymph-node involvement	M0: No distant metastasis
T1: Tumor invades submucosa	N1: Involvement of 1–3 regional lymph nodes	M1: Distant metastasis
T2: Tumor invades muscularis propria	N2: Metastasis in 4 or more regional lymph nodes	
T3: Tumor invades through muscularis propria into the subserosa or into nonperitonealized pericolic or perirectal tissues		
T4: Tumor perforates the visceral peritoneum and/or directly invades other organs or structures		

Stage I	T1	N0	M0
	T2	N0	M0
Stage II	T3	N0	M0
	T4	N0	M0
Stage III	Any T	N1	M0
	Any T	N2	M0
Stage IV	Any T	Any N	M1

[a]Modified from Sobin LH, Wittekind C (eds), Colon and rectum. In: *UICC International Union Against Cancer: TNM Classification of Malignant Tumours*, 5th edn. New York: Wiley, 1997: 67.

Table 18.5 Dukes staging system correlated with TNM[a]

Dukes A	T1 N0 M0
	T2 N0 M0
Dukes B	T3 N0 M0
	T4 N0 M0
Dukes C	T(any) N1 M0
	T(any) N2 M0
Dukes D	T(any) N(any) M1

Modified from Sobin LH, Wittekind C (eds), Colon and rectum. In: *UICC International Union Against Cancer: TNM Classification of Malignant Tumours*, 5th edn. New York: Wiley, 1997: 68.

Table 18.6 Five-year survival rates based on TNM disease stage

Disease stage	Survival rate (%)
Stage I	>90
Stage II	60–80
Stage III	20–50
Stage IV	<5

(M stage) (Table 18.4). The Dukes classification system (Table 18.5) was established in 1932, and is now rarely used. Neither system includes other important prognostic clinicopathologic variables, such as vascular and perineural invasion, tumor differentiation, and mucinous histology. Table 18.6 summarizes survival based on TNM stage.

Other factors associated with a poor prognosis include "signet ring" features, bowel perforation, elevated CEA levels, and aneuploid nuclei.

THERAPY

Colon cancer

Initial management of adenomatous polyps detected by endoscopy is polyp removal, since even adenomas less than 1 cm in diameter may harbor cancer.

The clinical significance of *small polyps* (<5 mm) is controversial. Techniques available for management include (1) biopsy, (2) ablation, and (3) removal with snare.

Table 18.7 Bowel preparation for colorectal surgery

	Diet	Laxatives	Antibiotics
Home bowel preparation			
2 days prior to surgery	Regular breakfast then clear liquids		
Day prior to surgery	Clear liquids No oral intake after midnight	10 a.m. – Fleet's Phospha Soda® 1.5 oz + 4 oz water Follow with 8 oz of clear liquid 4 p.m. – Fleet's Phospha Soda® 1.5 oz + 4 oz water Follow with 8 oz of clear liquid	3 p.m. – Metronidazole 250 mg tabs ×4, neomycin 500 mg tabs ×2 7 p.m. and 11 p.m. – Repeat above doses
In-hospital bowel preparation[a]			
Day prior to surgery	i.v. fluid: Ringer's lactate at 75 cc/hr Clear liquid diet No oral intake after midnight	One of the following three: bisacodyl 3–5 tabs on admission, or magnesium citrate (cold) 1 bottle, or Fleet's Phospha Soda® 45 cc plus soap suds enema ×2 or tap water enema ×2, until clear	3 p.m. – Neomycin 1 g, metronidazole 1 g 7 p.m. and 11 p.m. – Repeat above doses

Preoperative	
Colorectal surgery (CRS) prophylaxis	CRS prophylaxis: cefotetan 2 g, on call to OR
	CRS penicillin allergy prophylaxis: clindamycin 900 mg ×1, on call to OR
	tobramycin 1.5 mg/kg
	CRS SBE prophylaxis: ampicillin 2 g ×1, repeat 6 hrs after surgery clindamycin 900 mg ×1 tobramycin 1.5 mg/kg ×1
	CRS penicillin allergy and SBE: vancomycin 1 g, on call to OR metronidazole 500 mg, on call to OR tobramycin 1.5 mg/kg, on call to OR
	Should surgery be prolonged, repeat all doses in 4 hrs

aPossible reasons for preoperative-day admission:

- Bowel prep for clinical dehydration, tendency for bleeding or infection, or partial obstruction
- Pre-op antibiotics for immunosuppressed
- Conversion from oral to i.v. anticoagulation, with monitoring of PT/PTT
- Severe malnutrition or dehydration, not adequately managed by enteral support
- Labile hypertension, requiring treatment and monitoring
- Diabetes or other endocrine abnormality, requiring treatment and monitoring
- Angina or other cardiac abnormality, requiring treatment and monitoring
- Asthma or other pulmonary abnormality, requiring treatment and monitoring
- Renal failure or disease, requiring dialysis

For most *pedunculated polyps,* colonoscopic snare polypectomy is adequate treatment.

Large (>2 cm) sessile polyps frequently have villous histology and may harbor a focus of malignancy. Safe piecemeal removal of a benign-appearing lesion may be possible, especially with submucosal saline injection. If not feasible, a formal bowel resection is required. (See Table 18.7 for bowel preparation for colorectal surgery.)

In the case of *pedunculated malignant polyps,* colonoscopic polypectomy may be an option for invasive carcinomas with favorable pathologic features, since the risk of residual cancer or involved perirectal lymph nodes is minimal (0.3–1.5%). Follow-up colonoscopy is recommended 3–6 months after removal, to assess completeness of excision.

However, the existence of lymphovascular involvement, poor differentiation, or cancer within 2 mm of the resection margin are all indications for a formal bowel resection.

The major complications of colonoscopic polypectomy are perforation and bleeding, which occur in less than 2% of cases.

As a sessile polyp has no stalk, and the submucosa is immediately adjacent to the muscularis propria, sessile polyps with an invasive component require a formal colectomy.

Follow-up surveillance is important because of the increased risk of metachronous neoplasms, which occur at a rate of 29–60%, depending on interval of follow-up. Other risk factors include increasing dysplasia and villous histology. (See Table 18.3 for the surveillance schedule.)

In cases of lymphatic, vascular, or perineural invasion, operative intervention involving resection of the primary tumor and regional lymph nodes is required. A right hemicolectomy is appropriate for cancers located between the cecum and the hepatic flexure. Although transverse-colon cancers can be managed with a transverse colectomy, an extended right hemicolectomy with ligation of the middle colic artery and construction of an ileo-descending-colon anastomosis is preferred to prevent tension on the anastomosis and ensure adequacy of the blood supply. Cancers in the descending and sigmoid colon should be managed by a left hemicolectomy. With invasion of adjacent organs, an en bloc resection is required.

Adjuvant chemotherapy with 5-fluorouracil (5-FU) in combination with levamisole or leucovorin has been shown to have a significant benefit in terms of increased disease-free survival and overall survival, when administered postoperatively to patients with Stage III colon cancer who have no apparent residual disease.

Approximately 20% of patients with colon cancer have distant metastases at presentation. The 5-year survival rate in these cases is less than 5%. Palliative colon resection may prevent bleeding and obstruction, as well as alleviate symptoms related to local invasion.

Rectal cancer

Stage 0 cancers can be treated adequately with polypectomy.

Transanal excision is the technique most frequently used for local excision of selected rectal carcinomas. Local excision alone is appropriate for (1) early rectal tumors (T1 lesions without poor pathologic features), (2) relatively small tumors (<3–4 cm in diameter), (3) tumors located within 6 to 8 cm of the anal verge, and (4) tumors limited to one quadrant of the rectal circumference. For T1 lesions with adverse pathologic features (signet-ring type, poor differentiation, perineural invasion, lymphovasular invasion) and for more advanced lesions (T2 and above), formal resection should be recommended. When resection is not medically indicated or the patient has refused surgery, chemotherapy and/or irradiation may be added to lessen the chance of recurrence.

As 70–80% of rectal cancers present with disease beyond the rectal wall due to either direct extension or lymphatic spread, most rectal cancers require radical resection. Complete resection of low rectal cancers may be difficult, however, because of the narrow confines of the pelvis and proximity of delicate neurovascular structures.

Resection should encompass involved organs in an en bloc fashion. In addition, all resections should ensure adequate distal and circumferential margins of resection.

Adjuvant chemotherapy with 5-FU and leucovorin and radiation therapy has been found to be beneficial in patients with Stage II or III rectal cancer. 5-fluorouracil may have an additional role as a radiosensitizer. Chemoradiation therapy, when given preoperatively, may downstage a locally advanced cancer, making it resectable and possibly enhancing sphincter preservation. In approximately 10% of cases, a pathologic complete response to chemoradiation occurs (no evidence of tumor in the final pathologic specimen). These patients appear to have an improved prognosis compared with those without a complete response.

In the case of Stage IV cancers, surgical resection or bypass of obstructing lesions should be performed when possible. Complete resection of isolated metastatic disease may prolong survival in some cases.

The proximity of a rectal cancer to the anal sphincter mechanism is an important surgical consideration. If the lesion is located at least 2 cm above the upper part of the anorectal ring, then a *low anterior resection (LAR)* can be performed. This operation involves removal of portions of rectum, mesorectum, sigmoid colon, and sigmoid mesocolon, and the formation of an anastomosis between the descending colon and the lower rectum or anal canal. In the case of a very low colorectal or coloanal anastomosis, a protecting temporary loop ileostomy may be indicated.

If the cancer involves the sphincter mechanism, an *abdomino-perineal resection (APR)* must be performed. This involves removing the entire rectum, mesorectum, and sphincter complex, as well as part of the sigmoid colon, with the remaining proximal colon being used to create a permanent colostomy.

A *total mesorectal excision (TME)* in conjunction with LAR or APR involves removal of the entire rectal mesentery (mesorectum), including that distal to the tumor, as an intact unit. The advantages of this technique are (1) facilitation of autonomic nerve preservation, (2) decreased risk of tumor spillage from a disrupted mesentery, leading to decreased rates of local recurrence, and (3) possible avoidance of adjuvant therapy in carefully selected patients.

The overall 5-year survival rate after LAR or APR is approximately 50%. The overall local-recurrence rate is approximately 30%, with the pelvis being the most common site of recurrence. Overall, the risk of pelvic recurrence increases while the probability of survival decreases, with increasing stage of disease. There is no significant difference in recurrence rates between LAR and APR.

In the case of rectal cancer, the major risk factors for relapse are (1) the number of regional lymph nodes involved, (2) the extent of transmural penetration, (3) tumor grade, and (4) the experience of the surgeon.

POSTOPERATIVE SURVEILLANCE

The American Society of Clinical Oncology (ASCO) recommended postoperative surveillance strategy is given in Table 18.8.

PERSISTENT/RECURRENT DISEASE

An estimated 30–40% of patients with CRC treated with potentially curative surgery relapse, with 80% of recurrences being detected within 3 years of surgical treatment. The most common sites of relapse include the liver, the peritoneal cavity, the pelvis, the retroperitoneum, and the lungs. Metastases are

Table 18.8 American Society of Clinical Oncology (ASCO) postoperative surveillance recommendations

Test	Interval	Comments
Serum CEA	Every 2–3 months for >2 years after diagnosis	In patients with Stage II or III disease
History and physical exam, test coordination, physician counseling	Every 3–6 months for the first 3 years, then annually	
Colonoscopy	Every 3–5 years	
Direct imaging (flexible proctosigmoidoscopy)	Periodically	In patients with Stage II or III rectal disease who did not receive pelvic irradiation

often multifocal, and are treated palliatively with systemic chemotherapy. Patients who present with isolated sites of recurrence are candidates for surgical resection.

For rectal cancer, recurrence is most often local. In these cases, chemoradiation should be employed if it has not been used previously. Resection should include all involved organs. Palliation and salvage rates for recurrent rectal cancer are very low.

FUTURE/OTHER THERAPY

Laparoscopically assisted procedures remain a controversial option. Potential advantages may include reduced pain, shortened hospitalization, and improved aesthetics, although conflicting results exist. Questions remain about increased incidence of unrecognized injury to the small intestine, ureters, anastomotic leaks, postoperative bowel obstruction, and port-site herniation. Initial reports of trocar-site recurrences caused alarm, but more recent evidence suggests that wound recurrences in laparoscopic surgery are no more common than in open surgery. For now, performance of laparoscopic resection for invasive colorectal cancer is generally performed in the context of clinical trials.

SELECTED READING

Benson AB, Desch CE, Flynn PJ et al, 2000 update of American Society of Clinical Oncology colorectal cancer surveillance guidelines. *J Clin Oncol* 2000; **18**: 3586.

Corman ML, *Colon and Rectal Surgery*, 4th edn. Philadelphia: Lippincott-Raven Publishers, 1998.

Giardiello FM, Brensinger JD, Petersen GM, AGA technical review on hereditary colorectal cancer and genetic testing. *Gastroenterology* 2001; **121**: 198.

Gordon PH, Nivatvongs S, *Principles and Practice of Surgery for the Colon, Rectum and Anus*, 2nd edn. St Louis: Quality Medical Publishing, 1998.

Greenlee RT, Hill Harmon MB, Murray T, Thun M, Cancer statistics, 2001. *CA Cancer J Clin* 2001; **51**: 15.

Guillem, JG, Cohen AM, Treatment options for mid- and low-rectal cancers. In: *Advances in Surgery*, Vol 34 (Cameron JL, ed). St Louis: Mosby, 2000: 43.

Guillem JG, Cohen AM, Current issues in colorectal cancer surgery. *Semin Oncol* 1999; **26**: 1.

Guillem JG, Smith AJ, Puig-La Calle J, Rou L, Gastrointestinal polyposis syndromes. *Curr Probl Surg* 1999; **36**: 217.

Kodner IJ, Fry RD, Fleshman JW, Birnbaum EH, Read TE, Colon, rectum, and anus. In: *Principles of Surgery*, 7th edn (Schwartz SI, Fischer JE, Spencer FC et al, eds). New York: McGraw-Hill, 1998: 1328.

Rolandelli RH, Roslyn JJ, Colon and rectum. In: *Textbook of Surgery: The Biological Basis of Modern Surgical Practice*, 16th edn (Townsend CM, ed). Philadelphia: WB Saunders, 2001: 929.

Ruo L, Guillem JG, Major 20th century advancements in the management of rectal cancer. *Dis Colon Rectum* 1999; 42: 563.

Sobin LH, Wittekind C (eds), Colon and rectum. In: *UICC International Union Against Cancer: TNM Classification of Malignant Tumours*, 5th edn. New York: Wiley, 1997: 66.

19

Gestational trophoblastic disease

Carol A Aghajanian

The term *gestational trophoblastic disease (GTD)* applies to tumors that arise in the fetal chorion during pregnancy. They are unique among human malignancies in that the tumor arises in fetal tissue that is genetically foreign to the host. Gestational trophoblastic diseases include benign partial and complete hydatidiform (*hydatiform*) moles, persistent invasive or metastatic moles, placental-site trophoblastic tumors, and gestational choriocarcinomas. These tumors are of great interest because of the ability to cure them with chemotherapy, even in advanced stages of disease. Human chorionic gonadotropin (hCG), a tumor marker that accurately measures extent of disease, is produced by most of these tumors.

EPIDEMIOLOGY

The incidence of complete hydatidiform moles is estimated to be between 0.26 and 2.1 per 1,000 pregnancies. There is an apparent twofold increased risk in Saudi Arabia and Japan compared with other populations. There appears to be an increased risk of hydatidiform moles for women at each end of the range of reproductive life. A prior hydatidiform mole increases the risk of subsequent moles by approximately tenfold.

Risk factors for the development of gestational choriocarcinoma are less well defined. A hydatidiform mole in the prior pregnancy is the single greatest risk factor. As with complete hydatidiform moles, the incidence appears to be increased at the extremes of reproductive age. In addition, there appears to be a twofold increase in non-Caucasians as compared with Caucasians.

HISTOLOGIC TYPES AND CLINICAL CHARACTERISTICS

Complete hydatidiform moles are diploid conceptions of paternal origin. They are characterized by generalized diffuse hyperplasia of both cytotrophoblast and syncytiotrophoblast elements. Generalized edema of the chorionic villi with central cistern formation leads to a gross appearance classically described as a "bunch of grapes." Complete hydatidiform moles are often evident clinically (large for dates) or sonographically because of these hydropic changes. An embryo is generally not seen. No fetal or nucleated red blood cells are seen, since embryonic resorption occurs prior to the development of a fetal circulation. Vaginal bleeding is the most common clinical presenting symptom. Anemia is often present. Theca lutein cysts are present in approximately one-quarter to one-third of patients. Preeclampsia and hyperemesis occur in approximately 25% of patients. Both theca lutein cysts and preeclampsia are associated with high hCG levels (usually >100,000 mIU/ml). Elevated thyroid hormone levels are frequently seen, but clinical hyperthyroidism is rare. Malignant sequelae following evacuation of a complete hydatidiform mole occur in approximately 20% of patients. In most patients, the malignant sequela is the diagnosis of invasive or persistent mole, although one-quarter to one-third of patients with malignant sequelae following a complete hydatidiform mole will have gestational choriocarcinoma.

Invasive hydatidiform moles have the histopathologic features of complete hydatidiform moles, but with invasion beyond the normal placental implantation site directly into the myometrium. They often penetrate the venous system. Venous penetration can lead to the development of vaginal and lung metastasis and symptoms of bleeding. Deep penetration can lead to uterine perforation. It is a difficult diagnosis to make on specimens derived from endometrial curettage, and as hysterectomies are done so infrequently in GTD, it is not a common diagnosis. In the spectrum of malignant potential, they are intermediate between hydatidiform moles and choriocarcinomas.

Partial hydatidiform moles are triploid conceptions. They have a more subtle histologic appearance. There is only focal, slight trophoblastic hyperplasia and focal, variable hydropic villi. There is scalloping of the villi with trophoblastic inclusions within chorionic villi. The embryo survives longer than in complete hydatidiform moles, usually approximately 8 weeks. Therefore, there is frequently either gross or microscopic evidence of a fetus. In addition, fetal red blood cells can be identified within fetal vessels. Owing to both the presence of a fetus and the minimal hydropic changes in the villi, partial hydatidiform moles can be easily underdiagnosed without histologic and/or cytogenetic studies. Clinically, patients have uterine sizes either small or appropriate for dates. Sonographic appearance is often that of missed or spontaneous abortion. Pre-evacuation hCG levels are usually low. Patients usually do not have theca lutein cysts. Malignant sequelae are uncommon, compared with complete hydatidiform moles, and almost always consist of nonmetastatic postmolar GTD.

Gestational choriocarcinomas are a malignant transformation of molar tissue or a de novo lesion arising spontaneously from the placenta of a term pregnancy, abortion, or ectopic pregnancy. They are characterized histologically by a dimorphic population of cytotrophoblast and syncytiotrophoblast elements. Varying degrees of pleomorphism and anaplasia are seen. Chorionic villi are not seen. If villous structures are seen in either the primary uterine site or metastatic deposits, the diagnosis is invasive mole. Tumors often have cental necrosis and can give rise to massive local hemorrhage.

Placental-site trophoblastic tumors are predominately composed of intermediate cytotrophoblastic cells arising from the placental implantation site. Production of hCG by these tumors is scant, owing to the disproportionately small population of syncytiotrophoblast elements, and is therefore a less reliable marker of tumor volume than in other forms of GTD. Patients usually present with amenorrhea or irregular vaginal bleeding months or years after a normal pregnancy, abortion, or complete hydatidiform mole. Approximately 10% of patients have nephrotic syndrome that resolves following eradication of the tumor. These tumors are characterized by resistance to the conventional chemotherapy used in the treatment of GTD. Hysterectomy should therefore be considered early in the course of treatment.

MANAGEMENT OF HYDATIDIFORM MOLE

The management of a patient with a hydatidiform mole is the same regardless of whether it is felt to be partial or complete, and consists of a surgical evacuation, followed by close monitoring of the postevacuation hCG levels. Prior to proceeding with evacuation, an ultrasound exam is performed to confirm the diagnosis, evaluate for the presence of a fetus, and access the presence or absence of theca lutein cysts. Other preoperative evaluations include a complete history and physical exam, baseline hCG level, chest x-ray, complete blood count and coagulation profile, renal- and liver-function tests, and thyroid-function tests. If a patient is found to have anemia, pregnancy-induced hypertension, or clinically evident hyperthyroidism, these problems should be stabilized preoperatively. Special care must be taken with patients with large uterine size (>14- to 16-week size) because of the risk of perioperative complications, including respiratory distress syndrome. Evacuation of the mole can be accomplished by either hysterectomy with the mole in situ, or cervical dilatation and suction curettage in women desiring preservation of fertility. Evacuation by simple hysterectomy reduces the rate of malignant sequelae in women with complete hydatidiform mole to approximately 3.5% from 20%, the rate when suction dilation and curettage (D&C) is performed. Uterine perforation is a rare complication of suction D&C. The curettings from suction and sharp curettage should be submitted separately for pathologic review, since the trophoblastic tissue in contact with the myometrium is more likely to contain the worst histologic elements, such as choriocarcinoma, and might yield the diagnosis of invasive mole.

Following evacuation, surveillance with serial serum hCG determinations is begun. A baseline hCG level should be drawn within 48 hours of evacuation. Levels are then performed weekly until normal. Pelvic exams should also be performed every 2–4 weeks during this time. If vaginal bleeding redevelops after a period of cessation, care should be taken during examinations; there is the potential for promotion of significant bleeding in patients who have developed vaginal metastases. Monthly hCG determinations are then performed for 6–12 months. Patients should practice an effective form of contraception during the monitoring period to avoid the confusion caused by pregnancy-related elevations in hCG levels. Oral contraceptive pills are a safe and effective choice.

A diagnosis of malignant postmolar GTD is made if, during the surveillance period, the hCG levels rise, a plateau in hCG level ($\pm 10\%$) for 3 or more consecutive weeks is observed, metastases appear, or there is histologic evidence of choriocarcinoma, placental-site trophoblastic tumor, or invasive mole. Patients who meet these criteria for malignant postmolar GTD generally require treatment. One can individualize the indications for treatment in a reliable patient with low-hCG-level plateaus. In the UK, where patient follow-up and treatment is centralized such that decisions are made by a group of highly experienced physicians, more conservative treatment guidelines are often employed.

It should be noted that laboratory assays for hCG may yield false-positive results. The cause of these false-positive results may be numerous; human anti-mouse antibodies (HAMA), heterophile antibodies, and nonspecific protein interference are most common. There have been patients who have received unnecessary therapy, both surgical interventions and chemotherapy, based on phantom hCG results. When a clinical situation presents where therapy is based on the abnormal hCG value only, with no other evidence of disease confirmation, it is advisable to consider taking steps to confirm the reliability of the hCG result. Keeping in mind that multiple assays may report similar false-positive results, a prime consideration is to obtain a urinary hCG, since the interfering substances do not appear to be excreted in their interfering form into the urine. While performing a urinary assay for hCG is the simplest method to resolve a false-positive assay, alternative considerations include requesting the clinical laboratory to confirm the reliability of the assay by sending the serum of the patient in question to a national hCG reference laboratory.

MALIGNANT GESTATIONAL TROPHOBLASTIC DISEASE

The diagnosis of malignant gestational trophoblastic disease is generally made when a patient has a rising or plateauing hCG after evacuation of a hydatidiform mole or upon development of metastases after evacuation of a hydatidiform mole. Histologic evidence of choriocarcinoma, placental-site trophoblastic tumor, or invasive mole is also consistent with this diagnosis. About one-half to two-thirds of patients with malignant GTD present after molar evacuation. The majority of the remaining patients have choriocarcinoma derived from a term pregnancy, spontaneous abortion, or tubal pregnancy.

Once the diagnosis of malignant GTD has been made, a complete staging evaluation is done. Patients should have a computed tomography (CT) scan of the chest, abdomen, and pelvis. A magnetic resonance imaging (MRI) scan of the brain should also be obtained. With modern imaging techniques, lumbar puncture with simultaneous serum and cerebral spinal fluid hCG levels is no longer routinely needed.

Staging of malignant gestational trophoblastic disease

The three most frequently used systems for staging malignant GTD are the International Federation of Obstetrics and Gynecology (FIGO) staging system (see Appendix 3 of this handbook), the clinical classification system (Table 19.1), and the World Health Organization (WHO) prognostic index scoring system (Table 19.2). The clinical classification system is based on the prognostic factors that correlated with success or failure of single-agent therapy in NCI studies. Unlike standard staging systems, all three systems allow re-evaluation of previously treated patients at the time of secondary treatment. The hCG level in all three systems is the immediate prechemotherapy level (not the highest level ever measured for that patient). The duration of disease is measured as the time from either termination of the antecedent pregnancy or the beginning of symptoms to the initiation of treatment. When using the WHO prognostic scoring system, two modifications are generally made: the ABO blood groups are removed (because of lack of available data) and liver metastases are assessed as score 4.

Therapy for nonmetastatic malignant GTD

Patients who are found to have no evidence of metastatic disease on extent-of-disease evaluation have essentially a 100% chance of sustained remission with

---

Table 19.1 Clinical classification of malignant gestational trophoblastic disease

I   Nonmetastatic GTD: No evidence of disease outside of uterus; not assigned to prognostic category
II Metastatic GTD: Any metastases
    A. Good-prognosis metastatic GTD
       1. Short duration (<4 months)
       2. Low hCG level (<40,000 mIU/ml serum)
       3. No metastases to brain or liver
       4. No antecedent term pregnancy
       5. No prior chemotherapy
    B. Poor-prognosis metastatic GTD: Any high-risk factor
       1. Long duration (>4 months since last pregnancy)
       2. High pretreatment hCG level (>40,000 mIU/ml serum)
       3. Brain or liver metastases
       4. Antecedent term pregnancy
       5. Prior chemotherapy

The EP/EMA regimen is difficult to administer owing to both myelosuppression and the fact that even minor impairments in renal function caused by cisplatin can escalate the toxicities associated with methotrexate, which is renally excreted. Cytokines are often necessary. Other salvage regimens to consider are the vinblastine–ifosfamide–cisplatin (VeIP) regimen used in patients with refractory testicular cancer, taxane therapy, and high-dose chemotherapy with stem-cell rescue. The amount of data available on the potential efficacy of these treatments is very limited. Therefore, EP/EMA is the recommended salvage therapy for patients failing EMA/CO.

Placental-site trophoblastic tumors provide a particular challenge among patients with malignant GTD. These tumors are not as responsive to chemotherapy, and hCG is not a reliable marker of either extent of disease or response to treatment. These tumors are either diagnosed histologically or suspected on the basis of bulky intrauterine disease in conjunction with a relatively low hCG level. Single-agent therapy with either methotrexate or dactinomycin is not active. Hysterectomy is the mainstay of treatment for patients with nonmetastatic disease. Combination chemotherapy should be used in metastatic disease. Options are EMA/CO or EP/EMA. The therapeutic efficacy of chemotherapy is probably increased with the early introduction of cisplatin.

The two highest-risk sites of metastatic disease in GTD are the brain and liver. The presence of simultaneous central-nervous-system and liver metastases carries an even worse prognosis. Patients with brain metastases are treated with high-dose intravenous methotrexate infusions, since these infusions produce therapeutic drug levels in the cerebral spinal fluid. Routine radiation therapy to the brain is generally not recommended. Neurologic and/or neurosurgical consultation should be obtained early in the course of treatment. Patients may have neurologic decompensation caused by cerebral edema and acute hemorrhage into these highly vascular and often centrally necrotic lesions. Dexamethasone is often used to minimize cerebral edema. Emergency neurosurgery for decompression may be required. Surgical resection may also be part of the salvage therapy for these patients. Hepatic metastases can also be highly vascular and result in fatal intra-abdominal hemorrhage. Treatment with whole-liver irradiation, hepatic embolization, or hepatic ligation has been reported to control hemorrhage from hepatic metastases.

Surgery during the primary therapy of poor-risk metastatic GTD is employed in carefully selected patients exhibiting signs of drug-resistant disease. There is no role for surgical resection of sites of metastatic disease in patients exhibiting satisfactory hCG level response to systemic chemotherapy. Thoracotomy with pulmonary wedge resection is the most commonly performed procedure. A careful extent-of-disease evaluation to rule out other sites of disease should be performed prior to proceeding with surgery. This evaluation should include CT scans of the chest, abdomen, and pelvis, and MRI scanning of the brain. Hysterectomy, after careful exclusion of other potential sites of metastatic disease, may also benefit selected patients.

Patients with malignant GTD need to be monitored closely with serial serum hCG levels. It is generally recommended that hCG levels be drawn every 2 weeks for the first 3 months after completing chemotherapy and at least monthly for the remainder of the first year of surveillance. Levels should then be monitored indefinitely at 6-month intervals. Recurrence after 1 year is uncommon, but can occur. If a patient develops an elevated hCG level during follow-up, the first step is always to rule out pregnancy.

Pregnancies following successful treatment for malignant GTD are at no increased risk for complications or congenital malformations. The main risk is the increased risk of repeat molar gestation, and patients need to be counseled about this risk. Pregnancy should not be attempted until the 1-year follow-up period has been completed secondary to the interruption in monitoring caused by pregnancy-induced elevations in hCG. Patients should have an ultrasound at 6–8 weeks of gestation in order to exclude the possibility of a repeat molar pregnancy and to confirm a viable fetus. The placenta should be examined at the time of delivery to exclude choriocarcinoma. Serum hCG levels should also be followed postpartum.

SELECTED READING

Bagshawe KD, Dent J, Newlands ES et al, The role of low-dose methotrexate and folinic acid in gestational trophoblastic tumors (GTT). Br J Obstet Gynaecol 1989; 96: 795.

Bagshawe KD, Risk and prognostic factors in trophoblastic neoplasia. Cancer 1976; 38: 1373.

Bower M, Newlands ES Holden L et al, EMA/CO for high-risk gestational trophoblastic tumors: results from a cohort of 272 patients. J Clin Oncol 1997; 15: 2636.

Cole LA, Shahabi S, Butler SA et al, Utility of commonly used commercial human chorionic gonadotropin immunoassay in the diagnosis and management of trophoblastic diseases. Clin Chem 2001; 47: 308.

FIGO Oncology Committeee, Report. Int J Gynecol Obstet 1992; 39: 149.

Kohorn EI, The new FIGO 2000 staging and risk factor scoring system for gestational trophoblastic disease: description and critical assessment. Int J Gynecol Cancer 2001; 11: 73.

Newlands ES, Paradinas FJ, Fisher RA, Recent advances in gestational trophoblastic disease. Hematol Oncol Clin North Am 1999; 13: 225.

Pecorelli S, Benedet JL, Creasman WT, Shepherd JH, FIGO staging of gynecologic cancer. 1994–1997 FIGO committee on gynecologic oncology. International Federation of Gynecology and Obstetrics. Int J Gynaecol Obstet 1999; 64: 5.

Petrilli ES, Twiggs LB, Blessing JA et al, Single-dose actinomycin D treatment for nonmetastatic gestational trophoblastic disease. A prospective phase II trial of the Gynecologic Oncology Group. Cancer 1987; 60: 2173.

Soper JT, Evans AC, Conoway MR et al, Evaluation of prognostic factors and staging in gestational trophoblastic tumors. Obstet Gynecol 1994; 84: 969.

World Health Organization Scientific Group on Gestational Trophoblastic Diseases, Technical Report Series No. 692. Geneva: World Health Organization, 1983.

Appendices

APPENDIX 1
Normal anatomy

Anterior abdominal wall
Posterior abdominal wall
Arteries and veins of the perineum
Arteries and veins of pelvic organs
Arteries and veins of abdominal organs
Urogenital diaphragm
Perineum
Pelvic spaces
Pelvic diaphragm
Nerves of posterior abdominal wall
Femoral triangle
Lymphatics

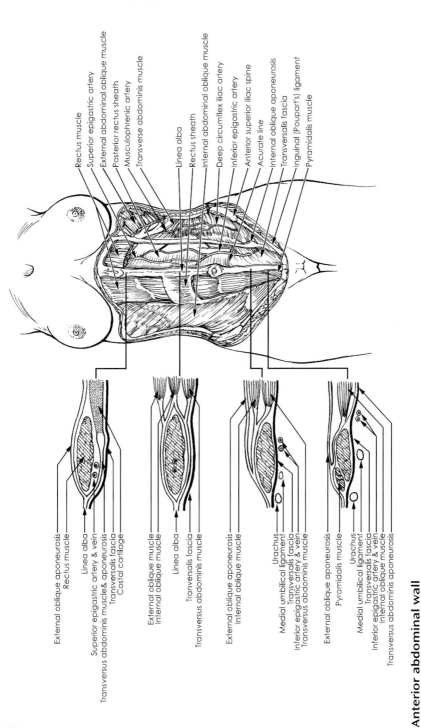

Rectus muscle
Superior epigastric artery
External abdominal oblique muscle
Posterior rectus sheath
Musculophrenic artery
Transverse abdominis muscle
Linea alba
Rectus sheath
Internal abdominal oblique muscle
Deep circumflex iliac artery
Inferior epigastric artery
Anterior superior iliac spine
Acurate line
Internal oblique aponeurosis
Transversalis fascia
Inguinal (Poupart's) ligament
Pyramidalis muscle

External oblique aponeurosis
Rectus muscle
Linea alba
Superior epigastric artery & vein
Transversus abdominis muscle& aponeurosis
Transversalis fascia
Costal cartilage

External oblique muscle
Internal oblique muscle
Linea alba
Tranversalis fascia
Transversus abdominis muscle

External oblique aponeurosis
Internal oblique muscle
Urachus
Medial umbilical ligament
Transversalis fascia
Inferior epigastric artery & vein
Transversus abdominis muscle

External oblique aponeurosis
Pyramidalis muscle
Urachus
Medial umbilical ligament
Transversalis fascia
Inferior epigastric artery & vein
Internal oblique muscle
Transversus abdominis aponeurosis

Anterior abdominal wall

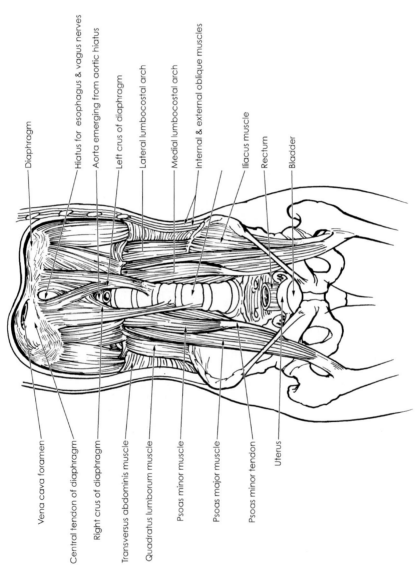

Diaphragm

Hiatus for esophagus & vagus nerves

Aorta emerging from aortic hiatus

Left crus of diaphragm

Lateral lumbocostal arch

Medial lumbocostal arch

Internal & external oblique muscles

Iliacus muscle

Rectum

Bladder

Vena cava foramen

Central tendon of diaphragm

Right crus of diaphragm

Transversus abdominis muscle

Quadratus lumborum muscle

Psoas minor muscle

Psoas major muscle

Psoas minor tendon

Uterus

Posterior abdominal wall

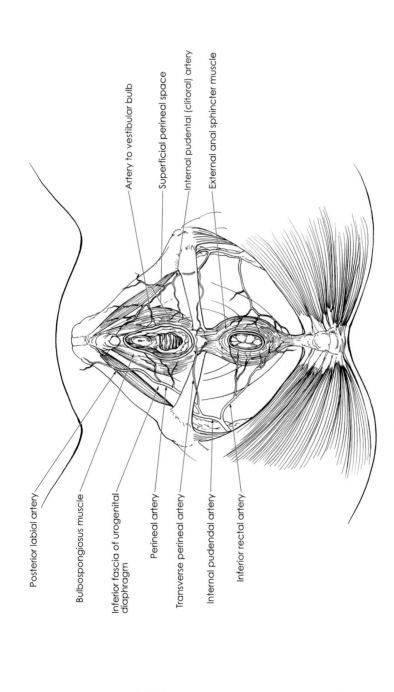

Posterior labial artery

Bulbospongiosus muscle

Inferior fascia of urogenital diaphragm

Perineal artery

Transverse perineal artery

Internal pudendal artery

Inferior rectal artery

Artery to vestibular bulb

Superficial perineal space

Internal pudendal (clitoral) artery

External anal sphincter muscle

Arteries and veins of the perineum

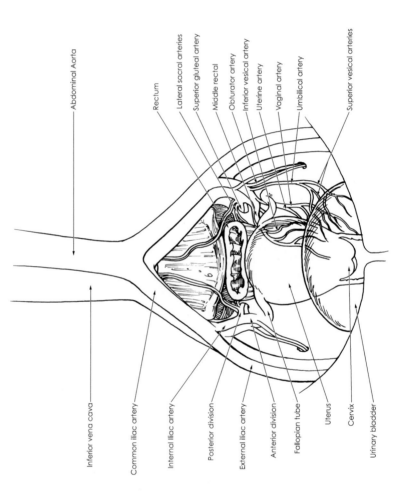

Arteries and veins of pelvic organs

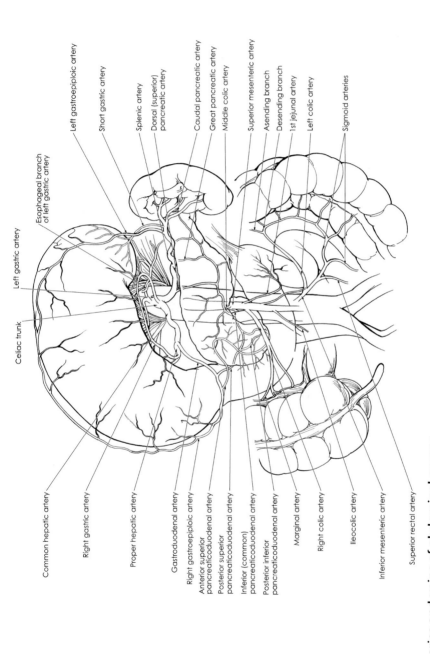

Left gastroepiploic artery

Short gastric artery

Splenic artery

Dorsal (superior) pancreatic artery

Caudal pancreatic artery

Great pancreatic artery

Middle colic artery

Superior mesenteric artery

Asending branch

Desending branch

1st jejunal artery

Left colic artery

Sigmoid arteries

Esophageal branch of left gastric artery

Left gastric artery

Celiac trunk

Common hepatic artery

Right gastric artery

Proper hepatic artery

Gastroduodenal artery

Right gastroepiploic artery

Anterior superior pancreaticoduodenal artery

Posterior superior pancreaticoduodenal artery

Inferior (common) pancreaticoduodenal artery

Posterior inferior pancreaticoduodenal artery

Marginal artery

Right colic artery

Ileocolic artery

Inferior mesenteric artery

Superior rectal artery

Arteries and veins of abdominal organs

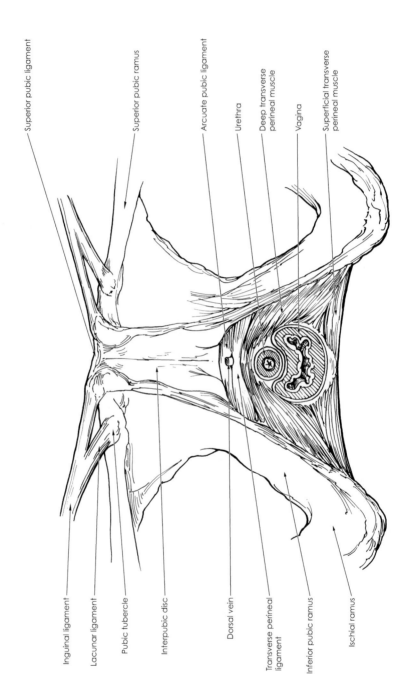

Superior pubic ligament

Superior pubic ramus

Arcuate pubic ligament

Urethra

Deep transverse
perineal muscle

Vagina

Superficial transverse
perineal muscle

Inguinal ligament

Lacunar ligament

Pubic tubercle

Interpubic disc

Dorsal vein

Transverse perineal
ligament

Inferior pubic ramus

Ischial ramus

Urogenital diaphragm

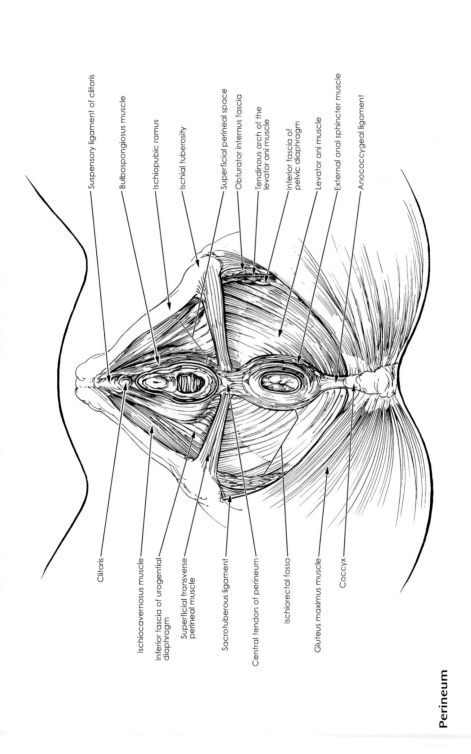

Suspensory ligament of clitoris

Bulbospongiosus muscle

Ischiopubic ramus

Ischial tuberosity

Superficial perineal space

Obturator internus fascia

Tendinous arch of the levator ani muscle

Inferior fascia of pelvic diaphragm

Levator ani muscle

External anal sphincter muscle

Anococcygeal ligament

Clitoris

Ischiocavernosus muscle

Inferior fascia of urogenital diaphragm

Superficial transverse perineal muscle

Sacrotuberous ligament

Central tendon of perineum

Ischiorectal fossa

Gluteus maximus muscle

Coccyx

Perineum

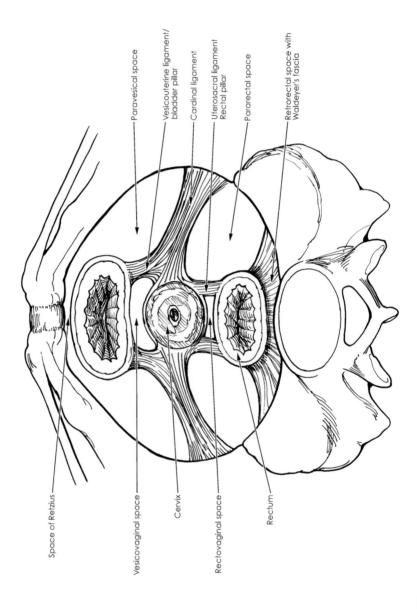

Paravesical space

Vesicouterine ligament/
bladder pillar

Cardinal ligament

Uterosacral ligament
Rectal pillar

Pararectal space

Retrorectal space with
Waldeyer's fascia

Space of Retzius

Vesicovaginal space

Cervix

Rectovaginal space

Rectum

Pelvic spaces

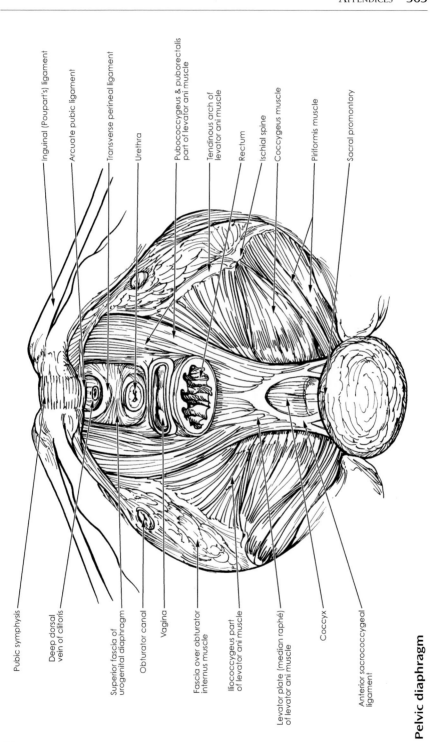

Pubic symphysis

Deep dorsal
vein of clitoris

Superior fascia of
urogenital diaphragm

Obturator canal

Vagina

Fascia over obturator
internus muscle

Iliococcygeus part
of levator ani muscle

Levator plate (median raphé)
of levator ani muscle

Coccyx

Anterior sacrococcygeal
ligament

Inguinal (Poupart's) ligament

Arcuate pubic ligament

Transverse perineal ligament

Urethra

Pubococcygeus & puborectalis
part of levator ani muscle

Tendinous arch of
levator ani muscle

Rectum

Ischial spine

Coccygeus muscle

Piriformis muscle

Sacral promontory

Pelvic diaphragm

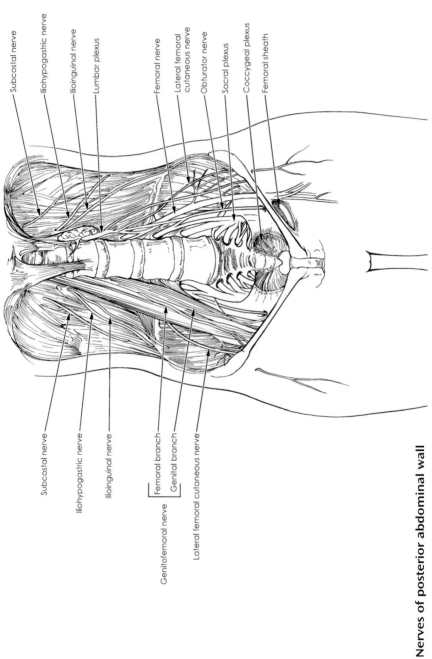

Subcostal nerve

Iliohypogastric nerve

Ilioinguinal nerve

Lumbar plexus

Femoral nerve

Lateral femoral cutaneous nerve

Obturator nerve

Sacral plexus

Coccygeal plexus

Femoral sheath

Subcostal nerve

Iliohypogastric nerve

Ilioinguinal nerve

Genitofemoral nerve

Femoral branch

Genital branch

Lateral femoral cutaneous nerve

Nerves of posterior abdominal wall

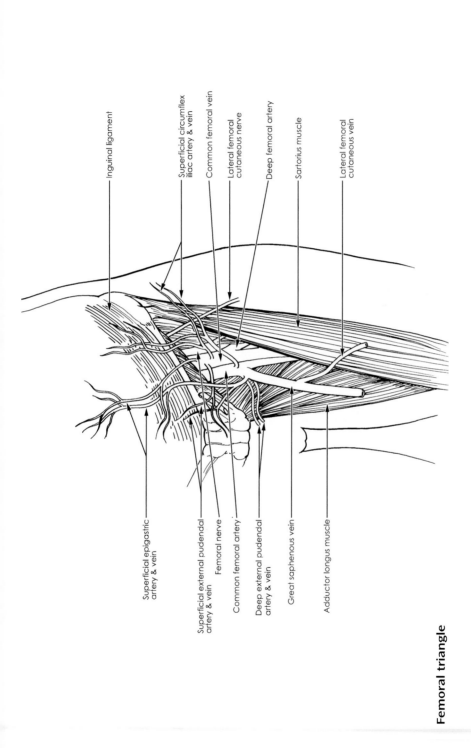

Inguinal ligament

Superficial circumflex iliac artery & vein

Common femoral vein

Lateral femoral cutaneous nerve

Deep femoral artery

Sartorius muscle

Lateral femoral cutaneous vein

Superficial epigastric artery & vein

Superficial external pudendal artery & vein

Femoral nerve

Common femoral artery

Deep external pudendal artery & vein

Great saphenous vein

Adductor longus muscle

Femoral triangle

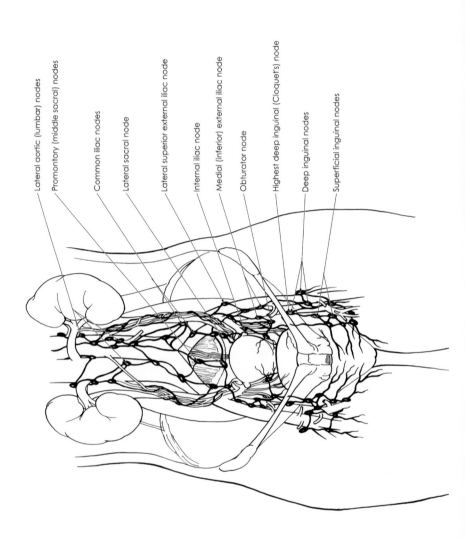

Lateral aortic (lumbar) nodes

Promontory (middle sacral) nodes

Common iliac nodes

Lateral sacral node

Lateral superior external iliac node

Internal iliac node

Medial (inferior) external iliac node

Obturator node

Highest deep inguinal (Cloquet's) node

Deep inguinal nodes

Superficial inguinal nodes

Lymphatics

APPENDIX 2
American Cancer Society screening recommendations

General

- Cancer-related checkup, including skin examination, every 3 years for people between 20 and 40 years of age, and every year for anyone age 40 and older.

Breast

- Women age 40 and older should have a screening mammogram every year.
- Between the ages of 20 and 39, women should have a clinical breast examination by a health professional every 3 years. After age 40, women should have a breast exam by a health professional every year.
- Women age 20 or older should perform a breast self-examination (BSE) every month. By doing the exam regularly, you get to know how your breasts normally feel and you can more readily detect any signs or symptoms.
- If a change occurs, such as development of a lump or swelling, skin irritation or dimpling, nipple pain or retraction (turning inward), redness or scaliness of the nipple or breast skin, or a discharge other than breast milk, you should see your health-care provider as soon as possible for evaluation. However, remember that most of the time, these breast changes are not cancer.
- Although there are some features of a mass that suggest whether it is likely to be benign or cancerous, women examining their own breasts should discuss any new lump with their health-care professionals. Experienced health-care professionals can examine the breast and determine whether the changes you have noticed are probably benign or whether there is a possibility they may be due to a breast cancer. They can determine when additional tests are appropriate to rule out a cancer and when follow-up exams are the best strategy. If there is any suspicion of cancer, a biopsy will be done.

Colorectal and anal

Beginning at age 50, both men and women should follow one of the three screening options below:

- yearly fecal occult-blood test plus flexible sigmoidoscopy every 5 years;* or

- colonoscopy every 10 years;* or
- double-contrast barium enema every 5–10 years.*

*Digital rectal examination should be performed at the time of each screening sigmoidoscopy, colonoscopy, or barium-enema examination.

People should begin colorectal-cancer screening earlier and/or undergo screening more often if they have any of the following colorectal-cancer risk factors:

- a strong family history of colorectal cancer or polyps (cancer or polyps in a first-degree relative younger than 60 or in two first-degree relatives of any age);
- families with hereditary colorectal cancer syndromes (familial adenomatous polyposis and hereditary nonpolyposis colon cancer);
- a personal history of colorectal cancer or adenomatous polyps; or
- a personal history of chronic inflammatory bowel disease.

Female reproductive tract

- Yearly Pap tests and pelvic examinations beginning at age 18 or when a woman becomes sexually active, whichever occurs earlier. If a woman has had three satisfactory negative annual Pap tests in a row, this test may be done less often at the judgment of a woman's health-care provider. But, the annual pelvic exam should be continued, regardless of how often the Pap test is done.
- This recommendation also applies to women who are postmenopausal. If a hysterectomy was done for cancer, more frequent Pap tests may be recommended.
- Women who have had a hysterectomy should talk with their doctor about whether to continue to have regular Pap tests. If the hysterectomy was performed for treatment of a precancerous or cancerous condition, the end of the vaginal canal still needs to be sampled for abnormal changes. If the uterus (including the cervix) was removed because of a noncancerous condition such as fibroids, routine Pap tests may not be necessary. However, it is still important for a woman to have regular gynecologic examinations as part of her health care.
- It is important to remember that while the Pap test has been more successful than any other screening test in preventing a cancer, it is not perfect. Because some abnormalities may be missed (even when samples are examined in the best laboratories), it is not a good idea to have this test less often than ACS guidelines recommend.

Skin

- Cancer-related checkup, including skin examination, every 3 years for people between 20 and 40 years old and every year for anyone age 40 and older.

- It is also important for the patient to check her own skin for melanoma and nonmelanoma skin lesions – preferably once a month.
- The **ABCD** rule can help distinguish a normal mole from a melanoma:
  Asymmetry: One half of the mole does not match the other half.
  Border irregularity: The edges of the mole are ragged or notched.
  Color: The color over the mole is not the same. There may be differing shades of tan, brown, or black, and sometimes patches of red, blue, or white.
  Diameter: The mole is wider than 6 millimeters (about 1/4 inch), although doctors are finding more melanomas between 3 and 6 millimeters in recent years.

Other important signs of melanoma include changes in size, shape, or color of a mole. Some melanomas do not fit the ABCD rule described above, so it is particularly important to be aware of changes in skin lesions.

APPENDIX 3
FIGO staging classifications

FIGO STAGING CLASSIFICATION: VULVA

0   Carcinoma in situ; preinvasive carcinoma

I   Tumor confined to vulva or vulva and perineum, 2 cm or less in greatest dimension, nodes are negative

IA   Stromal invasion no greater than 1 mm

IB   Stromal invasion greater than 1 mm

II   Tumor confined to vulva or vulva and perineum, more than 2 cm in greatest dimension, nodes are negative

III   Tumor of any size with adjacent spread to the lower urethra, vagina, or the anus and/or with unilateral regional lymph-node metastasis

IVA   Tumor invades upper urethra, bladder mucosa, rectal mucosa, or pelvic bone, and/or bilateral regional node metastases

IVB   Distant metastasis

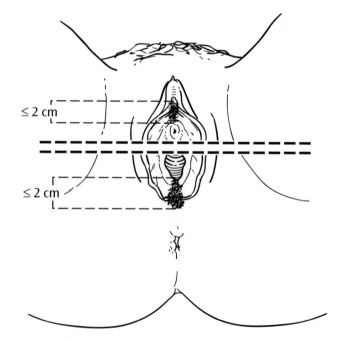

Vulva: FIGO Stage I.

370

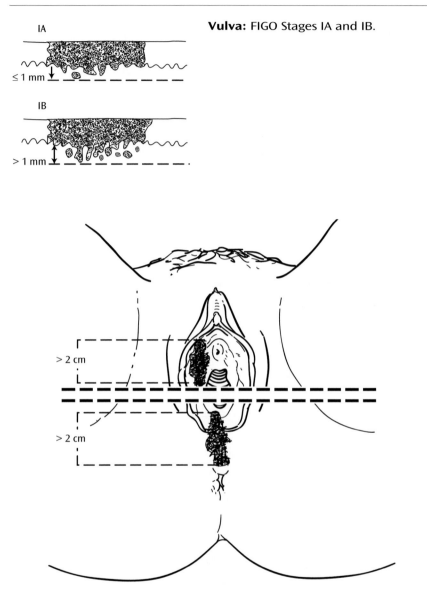

Vulva: FIGO Stages IA and IB.

Vulva: FIGO Stage II.

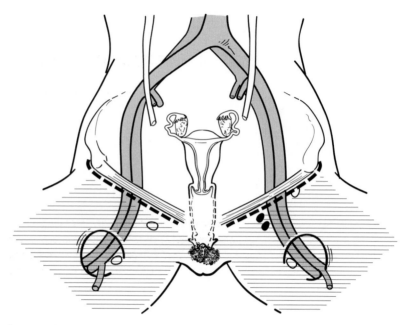

Vulva: FIGO Stage III.

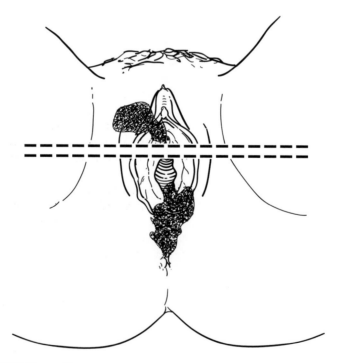

Vulva: FIGO Stage III.

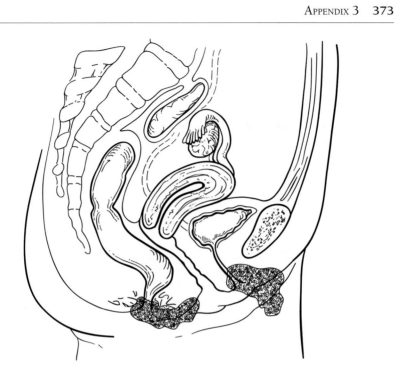

Vulva: FIGO Stage III.

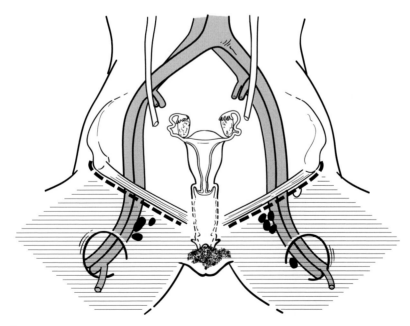

Vulva: FIGO Stage IVA.

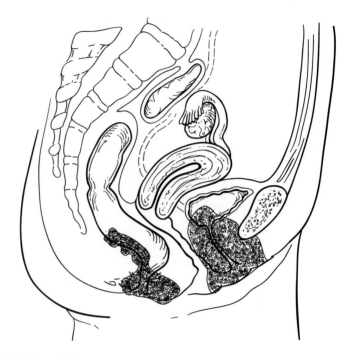

Vulva: FIGO Stage IVA.

FIGO STAGING CLASSIFICATION: VAGINA

0   Carcinoma in situ, intraepithelial carcinoma

I   Tumor confined to vaginal wall

II   Tumor involves subvaginal tissues but does not extend to pelvic wall

III   Tumor extends to pelvic wall

IVA   Tumor invades *mucosa* of bladder or rectum and/or extends beyond the true pelvis

IVB   Distant metastasis

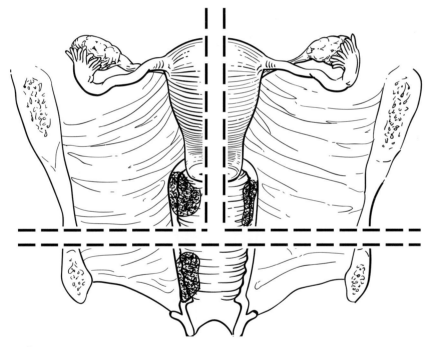

Vagina: FIGO Stage I.

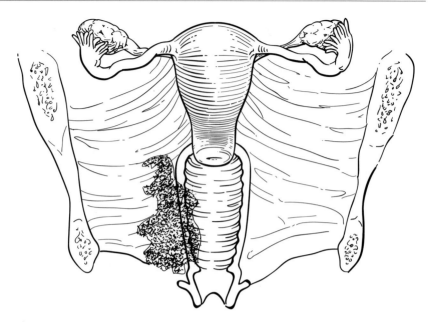

Vagina: FIGO Stage II.

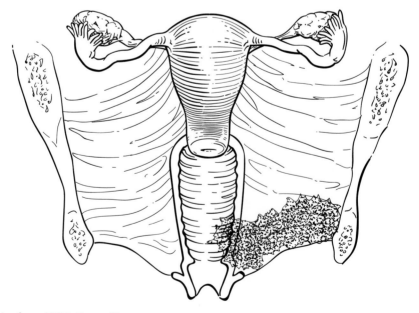

Vagina: FIGO Stage III.

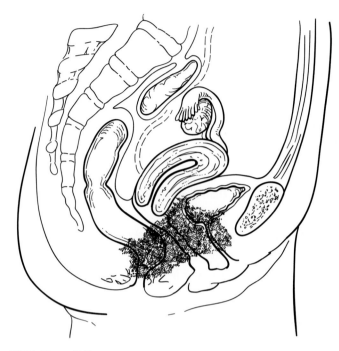

Vagina: FIGO Stage IVA.

FIGO STAGING CLASSIFICATION: CERVIX UTERI

0   Carcinoma in situ, intraepithelial carcinoma

I   Carcinoma confined to the cervix (extension to corpus should be disregarded)

IA   Invasive carcinoma diagnosed only by microscopy. All macroscopically visible lesions – even with superficial invasion – are Stage IB

IA1   Stromal invasion no greater than 3 mm in depth and 7 mm or less in horizontal spread

IA2   Stromal invasion more than 3 mm and not more than 5 mm, with a horizontal spread 7 mm or less

IB   Clinically visible lesion confined to the cervix or microscopic lesion greater than IA2

IB1   Clinically visible lesion 4 cm or less in greatest dimension

IB2   Clinically visible lesion more than 4 cm in greatest dimension

II   Tumor invades beyond uterus but not to pelvic wall or to lower third of the vagina

IIA   Without parametrial invasion

IIB   With parametrial invasion

III   Tumor extends to pelvic wall and/or involves the lower third of the vagina and/or causes hydronephrosis or nonfunctioning kidney

IIIA   Tumor involves lower third of vagina, no extension to pelvic wall

IIIB   Tumor extends to pelvic wall and/or causes hydronephrosis or nonfunctioning kidney

IV   Carcinoma has extended beyond the true pelvis or has clinically involved the mucosa of the bladder or rectum

IVA   Tumor invades *mucosa* of bladder or rectum and/or extends to adjacent organs

IVB   Distant metastasis

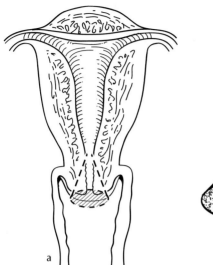
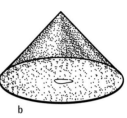

Cervix: FIGO Stage IA.

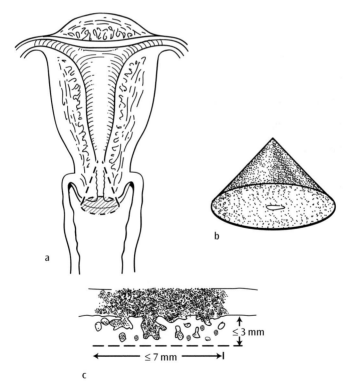

Cervix: FIGO Stage IA1.

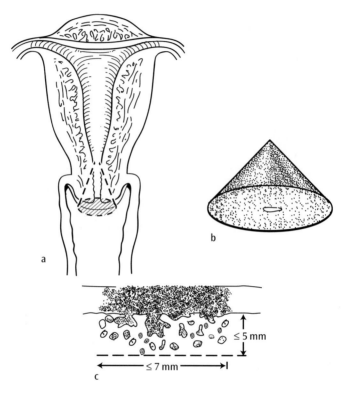

Cervix: FIGO Stage IA2.

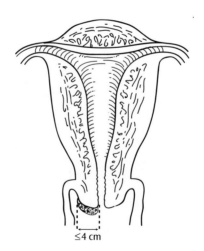

Cervix: FIGO Stage IB1.

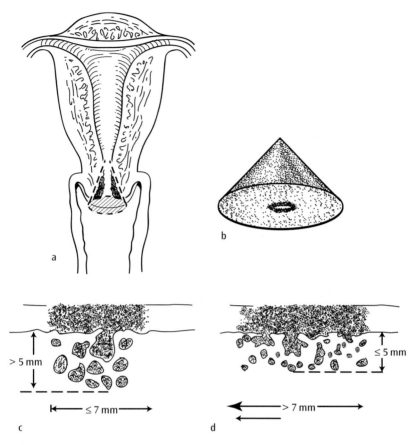

Cervix: FIGO Stage IB1.

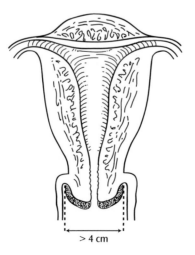

Cervix: FIGO Stage IB2.

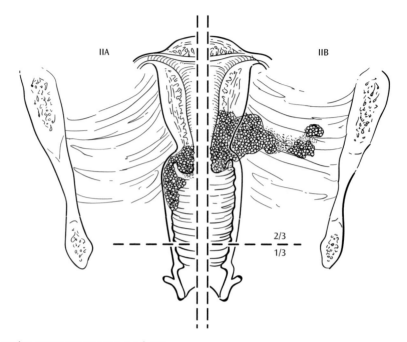

Cervix: FIGO Stages IIA and IIB.

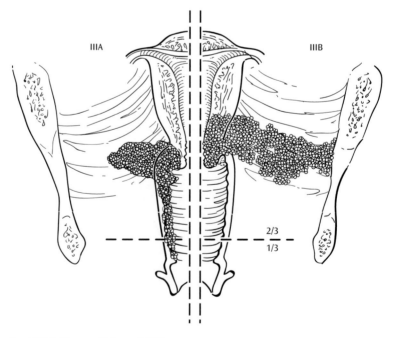

Cervix: FIGO Stages IIIA and IIIB.

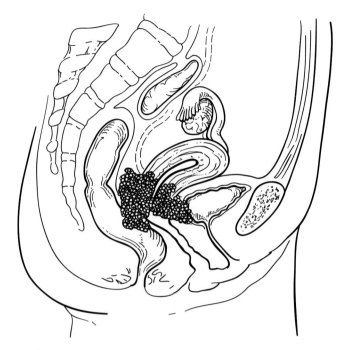

Cervix: FIGO Stage IVA.

FIGO STAGING CLASSIFICATION: OVARY

I   Growth limited to the ovaries

IA   Tumor limited to one ovary; capsule intact, no tumor on ovarian surface; no malignant cells in ascites or peritoneal washings

IB   Tumor limited to both ovaries; capsules intact, no tumor on ovarian surface: no malignant cells in ascites or peritoneal washings

IC   Tumor limited to one or both ovaries with any of the following: capsule ruptured, tumor on ovarian surface; malignant cells in ascites or peritoneal washings

II   Tumor involves one or both ovaries with pelvic extension

IIA   Extension and/or implants on uterus and/or tube(s); no malignant cells in ascites or peritoneal washings

IIB   Extension to other pelvic tissues; no malignant cells in ascites or peritoneal washings

IIC   Pelvic extension with malignant cells in ascites or peritoneal washings

III   Tumor involves one or both ovaries with peritoneal metastasis outside the pelvis and/or retroperitoneal or inguinal node metastasis

IIIA   Microscopic peritoneal metastasis beyond pelvis

IIIB   Macroscopic peritoneal metastasis beyond pelvis 2 cm or less in greatest dimension

IIIC   Peritoneal metastasis beyond pelvis more than 2 cm in greatest dimension and/or regional lymph node metastasis

IV   Distant metastasis (excludes peritoneal metastasis) to liver parenchyma or malignant pleural effusion

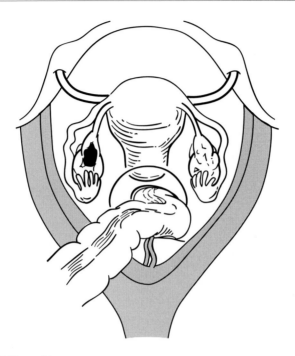

Ovary: FIGO Stage IA.

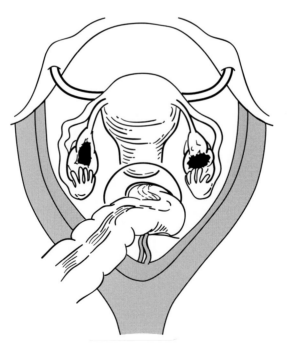

Ovary: FIGO Stage IB.

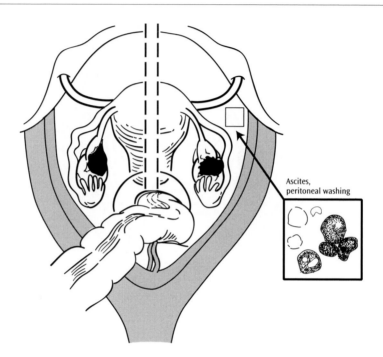

Ascites, peritoneal washing

Ovary: FIGO Stage IC.

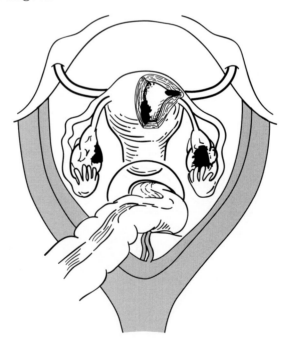

Ovary: FIGO Stage IIA.

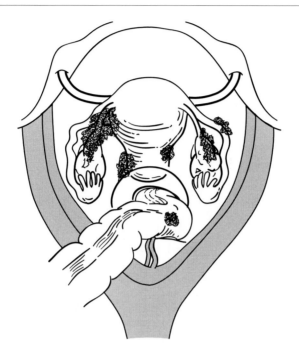

Ovary: FIGO Stage IIB.

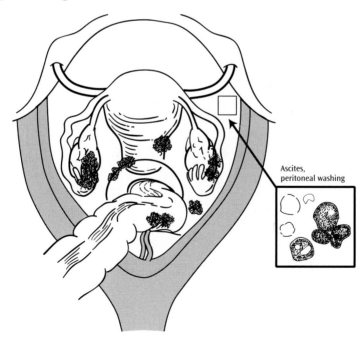

Ascites,
peritoneal washing

Ovary: FIGO Stage IIC.

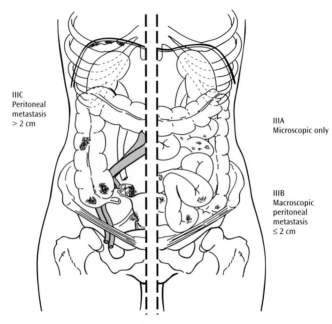

IIIC
Peritoneal
metastasis
> 2 cm

IIIA
Microscopic only

IIIB
Macroscopic
peritoneal
metastasis
≤ 2 cm

Ovary: FIGO Stages IIIA, IIIB, and IIIC.

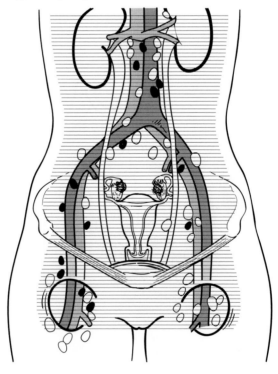

Ovary: FIGO Stage IIIC.

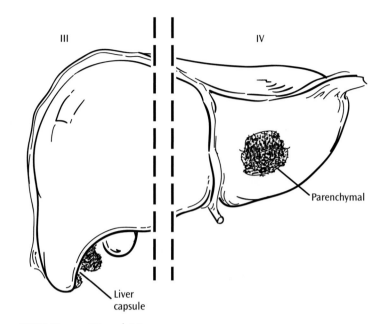

Ovary: FIGO Stages III and IV.

FIGO STAGING CLASSIFICATION: FALLOPIAN TUBE

0   Carcinoma in situ

I   Tumor confined to fallopian tube(s)

IA   Tumor limited to one tube, without penetrating the serosal surface; no ascites

IB   Tumor limited to both tubes, without penetrating the serosal surface; no ascites

IC   Tumor limited to one or both tube(s) with extension onto or through the tubal serosa, or with malignant cells in ascites or peritoneal washings

II   Tumor involves one or both fallopian tube(s) with pelvic extension

IIA   Extension and/or metastases to uterus and/or ovaries

IIB   Extension to other pelvic structures

IIC   Pelvic extension with malignant cells in ascites or peritoneal washings

III   Tumor involves one or both fallopian tube(s) with peritoneal implants outside the pelvis and/or positive retroperitoneal or inguinal nodes

IIIA   Microscopic peritoneal metastasis outside the pelvis

IIIB   Macroscopic peritoneal metastasis outside the pelvis 2 cm or less in greatest dimension

IIIC   Peritoneal metastasis more than 2 cm in greatest dimension and/or positive regional lymph nodes

IV   Distant metastasis (excludes peritoneal metastasis) to liver parenchyma or malignant pleural effusion

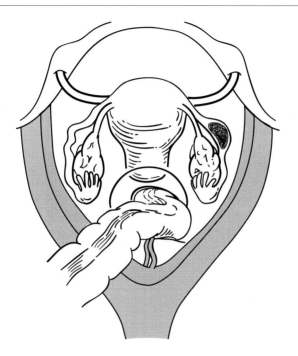

Fallopian tube: FIGO Stage IA.

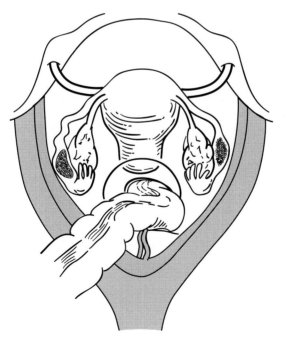

Fallopian tube: FIGO Stage IB.

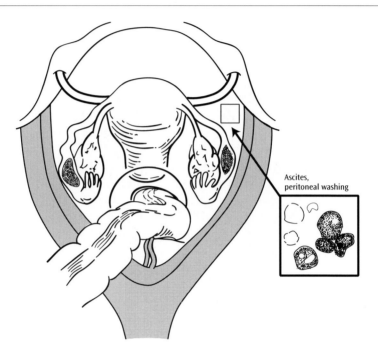

Ascites,
peritoneal washing

Fallopian tube: FIGO Stage IC.

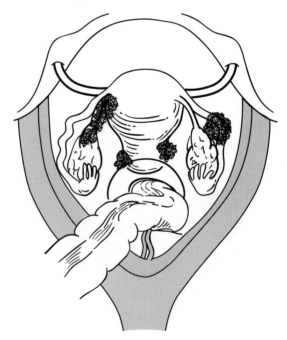

Fallopian tube: FIGO Stage IIA.

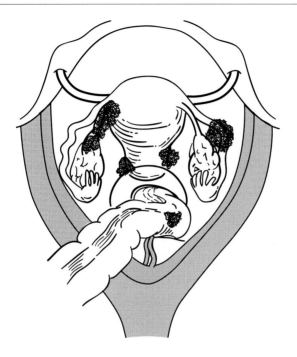

Fallopian tube: FIGO Stage IIB.

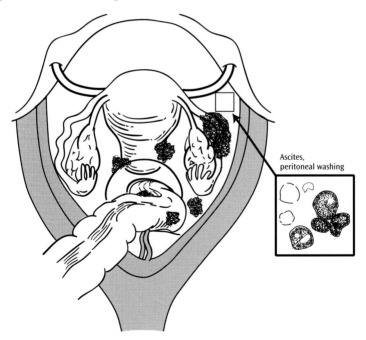

Ascites,
peritoneal washing

Fallopian tube: FIGO Stage IIC.

Fallopian tube: FIGO Stages III and IV – see figures for Ovary, Stages III and IV.

FIGO STAGING CLASSIFICATION: CORPUS UTERI

I   Tumor confined to corpus uteri

IA   Tumor limited to endometrium

IB   Tumor invades up to or less than one-half of myometrium

IC   Tumor invades more than one-half of myometrium

II   Tumor invades cervix but does not extend beyond uterus

IIA   Endocervical glandular involvement only

IIB   Cervical stromal invasion

III   Local and/or regional spread as specified in IIIA, B, C

IIIA   Tumor involves serosa and/or adnexa (direct extension or metastasis) and/or cancer cells in ascites or peritoneal washings

IIIB   Vaginal involvement (direct extension or metastasis)

IIIC   Metastasis to pelvic and/or para-aortic lymph nodes

IVA   Tumor invades bladder *mucosa* and/or bowel *mucosa*

IVB   Distant metastasis (including intra-abdominal and/or inguinal lymph nodes, excluding metastasis to pelvic serosa or adnexa)

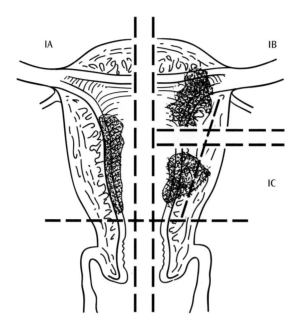

Corpus uteri: FIGO Stages IA, IB, and IC.

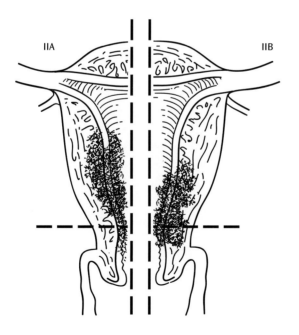

Corpus uteri: FIGO Stages IIA and IIB.

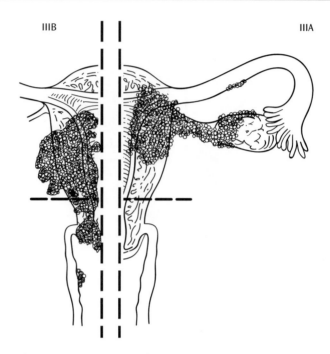

IIIB

IIIA

Corpus uteri: FIGO Stages IIIA and IIIB.

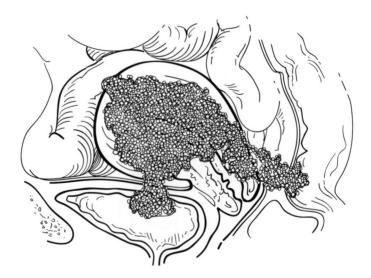

Corpus uteri: FIGO Stage IVA.

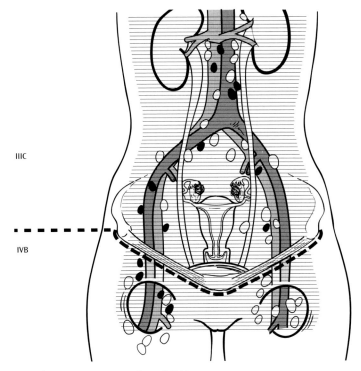

IIIC

IVB

Corpus uteri: FIGO Stages IIIC and IVB.

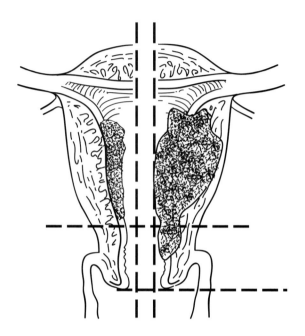

Gestational trophoblastic disease: FIGO Stage I.

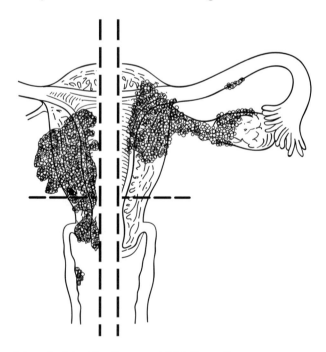

Gestational trophoblastic disease: FIGO Stage II.

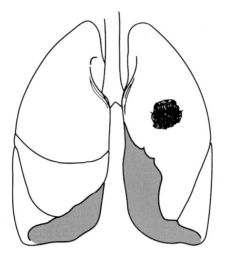

Gestational trophoblastic disease: FIGO Stage III (lung metastasis).

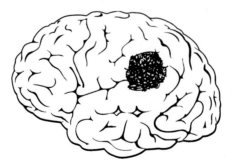

Gestational trophoblastic disease: FIGO Stage IV (brain metastasis).

APPENDIX 4
Common combination-chemotherapy regimens for gynecologic cancer

Regimen	Dose	Schedule	Indication
Doxorubicin	60 mg/m²	Once q 3 wks	Endometrial cancer
Cisplatin	50 mg/m²		
Ifosfamide	5,000 mg/m² over 24-hr continuous infusion	Once q 3 wks	Cervical cancer
Mesna	6,000 mg/m² as 30- to 36-hr infusion		Mixed mesodermal tumors or carcinosarcoma
Cisplatin	50 mg/m² bolus day 1 only		
Ifosfamide	1,500–2,500 mg/m² bolus	Daily × 3 days q 3 wks before, 4 hrs and 8 hrs after each ifosfamide	Leiomyosarcoma
Mesna	1,200–2,000 mg/m² bolus		
Doxorubicin	60–75 mg/m²	Day 1 only	
Paclitaxel	135 mg/m² over 24 hrs	Day 1 q 3 wks	Cervical cancer
Cisplatin	50 mg/m²	Day 2	Ovarian cancer
Paclitaxel	175 mg/m² over 3 hrs	Day 1 q 3 wks	Ovarian cancer
Carboplatin	AUC 5–6	Day 1	Endometrial cancer
Cyclophosphamide	600–750 mg/m²	Day 1	Ovarian cancer
Carboplatin	AUC 4–5	Day 1	
Cyclophosphamide	600 mg/m²	Day 1	Ovarian cancer
Doxorubicin	60 mg/m²	Day 1	
Cisplatin	60 mg/m²	Day 1	
EMA/CO			
EMA:			
Dactinomycin	0.5 mg i.v.p. (total dose)	Days 1 and 2	Gestational trophoblastic disease
Etoposide	100 mg/m²	Days 1 and 2	
Methotrexate	300 mg/m² as 12-hr continuous infusion	Day 1 only	
Leucovorin	15 mg p.o. or i.m. q 12 hrs × 48 hrs	Day 2	
CO:			
Cyclophosphamide	600 mg/m²	Day 8 (begun 24 hrs after beginning methotrexate)	
Vincristine	0.8 mg/m² (max 2 mg)	Day 8	
Bleomycin	30 units (total dose)	Day 1 only	Germ-cell tumors
Etoposide	100 mg/m²	Daily × 5	Stromal tumors
Cisplatin	20 mg/m²	Daily × 5	
Paclitaxel	175 mg/m² over 3 hrs	Day 1	Ovarian cancer
Cisplatin	75–100 mg/m² i.p.	Day 1	>1 cm

APPENDIX 5
Clinical research definitions

CLINICAL TRIAL DEFINITIONS

Phase I trial   Study conducted to estimate the maximum tolerated dose level of a new therapy.

Phase II trial   Study conducted to determine whether a new therapy has sufficient evidence of biologic activity to warrant further study in a randomized trial.

Phase III trial   Study conducted to provide an unbiased comparison of two or more therapeutic regimens.

Phase IV trial   Study conducted in a large-scale population to determine whether the results obtained in the clinical setting can be translated to the general population.

CLINICAL RESPONSE DEFINITIONS

Complete response   Total disappearance of all measurable and evaluable disease.

Partial response   50% decrease below baseline in the sum of the products of perpendicular diameters of all measurable lesions, no progression of evaluable disease, and no new lesions.

Stable disease   Disease that has neither progressed nor responded (complete or partial response).

Progression   50% increase in the sum of the products of measurable lesions over the smallest sum observed, the reappearance of any disease, the clear worsening of evaluable disease, the appearance of any new disease, or failure to return for evaluation owing to death or deteriorating condition (unless clearly unrelated to the disease under study).

SURVIVAL DEFINITIONS

Overall survival   Time from first day of treatment to time of death due to any cause.

Progression-free survival   Time from the first day of treatment to the first observation of disease progression or death due to any cause.

APPENDIX 6
Memorial Sloan-Kettering Surgical Complications Criteria (12/99)

For the Common Toxicity Criteria (CTC), the reader is referred to the *Common Toxicity Criteria Manual*, which can be downloaded from: http://ctep.info.nih.gov/

MEMORIAL SLOAN-KETTERING SURGICAL COMPLICATION CRITERIA 12/99

*Category	Grade	Grade criteria
Toxicity name		

*Cardiovascular

	Grade	Grade criteria
Angina	1	Oral or first-line medical therapy
	2	i.v. medical treatment for significant angina
	3	IR or operative intervention required
	4	Chronic, new disability due to angina
	5	Death due to complication
Arterial insufficiency	1	Supportive medical care
	2	i.v. medical treatment with resolution
	3	IR or operative intervention required
	4	Chronic, new disability (amputation, claudication) due to arterial insufficiency
	5	Death due to complication
Congestive heart failure	1	Responsive to oral medication
	2	i.v. medical treatment with resolution
	3	—
	4	Severe or refractory CHF or requiring intubation
	5	Death due to complication
Dysrhythmia	1	Monitoring or oral medical, acute or chronic
	2	Monitoring and i.v. medical treatment, acute or chronic
	3	Requiring IR or operation for pacemaker or other treatment
	4	Chronic functional disability as result of new or exacerbated dysrhythmia
	5	Death due to complication
Hyper- or hypotension	1	Requiring new or more intensive oral therapy
	2	Hypertensive crisis or shock requiring intensive medical therapy
	2	i.v. medical treatment with resolution
	4	—
	5	Death due to complication
Myocardial infarction	1	—
	2	Without hemodynamic change, requiring monitoring and standard treatment
	3	With hemodynamic change, radiologic or operative intervention required
	4	Chronic disability (angina, CHF, or reduction of EF > 20%) due to MI or intubation
	5	Death due to complication
Pericarditis, tamponade	1	Responsive to oral medication
	2	i.v. medical treatment, with resolution
	3	Needle decompress, IR, or operative intervention required

*Category	Grade	Grade criteria
Toxicity name		
	4	—
	5	Death due to complication
*Central nervous system		
CSF leak	1	Supportive care, oral antibiotics
	2	i.v. antibiotics, possible neurologic sequelae with resolution
	3	IR or reoperation required for CSF leak
	4	Chronic neurologic deficit as result of CSF leak
	5	Death due to complication
Cerebrovascular accident or CNS event	1	Transient ischemic attack <24 hrs, no neurologic sequelae
	2	Neurologic deficit lasting >24 hrs but with subsequent resolution or absence of long-term major deficit
	3	Interventional radiology or operation required for treatment
	4	Chronic neurologic deficit
	5	Death due to complication
Psychosis, confusion, or depression	1	Oral medication
	2	i.v. medication
	3	—
	4	New and chronic disability judged not to be situational and requiring treatment
*Endocrine		
Adrenal dysfunction	1	Replacement therapy or first-line medical treatment
	2	Intensive medical therapy or i.v. medication beyond first-line treatments
	3	—
	4	Endocrine cause of chronic disability or organ dysfunction
	5	Death due to complication
Pancreas dysfunction	1	Replacement therapy or first-line medical treatment
	2	Intensive medical therapy or i.v. medication beyond first-line treatments
	3	—
	4	Endocrine cause of chronic disability or organ dysfunction
	5	Death due to complication
Parathyroid dysfunction	1	Replacement therapy of first-line medical treatment
	2	Intensive medical therapy or i.v. medication beyond first-line treatments

*Category	Grade	Grade criteria
Toxicity name		
	3	—
	4	Endocrine cause of chronic disability or organ dysfunction
	5	Death due to complication
Pituitary dysfunction	1	Replacement therapy of first-line medical treatment
	2	Intensive medical therapy or i.v. medication beyond first-line treatments
	3	—
	4	Endocrine cause of chronic disability or organ dysfunction
	5	Death due to complication
Thyroid dysfunction	1	Replacement therapy of first-line medical treatment
	2	Intensive medical therapy or i.v. medication beyond first-line treatments
	3	—
	4	Endocrine cause of chronic disability or organ dysfunction
	5	Death due to complication
*Gastrointestinal		
Anastomotic leak	1	Oral antibiotics, supportive care
	2	i.v. antibiotics or TPN, drainage not required
	3	IR or operative intervention for drainage, resection
	4	Enteral diversion
	5	Death due to complication
Bowel perforation	1	—
	2	i.v. antibiotics
	3	IR or operative intervention required
	4	Organ resection or chronic disability resulting from bowel perforation
	5	Death due to complication
Cholecystitis	1	Oral antibiotics, supportive care
	2	i.v. antibiotics
	3	IR or operative intervention for cholecystostomy or cholecystectomy
	4	—
	5	Death due to complication
Delayed gastric emptying	1	Resolution with oral medical therapy
	2	Parenteral nutrition or enteral nutrition through G/J tube
	3	Reoperation required or endoscopic feeding tube

*Category	Grade	Grade criteria
Toxicity name		
	4	Chronic disability, home enteral or parenteral nutrition
	5	Death due to complication
Fistula	1	Resolution with supportive care
	2	Parenteral nutrition or prolonged tube feeding >POD #10
	3	IR or operative intervention
	4	Chronic disability or intensive medical therapy
	5	Death due to complication
Gastrointestinal bleeding	1	Diagnostic testing or stabilization with supportive care and monitoring without transfusion
	2	Transfusion
	3	Endoscopic, IR, or operative intervention for control of GI bleeding
	4	Organ resection or chronic disability
	5	Death due to complication
Hepatic failure	1	Resolution with supportive care or oral medical therapy
	2	Resolution with i.v. medical therapy
	3	Requiring intensive medical therapy, IR or operative intervention
	4	Chronic clinical evidence of liver dysfunction
	5	Death due to complication
Pancreatitis	1	Bowel rest, supportive care or oral medical therapy
	2	i.v. medical therapy
	3	IR or operative intervention for complication of pancreatitis
	4	Organ resection or chronic disability
	5	Death due to complication
Small-bowel obstruction	1	Resolution with bowel rest and supportive care
	2	Parenteral nutrition
	3	Operative intervention required
	4	Bowel resection required or chronic disability
	5	Death due to complication
Stoma dysfunction	1	Local wound care or antidiarrheals
	2	Major wound care or enterostomal therapy required or i.v. rehydration
	3	Reoperation required
	4	—
	5	Death due to complication

*Category	Grade	Grade criteria
Toxicity name		

*General

	Grade	Grade criteria
Anesthetic complication	1	Reversal of agent, supportive care or oral medication required for resolution
	2	Intensive medical therapy required for resolution of anesthetic secondary event
	3	Reoperation or interventional radiology required
	4	Chronic disability (e.g., cardiac, pulmonary, neurologic) as result of anesthesia SSE
	5	Death due to complication
Injury of organ or vessel	1	Repair at operation, no secondary effects
	2	Intensive medical therapy required for resolution of intraoperative injury of organ or vessel
	3	Reoperation or intervention for further treatment injury
	4	Resection of injured organ or major vascular repair with permanent prosthesis
	5	Death due to complication
Medication toxicity	1	Anaphylactic reaction or medication toxicity reversed with first-line medication or discontinuation
	2	Intensive medical therapy required
	3	Dialysis required
	4	Chronic disability resulting from education toxicity
	5	Death due to complication
Prosthetic device dysfunction	1	Resolution with surgical or medical therapy at bedside
	2	Intensive medical therapy required for resolution or device replaced or permanently nonfunctional
	3	Interventional radiology or operation required
	4	Chronic disability resulting from dysfunction
	5	Death due to complication
Retained foreign body	1	Removed at bedside with resolution
	2	Intensive medical therapy required as result of retained foreign body
	3	Interventional radiology or operation required for removal
	4	—
	5	Death due to complication
Wound dehiscence	1	Serous peritoneal fluid drainage, no operation required
	2	No procedure required, prolonged hospital stay
	3	Reoperation for abdominal wall closure
	4	—
	5	Death due to complication

*Category	Grade	Grade criteria
Toxicity name		

*Genitourinary

Category	Grade	Grade criteria
Erectile dysfunction	1	Transient or intermittent
	2	Medical management required, impotence
	3	Operative intervention required
	4	—
Incontinence	1	Intermittent and self limited
	2	—
	3	Operative intervention required
	4	Chronic disability
Renal failure	1	Resolution with supportive care or oral medical therapy
	2	i.v. medication
	3	ARF requiring dialysis
	4	Permanent renal failure, dialysis dependent
	5	Death due to complication
Urinary retention	1	Retention requiring reinsertion of Foley catheter
	2	Discharge with Foley catheter
	3	TURP required for resolution
	4	Permanent indwelling catheter required for dystonic bladder
	5	Death due to complication

*Hematologic

Category	Grade	Grade criteria
Deep venous thrombosis (clinical or radiologic dx)	1	—
	2	Anticoagulation required
	3	—
	4	Chronic extremity changes from DVT requiring treatment
	5	Death due to complication
Diffuse intravascular coagulation	1	DIC with no major bleeding, no medial intervention required with resolution
	2	Transfusion or intensive medical therapy required
	3	—
	4	—
	5	Death due to complication
Hematoma	1	Supportive care or bedside aspiration
	2	Transfusion or intensive medical therapy required
	3	Reoperation or IR drainage required
	4	—
	5	Death due to complication
Hemorrhage	1	Stable vital signs, patient observed without transfusion

*Category	Grade	Grade criteria
Toxicity name		
	2	Intensive medical therapy or monitoring required
	3	Intubation and ventilation required
	4	—
	5	Death due to complication
Electrolyte imbalance	1	Treated with replacement therapy or first-line medical therapy to resolve
	2	Intensive medical therapy or monitoring required
	3	Dialysis required
	4	Chronic disability or organ dysfunction due to electrolyte imbalance
	5	Death due to complication
Fluid imbalance	1	Treated with replacement therapy or first-line medical therapy to resolve
	2	Intensive medical therapy or monitoring required
	3	—
	4	—
Malnutrition	1	loss of >10% preoperative body weight
	2	Parenteral or enteral hyperalimentation required
	3	—
	4	Chronic disability or organ dysfunction or home TPN required due to malnutrition
	5	Death due to complication
*Musculoskeletal		
Arthritis	1	Oral medication, aspiration, or supportive care
	2	i.v. medication
	3	Operative or IR drainage required
	4	Chronic disability resulting from postoperative arthritis
Flap failure	1	Loss of <50% of flap or significant epidermolysis requiring local wound care
	2	Loss of >50% of flap, requiring debridement
	3	Reoperation to modify flap reconstruction
	4	Total loss of flap requiring additional reconstruction
Fracture/fall	1	Fracture requiring nonoperative treatment or injury resulting in wound care or change in neurologic status
	2	—
	3	Operation or IR required for treatment of injury
	4	Chronic disability or organ resection resulting from injury
	5	Death due to complication

*Category	Grade	Grade criteria
Toxicity name		
Lymphedema	1	Compression stockings required for symptomatic treatment and control
	2	—
	3	—
	4	Chronic, symptomatic disability requiring active compression treatment
Osteonecrosis	1	Oral antibiotics or supportive care
	2	Hyperbaric treatments or i.v. antibiotics
	3	Operation required for treatment of osteonecrosis
	4	Chronic disability or major bone resection required
	5	Death due to complication
Phlebitis	1	Oral antibiotics, anti-inflammatory medications, or bedside incision and drainage
	2	i.v. antibiotics, anticoagulation
	3	—
	4	Chronic disability from phlebitis
	5	Death due to complication
Seroma	1	Aspirations or supportive care
	2	—
	3	Operation or IR required for drainage
	4	—
*None at 30 days postop		
None	0	None
*Pain		
Acute pain syndrome	1	Oral or i.v. first-line medical treatment
	2	Complex treatment or diagnostic tests required or i.v. medication beyond first-line treatments
	3	Interventional radiology or operative procedure required for reversal
	4	—
Chronic pain syndrome	1	Oral or i.v. first-line medical treatment
	2	Complex treatment or diagnostic tests required or i.v. medication beyond first-line treatments
	3	Interventional radiology or operative procedure required for reversal
	4	Chronic disability changing performance status
*Pulmonary		
Adult respiratory-distress syndrome	1	—
	2	i.v. medical treatment required, rebreather or other supplemental oxygen
	3	—

*Category	Grade	Grade criteria
Toxicity name		
	4	Requiring intubation and intensive medical therapy
	5	Death due to complication
Apnea/hypoxia	1	Oxygen by rebreather
	2	—
	3	Requiring intubation for less than 24 hours
	4	Requiring intubation and intensive medical therapy
	5	Death due to complication
Atelectasis	1	Treatment at bedside, oral medications
	2	—
	3	—
	4	—
	5	Death due to complication
Pleural effusion	1	Therapeutic thoracentesis
	2	Tube thoracostomy or sclerosis required
	3	IR or operative intervention
	4	Requiring intubation and intensive medical therapy
	5	Death due to complication
Pneumonia	1	Oral antibiotics
	2	i.v. medical treatment with resolution
	3	—
	4	Requiring intubation and intensive medical therapy
	5	Death due to complication
Pneumothorax	1	Therapeutic needle aspiration or observation
	2	Tube thoracostomy
	3	IR or operative intervention
	4	—
	5	Death due to complication
Prolonged air leak	1	Tube thoracostomy treatment, possible sclerosis
	2	—
	3	IR or operative intervention
	4	—
	5	Death due to complication
Prolonged intubation	1	—
	2	Resolution within 72 hrs
	3	Resolution beyond 72 hrs or tracheostomy required
	4	Requiring intensive medical therapy and associated with chronic disability
	5	Death due to complication

*Category	Grade	Grade criteria
Toxicity name		
*Skin and peripheral nerve		
Neuropathy, motor	1	Motor dysfunction, unanticipated
	2	Rehabilitation required for acts of daily living
	3	—
	4	Permanent deficit requiring ambulatory assistance, bracing
	5	Death due to complication
Neuropathy, sensory	1	Sensory deficit only, unanticipated
	2	Difficulty with acts of daily living, ambulation
	3	—
	4	Associated chronic pain syndrome
	5	Death due to complication
Skin breakdown	1	Bedside debridement or local wound care
	2	Prolongation of hospital stay
	3	Operative debridement
	4	Flap, plastic surgical procedure
	5	Death due to complication
Skin-graft complication	1	Loss of >50% of skin graft
	2	—
	3	Total loss of graft, requiring reoperation
	4	—
	5	Death due to complication

APPENDIX 7
Laboratory values

CHEMISTRIES

Sodium	135–147 mEq/L
Potassium	3.5–5.5 mEq/L
Chloride	98–108 mEq/L
Bicarbonate	24–31 mEq/L
Anion gap: $Na - (Cl + HCO_3)$	8–12 mEq/L
BUN	8–20 mg/dl
Creatinine	0.8–1.5 mg/dl
Glucose	60–110 mg/dl
Calcium	8.0–10.4 mg/dl
Magnesium	1.8–2.9 mg/dl
Phosphorus	2.5–4.5 mg/dl
Uric acid	2.6–7.1 mg/dl
Total protein	6.0–8.2 gm/dl
Amylase	5–81 IU/L
Lipase	23–300 IU/L
Lactate	4–16 mg/dl
Osmolality	275–300 mOsm/kg

LIVER-FUNCTION TESTS

Albumin	3.5–4.7 gm/dl
Total bilirubin	0–1 mg/dl
Direct bilirubin	0–0.4 mg/dl
Alkaline phosphatase	38–126 IU/L
Aspartate aminotransferase (AST, SGOT)	15–46 IU/L
Alanine aminotransferase (ALT, SGPT)	7–56 IU/L
Gamma-glutamyl transpeptidase (GGT)	8–78 IU/L
Lactase dehydrogenase (LDH)	313–618 IU/L
Ammonia	11–35 mmol/L

CARDIAC

Creatine kinase
CK	20–170 IU/L
CK MB	0–12 IU/L
Troponin I	<0.7 ng/ml
LDH	313–618 IU/l

LIPIDS

Total cholesterol	**<200 mg/dl**
Borderline	200–239 mg/dl
High-risk	>239 mg/dl
LDL cholesterol	**<130 mg/dl**
Borderline high	130–159 mg/dl
High-risk	>159 mg/dl
HDL cholesterol	**>35–40 mg/dl**
High-risk	<35 mg/dl
Chol: HDL ratio	<4.5–6.0
Triglycerides	**30–200 mg/dl**
Borderline high	200–400 mg/dl
High-risk	400–1,000 mg/dl
Very high	>1,000 mg/dl

HORMONES

Cortisol	6–30 μg/dl
Follicle-stimulating hormone:	
FSH follicular	2.5–10.2 mIU/ml
FSH luteal	1.5–9.1 mIU/ml
FSH mid-cycle	3.4–33.4 mIU/ml
FSH menopausal	23–116.3 mIU/ml
Growth hormone	<10 ng/ml
17-Hydroxyprogesterone:	
Follicular	<80 ng/dl
Luteal	<285 ng/dl
Luteinizing hormone:	
LH follicular	0.5–16.9 mIU/ml
LH luteal	8.7–76.3 mIU/ml
LH mid-cycle	8.7–76.3 mIU/ml
LH menopausal	15.9–54 mIU/ml
Progesterone:	
Follicular	0.1–1.5 ng/ml

Luteal	2.5–28 ng/ml
Postmenopausal	<0.5 ng/ml
Prolactin:	
Nonpregnant	2.8–29.2 ng/ml
Postmenopausal	1.8–20.3 ng/ml
Testosterone (total)	14–76 ng/dl
Total thyroxine (T_4)	4.5–10.9 g/dl
Free thyroxine	0.8–2.7 ng/dl
T-uptake	0.72–1.24 units
Triiodothyronine (T_3)	59–174 ng/dl
Thyroid-stimulating hormone (TSH)	0.5–5.5 μU/ml

BLOOD GASES

pH	7.37–7.43
p_{CO_2}	37–43 mmHg
p_{O_2}	>80 mmHg
HCO_3	21–28 mmol/L

HEMATOLOGY

WBC	$(4–11) \times 10^3/\mu l$
Segs	42–66%
Bands	0–5%
Lymph	24–44%
Mono	2–7%
Eos	1–4%
Baso	0–1%
Hemoglobin	12–16 g/dl
Hematocrit	37–47%
RBC	$(4.1–5.5) \times 10^6/mm^3$
MCV	82–98 fl
MCH	27–31 pg
MCHC	32–36%
RDW	12–15.5%
Platelets	$(1.5–4) \times 10^5/\mu l$
Hgb_{A1c}	3–5%
Retic count	0.5–2.0%
Erythropoietin	4–25 mU/ml
Haptoglobin	30–221 mg/dl
Iron	37–170 μg/dl
Total iron-binding capacity (TIBC)	250–450 μg/dl
Iron % sat	20–55%

Ferritin   10–291 ng/ml
Folate   1.5–20 ng/ml

COAGULATION

Activated partial thromboplastin time (aPTT)   22–34 sec
Prothrombin time (PT)   10.4–13.5 sec
International normalized ratio (INR)   0.9–1.1
Thrombin time   14.1–17.7 sec
Bleeding time   2.5–8 min
Fibrinogen   200–400 mg/dl
Fibrin split products   <10 μg/ml

APPENDIX 8
Critical-care formulas

HEMODYNAMIC FORMULAS

Pulse pressure = Systolic BP − Diastolic BP

    Normal range 30–55 mmHg

Mean arterial pressure (MAP) = $\dfrac{SBP + 2(DBP)}{3}$

    Normal range 70–105 mmHg

Stroke volume (SV) = CO/HR = ml/beat

    Normal range 60–120 ml/beat

Cardiac output (CO) = SV × HR

    Normal range 3–7 L/min

Cardiac index (CI) = CO/BSA

    Normal range 2.5–4.0 L/min

Stroke volume index = (SV/BSA)1,000

    Normal range 30–65 ml/beat/m^2

Central venous pressure (CVP) = 0–8 mmHg

Right atrial pressure (RAP) = 0–8 mmHg

Right ventricular pressure = 25/5 mmHg

Pulmonary artery pressure (PAP):
  Diastolic = 5–12 mmHg
  Systolic = 15–30 mmHg
  Mean PAP = 5–10 mmHg

Pulmonary capillary wedge pressure (PCWP) = 5–12 mmHg

Pulmonary vascular resistance (PVR) = $\dfrac{(PAP - PCWP)80}{CO}$

    Normal range 150–250 dyne sec cm^{-5}

Systemic vascular resistance (SVR) $= \dfrac{(MAP - CVP)80}{CO}$

Normal range 800–1,200 dyne sec cm^{-5}

Arterial–venous oxygen content difference [(A − V)O$_2$ Diff]

$= Ca_{O_2} - Cv_{O_2}$

$= 1.36(Hgb)(Sa_{O_2} - Sv_{O_2})$

Normal range 3.5–5.5 mlO$_2$/dl

Oxygen delivery (D_{O_2}) = CO × Ca_{O_2}

$= 1.36(Hgb)(Sa_{O_2})(CO)(10)$

Normal range 800–1200 ml/min

Oxygen consumption (V_{O_2}) = CO$(Ca_{O_2} - Cv_{O_2})$

$= 1.36(Hgb)(Sa_{O_2} - Sv_{O_2})(CO)(10)$

Normal range 225–275 ml/min

RESPIRATORY FORMULAS

Shunt fraction (Q_s/Q_t):

$$\frac{Q_s}{Q_t} = \frac{Cc_{O_2} - Ca_{O_2}}{Cc_{O_2} - Cv_{O_2}} \times 100$$

Normal 5%

Cc_{O_2} = capillary oxygen content
Ca_{O_2} = arterial oxygen content
Cv_{O_2} = venous oxygen content

Calculation of capillary oxygen content (Cc_{O_2}):

$$Cc_{O_2} = (Hgb \times 1.34 \times Sc_{O_2}) + (Pc_{O_2} \times 0.003)$$

No established normal range

Sc_{O_2} = pulmonary capillary oxygen saturation
Pc_{O_2} = partial pressure of oxygen in capillary blood

Calculation of arterial oxygen content (Ca_{O_2}):

$$Ca_{O_2} = (Hgb \times 1.34 \times Sa_{O_2}) + (Pa_{O_2} \times 0.003)$$

Normal 20 mlO$_2$/dl

Calculation of venous oxygen content (Cv_{O_2})

$$Cv_{O_2} = (Hgb \times 1.34 \times Sv_{O_2}) + (Pv_{O_2} \times 0.003)$$

Normal 15 mlO$_2$/dl

Pv_{O_2} = partial pressure of oxygen in mixed venous blood
Sv_{O_2} = mixed venous oxygen saturation

Calculation of alveolar oxygen partial pressure (PA_{O_2})

$$PA_{O_2} = Pa_{O_2} - Fi_{O_2} \times (Pb - P_{H_2O}) - Pa_{O_2}/RQ$$

Normal range 60–100 mmHg

Pb = barometric pressure (=760 mmHg at sea level)
P_{H_2O} = water pressure in lungs (=47 mmHg)
RQ = respiratory quotient (=0.8)

Calculation of Pa_{O_2}/Fi_{O_2} ratio:

$$Pa_{O_2}/Fi_{O_2} \text{ ratio} = \frac{Pa_{O2}}{Fi_{O2}}$$

Normal >286

Calculation of alveolar–arterial gradient:

$$P(A - a)_{O_2} = PA_{O_2} - Pa_{O_2}$$

Normal range 0–20 mmHg

RENAL EQUATIONS

$$\text{Creatinine clearance} = \frac{\text{urine creatinine}}{\text{serum creatinine}} \times \text{urine volume (ml/min)} \times \frac{1.73\ (\text{m}^2)}{\text{BSA}}$$

Normal range 74–160 ml/min

$$\text{Fractional excretion of Na}^+ \text{ (FENa)} = \frac{\text{urine Na}}{\text{serum Na}} \times \frac{\text{serum creatinine}}{\text{urine creatinine}} \times 100$$

Free water clearance
$$= \text{urine volume (ml/min)} - \frac{\text{urine osmolality}}{\text{plasma osmolality}} \times \text{urine volume} \quad (\text{ml/min})$$

Water deficit in hypernatremia = $0.6 \times$ (body weight [kg]) $\times$ ([Na$^+$]/140 $-$ 1)

Water excess in hyponatremia = $0.6 \times$ (body weight [kg]) $\times$ (1 $-$ [Na$^+$]/140)

$$\text{Calculated serum osmolality} = 2(\text{Na}^+ + \text{K}^+) + \frac{\text{glucose}}{18} + \frac{\text{BUN}}{2.8}$$

Normal range: 275–290 mOsm/kg

Osmolal gap = measured osmolality $-$ calculated osmolality

Normal range: 0–5 mOsm/kg

APPENDIX 9
Advanced cardiac life-support algorithms

Adapted from Guidelines 2000 for Cardiopulmonary Resuscitation and Emergency Cardiovascular Care. *Circulation* 2000; **102**(Suppl I): I86.

PRIMARY AND SECONDARY ABCD SURVEY

1. Primary ABCD Survey (basic CPR and defibrillation)
   - Check responsiveness, activate emergency medical response system, call for defibrillator
   - **A** Airway: assess and manage the airway with noninvasive devices
   - **B** Breathing: assess and manage breathing. If the patient is not breathing, give two slow breaths
   - **C** Circulation: assess and manage the circulation; if no pulse, begin chest compressions
   - **D** Defibrillation: assess for and shock ventricular fibrillation/pulseless ventricular tachycardia, up to 3 times (200 J, 300 J, 360 J) if necessary.
2. Secondary ABCD Survey (advanced assessments and treatment)
   - **A** Airway: place airway device as soon as possible
   - **B** Breathing: assess adequacy of airway device placement and performance; secure airway device; confirm effective oxygenation and ventilation
   - **C** Circulation: establish IV access; administer drugs appropriate for rhythm and condition
   - **D** Differential diagnosis: search for and treat identified reversible causes

VENTRICULAR FIBRILLATION (VF) AND PULSELESS VENTRICULAR TACHYCARDIA (VT)

1. Primary ABCD
2. Assess rhythm after 3 shocks: continue CPR for persistent or recurrent VF/pulseless VT
3. Secondary ABCD
4. Epinephrine 1 mg i.v. push, repeat every 3–5 minutes, or vasopressin 40 U i.v., single dose, 1 time only
5. Resume attempts to defibrillate, 1 × 360 J, within 30–60 seconds

6. Consider antiarrhythmics:
    (a) Amiodarone 300 mg i.v. push. Consider second dose of 150 mg if VF/pulseless VT recurs
    (b) Lidocaine 1.5 mg/kg i.v. push, repeat every 3–5 minutes to a maximum cumulative dose of 3 mg/kg
    (c) Magnesium sulfate 1–2 g i.v. in polymorphic VT and suspected hypo-magnesemic states
    (d) Procainamide 30 mg/kg in refractory VF (maximum total dose of 17 mg/kg)
7. Defibrillate 360 J, 30–60 seconds after each dose of medication or after each minute of CPR
8. Sodium bicarbonate 1 mEq/kg is indicated for conditions known to provoke sudden cardiac arrest (hypoxic lactic acidosis, hypercarbic acidosis, tricyclic antidepressant overdose)

PULSELESS ELECTRICAL ACTIVITY (PEA)

1. Pulseless electrical activity on monitor, without detectable pulse
2. Primary ABCD survey
3. Secondary ABCD survey
4. Consider possible causes: hypovolemia, hypoxia, acidosis, hyperkalemia, hypokalemia, hypothermia, drug overdose, cardiac tamponade, tension pneumothorax, myocardial infarction, pulmonary embolism
5. Epinephrine 1 mg i.v. push, repeat every 3–5 minutes
6. Atropine 1 mg i.v. (if PEA rate is slow), repeat every 3–5 minutes as needed, to a total dose of 0.04 mg/kg

ASYSTOLE

1. Primary ABCD survey
2. Confirm asystole in two or more leads. If rhythm is unclear and possible VF, defibrillate for VF
3. Secondary ABCD survey
4. Consider transcutaneous pacing (if considered, perform immediately)
5. Epinephrine 1 mg i.v. push, repeat every 3–5 minutes
6. Atropine 1 mg i.v. push, repeat every 3–5 minutes up to a total of 0.04 mg/kg
7. If asystole persists, consider withholding or ceasing resuscitative efforts

BRADYCARDIA

1. Slow (absolute bradycardia < 60 BPM) or relatively slow (rate less than expected relative to underlying condition or cause)
2. Primary ABCD survey
3. Secondary ABCD survey and 12-lead ECG
4. If unstable if chest pain, shortness of breath, decreased level of consciousness, hypotension, shock, pulmonary congestion, congestive heart failure or acute myocardial are present. Intervention sequence:
   (a) Atropine 0.5–1.0 mg i.v. push, repeated every 3–5 minutes, up to 0.04 mg/kg
   (b) Transcutaneous pacing
   (c) Dopamine 5–20 μg/kg/min
   (d) Epinephrine 2–10 μg/min
5. If stable and not in Type II or Type III AV block, observe
6. If Type II or Type III AV block, prepare for transvenous pacer. If symptoms develop, use transcutaneous pacer

UNSTABLE SYMPTOMATIC TACHYCARDIA

1. Consider unstable if chest pain, hypotension, congestive heart failure, myocardial infarction, ischemia, decreased level of consciousness, shock, dyspnea, or pulmonary congestion are present
2. Assess ABCs, secure airway, administer oxygen, 12-lead ECG and obtain venous access
3. Prepare cardioversion
4. Consider brief trial of medications based on specific arrhythmia
5. Consider premedication for cardioversion with a sedative and analgesic agent
6. Synchronized cardioversion:
   (a) 50 J PSVT or atrial flutter only
   (b) 100 J
   (c) 200 J
   (d) 300 J
   (e) 360 J

APPENDIX 10
Useful Web addresses

FEDERAL

Agency for Health Care Policy and Research
    http://www.ahcpr.gov

Centers for Disease Control and Prevention
    http://cdc.gov
    Cancer Prevention and Control
        http://cdc.gov/nccdphp/dcpc/index.htm
    National Center for Health Statistics
        http://www.cdc.gov/nchswww
    National Program of Cancer Registries
        http://www.cdc.gov/nccdphp/dcpc/npcr/register.htm

Department of Defense Congressionally Mandated Medical Research Programs
    http://www.cdmrp.arm.mil

Food and Drug Administration
    http://www.fda.gov
    Center for Biologics Evaluation and Research
        http://www.fda.gov/cber/about.htm
    Center for Devices and Radiologic Health
        http://www.fda.gov/cdrh/about.htm
    Center for Drug Evaluation and Research
        http://www.fda.gov/cder/about.htm

Health Care Financing Administration
    http://www.hcfa.gov

Health Services Research Administration
    http://www.hrsa.gov

National Cancer Institute
    http://www.nci.nih.gov
    CancerNet (PDQ and Cancerlit)
        http://cancernet.nci.nih.gov
    Clinical trials
        http://www.cancertrials.nci.nih.gov

Cancer Genetics Network
> http://www-dccps.ims.nic.nih.gov/CGN

Cooperative Human Tissue Network
> http://www-chtn.ims.nci.nih.gov

State Cancer Legislation Database
> http://www.dcpps.nci.nih.gov/scld

Surveillance, Epidemiology, and End Results (SEER) program
> http://www-seer.ims.nci.nih.gov

National Institute of Child Health and Human Development
> http://nichd.gov

National Institutes of Health
> http://www.nih.gov

PubMed (Medline)
> http://www.ncbi.nlm.nih.gov/PubMed

The Visible Human Project®
> http://www.nlm.nih.gov/research/visible/visible_human.html

NON-FEDERAL

Professional societies and associations

American College of Obstetricians and Gynecologists
> http://www.acog.org

American College of Surgeons
> http://www.facs.org

American Medical Association
> http://www.ama-assn.org/home.htm

American Society for Clinical Oncology
> http://www.asco.org

Society of Gynecologic Oncologists
> http://www.sgo.org

General cancer information

American Cancer Society
> http://www.cancer.org

American Institute for Cancer Research
> http://www.aicr.org

@Cancer
> http://atcancer.com/cancer

CancerBacUp
> http://www.cancerbacup.org.uk

Cancer Care, Inc.
  http://www.cancercare.org
Cancer Information Network
  http://www.cancernetwork.com/index2.htm
Cochrane Cancer Network
  http://www.canet.demon.co.uk
Medicine Online
  http://www.meds.com
Medical Conferences and Meetings
  http://www.pslgroup.com/medconf.htm
MedWeb
  http://www.medwebplus.com
National Coalition for Cancer Survivorship
  http://www.cansearch.org
National Comprehensive Cancer Network
  http://www.cancernetwork.com
Network for Oncology Communication and Research
  http://www.nocr.com
OncoLink
  http://www.oncolink.upenn.edu
Oncology Online – Oncology Therapeutics Network
  http://205.239.179.160.81
WebMD
  http:///my.webmd.com
Yahoo
  http://dir.yahoo.com/Health/Medicine/Oncology

Gynecologic cancer

Women's Cancer Network
  http://www.wcn.org
Gynecologic Cancer Foundation
  http://www.sgo.org.gcf

Breast cancer

Breast Cancer Action
  http://www.bcaction.org
Susan G. Komen Breast Cancer Foundation
  http://www.komen.org
National Action Plan on Breast Cancer
  http://www.napbc.org
National Alliance of Breast Cancer Organizations
  http://www.nabco.org
National Breast Cancer Coalition
  http://www.natbcc.org

Y-ME National Breast Cancer Organization
        http://www.y-me.org

Breast and ovarian cancer

SHARE: Self Help for Women with Breast and Ovarian Cancer
        http://www.noah.cuny.edu/providers/cancare/html

Breast and cervical cancer

National Asian Women's Health Organization
        http://nawho.org

Cervical cancer

Center for Cervical Health
        http://cervicalhealth.org
The DES Cancer Network
        http://www.descancer.org
National Cervical Cancer Coalition
        http://www.nccc-online.org

Ovarian cancer

Conversations! The Newsletter for Women Fighting Ovarian Cancer
        http://www.geocities.com/HotSprings/7938
National Ovarian Cancer Coalition
        http://www.ovarian.org
Ovarian Cancer National Alliance: Ovar'coming Together
        http://wwww.ovariancancer.org
Ovarian Plus International: Gynecologic Cancer Prevention Quarterly
        http://www.monitor.net/ovarian

Oncology journals and publication information

American Journal of Obstetrics and Gynecology
        http://www1.mosby.com
Cancer Online
        http://www.canceronline.wiley.com
Gynecologic Oncology
        http://www.apnet.com/www/journal/go.htm
JAMA – The Journal of the American Medical Association
        http://jama.ama-assn.org
Journal of Clinical Oncology
        http://www.jco.org

MD Digests
  http://php2.silverplatter.com/physicians/digest.htm
Medscape Oncology
  http://www.medscape.com/home/topics/oncology/oncology.html
Merck Manual
  http://www.merck.com/pubs/mmanual
New England Journal of Medicine
  http://www.nejm.org/content/index.asp
Obstetrics and Gynecology ("The Green Journal")
  http://www-east.elsevier.com/ong
World Oncology Network
  http://www.worldoncology.net/oncology_journas.htm

MD Anderson Cancer Center

  http://www.mdanderson.org

Memorial Sloan-Kettering Cancer Center

  http://www.mskcc.org

Index